The Making of Modern
Chinese Medicine, 1850-1960

Contemporary Chinese Studies

This series provides new scholarship and perspectives on modern and contemporary China, including China's contested borderlands and minority peoples; ongoing social, cultural, and political changes; and the varied histories that animate China today.

A list of titles in this series appears at the end of this book.

The Making of
Modern Chinese Medicine,
1850-1960

BRIDIE ANDREWS

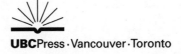

UBCPress · Vancouver · Toronto

21 20 19 18 17 16 15 14   5 4 3 2 1

Printed in Canada on FSC-certified ancient-forest-free paper
(100% post-consumer recycled) that is processed chlorine- and acid-free.

Library and Archives Canada Cataloguing in Publication

Andrews, Bridie, author
    The making of modern Chinese medicine, 1850-1960 / Bridie Andrews.

(Contemporary Chinese studies)
Includes bibliographical references and index.
Issued in print and electronic formats.
ISBN 978-0-7748-2432-3 (bound); ISBN 978-0-7748-2433-0 (pbk.)
ISBN 978-0-7748-2434-7 (pdf); ISBN 978-0-7748-2435-4 (epub)

1. Medicine, Chinese – China – History – 19th century. 2. Medicine, Chinese – China – History – 20th century. 3. Medical care – China – History – 19th century. 4. Medical care – China – History – 20th century. I. Title. II. Series: Contemporary Chinese studies

R601.A54 2013   610.951   C2013-905693-9
                                                          C2013-905694-7

Canadä

UBC Press gratefully acknowledges the financial support for our publishing program of the Government of Canada (through the Canada Book Fund) and the British Columbia Arts Council.

Financial support from the Chiang Ching-kuo Foundation, the Association for Asian Studies, and Bentley University is also greatly appreciated.

UBC Press
The University of British Columbia
2029 West Mall
Vancouver, BC V6T 1Z2
www.ubcpress.ca

For my brothers, and those they left behind.

Contents

Figures and Tables

Tables

Acknowledgments

I am humbled by the recollection of all the help and goodwill that I have received while working on this book, and it is my pleasure to acknowledge it here. My initial research was supervised by historian of medicine Andrew Cunningham at Cambridge, a kind and inspiring guide to academic life as well as a brilliant model of research and writing. I owe him my career, which is a debt not easily repaid, though I hope the appearance of this work will bring him some satisfaction.

After years of rewriting individual chapters to incorporate new material, it took the intervention of my friend and colleague at Bentley, David Schwarzkopf, to bring these efforts back into a coherent narrative. He heroically read multiple drafts and was often able to articulate my argument better than I could myself. The fact that both our names appear as authors of the final chapter here does not do justice to his contributions, for which I am profoundly grateful.

Other friends and colleagues to whom I am indebted for their comments on the entire manuscript at different times in its evolution include Linda Barnes, Miranda Brown, Benjamin Elman, Charlotte Furth, Marta Hanson, T.J. Hinrichs, Angela Leung, Charles Rosenberg, Nathan Sivin, Michael Worboys, and Yi-Li Wu. Individual chapters have benefited from the comments of the late and much missed Chris Gilmartin, also Chris Bayly, Chris Beneke, Francesca Bray, Bu Liping,

Christopher Cullen, Robert Culp, Gao Xi, Elisabeth Hsu, Eric Jacobson, Ted Kaptchuk, Cathy Kerr, Geoffrey Lloyd, David Luesink, David McMullen, Georges Métailié, Katy Park, Caroline Reeves, Volker Scheid, Darwin Stapleton, Eddy U., Cyrus Veeser, Yip Ka-che, and Yu Xinzhong. Marc Stern was the best department chair imaginable – at once urging me on (sternly!) and acting as a steadfast advocate.

The materials for this book were collected from several libraries and archives. I particularly wish to acknowledge John Moffett, librarian at the Needham Research Institute in Cambridge, who provided me with many sources essential to this project, as did Gao Chuan and Hilary Chung. I also owe thanks to Charles Aylmer at Cambridge University Library, Martha Smalley at the Yale Divinity School Missionary Archives, Martin Heijdra at Princeton University Library, Nobuhirō Abe, Ellen McGill, and the staffs of the Harvard-Yenching Library, the School of Oriental and African Studies Library, and the Wellcome Library in London, the Beijing University of Chinese Medicine (*Beijing zhongyi xueyuan*), the Chinese Academy of Chinese Medicine (*Zhongguo zhongyi yanjiu yuan*), Beijing Municipal Library, Shanghai Municipal Library, Hong Kong University Library, and the Fu Sinian Library at Academia Sinica, Taiwan.

For generously sharing research materials I wish to remember the late Wu Sunquan and his wife Xiong Zina in Xiamen and the late Zhao Pushan in Beijing, who selflessly shared much of his collection of Chen Yuan's early published articles. At the Beijing University of Chinese Medicine I was mentored by Zhen Zhiya, whose support allowed me access to many other rare materials. Colleagues who have kindly provided me with books and photocopies include Florence Brételle-Establet, Fang Xiaoping, Gao Xi, Marta Hanson, T.J. Hinrichs, Sean Hsiang-lin Lei, Mike Shi-yung Liu, David Luesink, Ruth Rogaski, Shen Guowei, Kim Taylor, Toshihiro Tōgō, Tōgō Tsukahara, Cyrus Veeser, and Junsei Watanabe: many thanks to you all. I would also like to acknowledge the research assistance of Dai Chen, Atsushi Koike, Elizabeth Lee, Grace Y. Shen, and Weicong Tian.

I have been sustained and delighted in academic life by many fellow-travellers whose contributions, though indirect, were nonetheless essential to my well-being. For their tolerant ears, wise words, and great sense of humour, I would like to thank T.J. Hinrichs, Caroline Reeves, Molly Sutphen, Peter Buck, Mary Brown Bullock, Lu Yan, Zhang Qiong, Vivienne Lo, Cathérine Jami, Fan Ka-wai, Volker Scheid, Michele Thompson, Monica Green, Katy Park, Charles Rosenberg, Fred Ledley, and the entire Bentley University history department.

Financial support for this research was provided along the way by the Wellcome Trust, the British Council, the Chiang Ching-kuo Foundation, an Andrew W. Mellon Foundation Fellowship at the University of Pennsylvania, the Radcliffe Institute for Advanced Study at Harvard University, and the Jeanne and Dan Valente Center for Arts and Sciences at Bentley University. Travel assistance was provided by the British Council, the Whiting Foundation, and the Bentley University Deans' Fund for International Travel. Publication subventions were provided by the Association for Asian Studies, the Chiang Ching-kuo Foundation for International Scholarly Exchange, and Bentley University.

At UBC Press, I was fortunate to have the editorial guidance and professionalism of Emily Andrew and the production team headed by Megan Brand. David Luesink first mentioned my project to Timothy Brook, who invited me to submit my manuscript to this series; for both these kind acts I am much indebted.

My children have been hearing about this research their whole lives, and they, my mother Marion Cooke, my sister Beth Andrews-Dawson, and Tom Minehan provided the love and encouragement that made it possible. If there are others whose help has gone unacknowledged here, I apologize for the oversight. Other oversights and errors in this book are, naturally, my responsibility.

I am deeply grateful to be sustained by such wonderful friends, colleagues, and family. Thank you all.

Conventions and Abbreviations

Chinese is romanized using the pinyin romanization system developed in the People's Republic of China, with the exception of a few proper names (such as Chiang Kai-shek, Wu Lien-teh, Peking in the name of Peking Union Medical College).

Chinese characters are given after first use, simplified characters are given for names and institutions after 1949, and traditional (unsimplified) characters are given for names and institutions in the Republic of China. Occasionally, as in the case of Cheng Dan'an, it has been necessary to give names in both traditional and simplified forms because they differ significantly.

Abbreviations are as follows:

CMJ	*China Medical Journal* (1907-31), renamed *Zhonghua yixue zazhi* (*Chinese Medical Journal*) (1931-66)
CMMJ	*China Medical Missionary Journal* (1887-1907)
CR	*Chinese Recorder*
GYPL	*Guoyi pinglun* 國醫評論 (*National Medicine Critic*)
JNCBRAS	*Journal of the North China Branch of the Royal Asiatic Society*

MGYXZZ	*Minguo yixue zazhi* 民國醫學雜誌 *(Republican Medical Journal)*
NCH	*North-China Herald and Supreme Court and Consular Gazette*
NMJC	*National Medical Journal of China* (English-language edition of *CMJ* from 1907 to 1931, thereafter absorbed into *CMJ*)
SXYYXB	*Shaoxing yiyao xuebao* 紹興醫藥學保 *(Shaoxing Journal of Medicine and Pharmacy)*
YXB	*Yixue bao* 醫學報 *(Medical News)*
YXWSB	*Yixue weisheng bao* 醫學衛生報 *(Journal of Medicine and Hygiene)*
ZHYSZZ	*Zhonghua yishi zazhi* 中华医史杂志 *(Chinese Journal of Medical History)*
ZXYY	*Zhong-xi yiyao* 中西醫藥 *(Sino-Western Medicine and Pharmacy)*
ZXYXB	*Zhong-xi yixue bao* 中西醫學報 *(Journal of Sino-Western Medicine)*
YXZZ	*Yixue zazhi* 醫學雜誌 *(Journal of Medicine)*

The Making of Modern Chinese Medicine, 1850-1960

Modernities and Medicines 1

You wouldn't expect to find Chinese medicine in the home of Dr. Wu Lien-teh 伍連德 (1879-1960). Dr. Wu, born in British Malaya, was one of the first ethnic Chinese to study modern medicine in England. After graduating from Cambridge University, he studied in Britain, France, and Germany with some of the world's leading medical researchers. In 1908, he was hired to be vice-director of the Imperial Army Medical College in Tianjin, a treaty port just eighty miles/one hundred and thirty kilometres from the Chinese capital, Beijing. Two years later, when pneumonic plague broke out in northern Manchuria, he was sent to direct the government's control and eradication effort. (Pneumonic plague is caused by the same bacterium that causes bubonic plague, but it spreads like influenza in droplets exhaled by its victims.) In the aftermath, he organized China's first international research conference then set up the North Manchuria Plague Prevention Service, the Chinese government's first modern public health organization. In 1915, he was instrumental in establishing the Chinese Medical Association, becoming its president in 1916. He was appointed head of the new Central Epidemic Bureau in Beijing in 1919, and in 1930 he became director-general of China's National Quarantine Service. As a man of science, he insisted that his family use only Western medicine. But behind his back, his wife persisted in administering Chinese-medical tonics and even treating the children with traditional remedies when they got sick.[1] The irony that China's most celebrated MD was unable to curtail the use of Chinese medicine even in his own home is a salutary reminder that the modernization of medicine in China is a story that interweaves many strands of human and group agency, including gender roles, domestic and regional cultures, battles for influence between newly organized professional elites and the new politicians of post-Imperial China, and international relations. The resulting fabric becomes a kind of magic carpet from which to observe the battles over, and the creation of, Chinese medical modernity.

The elements of modernity are familiar to European and American history: the overthrow of monarchical rule in favour of popular sovereignty; the rise of the nation-state, secularism, and science; industrialization and rapid technological change; the development of a sense of time as progressive and linear; the global spread of capitalism; and the emergence and celebration of the autonomous individual as the unit of society, replacing the extended family, clan, or village. Thus the tendency when Westerners discuss modernity in other parts of the world is to measure the degree to which 'they' resemble 'us.' That was why Ralph Croizier sought to explain 'why twentieth-century intellectuals, committed in so many ways to science and modernity, have insisted on upholding China's pre-scientific medical tradition.'[2] Chinese medicine was, by definition, not modern, so its survival in a modernizing China required explanation.

This idea of a single, normative modernity was widely accepted by elites around the world in the mid-twentieth century but has recently come in for increasing criticism. Many of the markers of modern progress turned out, on examination, to be chimerical. For example, does the increasing influence of Christian fundamentalism in the United States make that country less modern? When scientific communities deny access to scientists with startling new findings, does that make them less scientific? When it turns out that individuals in industrialized societies may still subordinate their interests to those of their extended families, does the modern nation suffer? Sociologist Bruno Latour argues that such events are not really anomalies because modernity is an illusion created by translating the messy hybrid relationships or networks between humans and the natural world into the 'modern' institutions of science, law, society, and so on. The maintenance of the illusion of these independent realms, he argues, requires constant vigilance, a work he labels 'purification.' To be modern is to believe in the purified realms as though they function independently of one another. But since none of them can really be independent of the others, 'we have never been modern.'[3]

We might interpret the contrast between Dr. Wu Lien-teh's public persona and the continued use of traditional medicine in his home as an example of such a messy, hybrid, non-modern network. But by the 1940s and 1950s, when Dr. Wu and his wife were disagreeing over how to treat their children, Chinese medicine had already acquired many of the hallmarks of modernity. It was democratic in that anyone could study it in medical school. Its practice was usually secular and professionalized, and Chinese-medical research was increasingly conducted scientifically, with laboratory testing of drugs and with journals publishing the results of clinical observations.

This is more than a matter of terminology. It is fruitful to look at the battles between 'modern' and 'traditional' medicine as part of a larger struggle over sovereignty. One of the strongest arguments for Western-style medicine was that it was essential to the recovery of national sovereignty. Dr. Wu Lien-teh's efforts to control the spread of plague in 1910 were intended to stave off Russian and Japanese military-led sanitary interventions, and his tenure at the National Quarantine Service aimed to demonstrate that the Chinese government could be trusted with the management of its own international trade: the 'unequal treaties' created in the nineteenth century were no longer necessary to protect foreign interests. This struggle to regain national sovereignty was conducted in the international arena. Within China, it was inappropriate as well as unrealistic to expect ordinary people to replace their culture with foreign behavioural norms, yet this is what many of the most outspoken and famous Chinese modernizers – and, after 1928, the Nationalist government – set out to achieve.

The resulting battles over whether the Nationalist state should support modern over Chinese medicine can also be understood as a struggle over the limits of state control, this time internally. While many in government wanted to legislate Chinese medicine out of existence on the grounds that it was superstitious, unscientific, and unhygienic – a threat to the health of the nation – they encountered so much opposition that the Nationalists ended up capitulating and supporting the Institute of National Medicine, which was established in 1931. From this we can see that the argument that Western medicine and Chinese medicine represented mutually exclusive practices was harder to make – and impossible to enforce. Instead, the Institute of National Medicine's founders worked to create a modern Chinese medicine, in 1936 winning the right to have licensed Chinese-medical doctors practise legally. The subjects that were to be examined for the licence were strictly secular but did not include acupuncture, an omission to which we return in Chapter 8. Apparently some aspects of earlier native medical practice had been accepted as modern enough to be folded into the new Chinese polity while others had not.

It may seem odd to see this controversy because today, in the West, Chinese medicine is successful in large part because people perceive it as embodying the accumulated wisdom of a five-thousand-year-old culture, able to communicate eternal truths about the body, unlike the seemingly fickle here-today-outdated-tomorrow approach of scientific medicine. It is also seen as a holistic practice that considers the individual patient, unlike the reductionist, over-specialized practice of modern medicine, which considers mainly diseases. As we shall see, these stereotypes, while not entirely incorrect, obscure the immense changes that have occurred in the theory and practice of Chinese medicine in the last hundred years.

The contrast between the rhetoric of Chinese medicine as backward, as seen by Chinese modernizers in the early twentieth century, and Chinese medicine as authentic and holistic, as seen by 'alternative' healers in the contemporary West, also indicates that the term 'culture' is as contested and agonistic as are the terms 'modern' and 'traditional.' As Leach and Englund observe, the concept of discrete cultures is one of the artefacts of the discourse of modernity.[4] Modernizers need to be modernizing something, and that something is often framed in terms of culture. Here, too, a purification process has been at work, attempting to identify 'Chinese' and 'Western' when, as we shall see for medicine, both cultures are hopelessly entangled.

In the West today there is understandable confusion about the age and authenticity of Chinese medicine because few people know its recent history, and the supposed longevity of Chinese medicine is an important aspect of its appeal. By contrast, when studying Chinese medicine in China in the 1980s, I noticed that bookstores carried a substantial number of titles devoted to something called 'Combined Chinese and Western medicine' (*Zhong-xi yi jiehe* 中西医结合). This phrase originally referred to People's Republic of China chairman Mao Zedong's 1956 policy requiring doctors of Western medicine to study Chinese medicine, with the explicit goal of creating a new medicine that would combine the best of Chinese and Western medical culture and be a contribution to the world. At the time, this enforced cross-fertilization was also one of the ways in which the Chinese Communist Party under Mao attempted to discipline 'bourgeois' Western-influenced doctors. It was a reversal of the previous policy of requiring doctors of Chinese medicine to study Western medicine in order to promote the scientization (*kexuehua* 科学化) of their practice.[5] I call this phenomenon 'Combined Medicine,' with the capital letters indicating its official status. The most famous example of Combined Medicine is the use of acupuncture analgesia for major internal operations during the Cultural Revolution (1966-76).[6] In its broadest sense the term refers to the use of Chinese therapies by doctors of Western medicine and (more commonly) the use of Western medicine by doctors of Chinese medicine. In 1980, the Chinese Ministry of Health started to refer to the 'three paths' of medical practice in China: Western medicine, Combined Medicine, and Chinese medicine.[7] In recent years, the institutionalization of Combined Medicine has continued, and it is reflected in the establishment of hospitals of Combined Medicine in major cities. A similar development in the West has been the creation of short training programs in acupuncture for doctors with an MD degree.

The fact that both 'Chinese' medicine and 'Western' medicine are important components of the Chinese health care delivery system is partly a matter of national policy. Article 21 of the 1982 Constitution of the People's Republic of China states:

The state develops medical and health services, promotes modern medicine and traditional Chinese medicine, encourages and supports the setting up of various medical and health facilities by the rural economic collectives, state enterprises and undertakings and neighborhood organizations, and promotes sanitation activities of a mass character, all to protect the people's health.[8]

Anyone with even a passing knowledge of Chinese medical ideas, such as *yin* and *yang*, the Five Phases (*wuxing* 五行, also translated as Five Elements or Five Agents), or the system of channels (*jingluo* 經絡, meridians) for the movement of vital energy, or *qi* 氣/气, around the body, will realize that the two systems cannot readily be integrated on a theoretical level. At the same time, no one suggests that Western medicine adopt the concepts of Chinese medicine. Thus, Combined Medicine is mostly a way of assuring patients that Chinese medicine is operating within limits determined by the dominant biomedical paradigm. This has clinical consequences: for example, where a practitioner of Chinese medicine might describe an ailment as *xiao ke* (消渴, wasting and thirsting), in combined practice it is necessary to identify the syndrome as diabetes mellitus so that communication is possible. Chinese medicine loses much of its epistemological authority in the process. The same is true of the burgeoning 'integrated health care' practices in the West, where chiropractors, nutritionists, acupuncturists, and other complementary therapists may be employed to work in tandem with biomedical clinicians. The MDs are usually in the front seats.

A hundred and fifty years ago, the situation was very different. At that time it was not necessary to speak of 'Chinese' medicine – medicine in China was simply 'medicine.' In port cities like Shanghai and Canton, a handful of Western medical missionaries were opening dispensaries and tiny hospitals of a few beds each, but most of the general population was wary of foreign drugs and suspicious of the motives of the medical missionaries. Some medical missionaries did run busy clinics, gaining the trust of local populations due to their skill with regard to particular interventions, such as cataract surgery or the excision of tumours. In terms of drug therapies, quinine was the single obvious improvement on the Chinese pharmacopeia, but it was initially very expensive and so was dispensed sparingly. The missionary example did not lead to general acceptance of the new medicine from the West, and medical missionaries were even less successful at converting patients into Christians.[9]

How, then, did Western medicine become transformed from a dubious curiosity in mid-nineteenth-century China into its current status as the dominant medical system? Perhaps more intriguing, how were the competing approaches to therapy organized into the contrasting categories of 'Chinese' and 'Western' and then integrated into the official health system? Addressing these questions in the history of medicine can provide insight into the history of Western influence in non-Western countries, the ways in which science is perceived and performed as a marker of modernity, and the relationship of the discourses of modernity to cultural change and the construction of national identities. That is what this book hopes to achieve.

In keeping with this ambition to fit the history of medicine into these larger narratives of change, I do not attempt an exhaustive account of the medical history of the period, which would require a much longer book; nor do I offer a microhistory, hoping to illuminate broad trends through a narrow focus on a single individual or institution. Instead, I focus on key issues and important agents of change to illuminate the motives driving the active assimilation of some aspects of Western medicine and the reasons for the forging of a new Chinese medicine. This approach is designed to demonstrate the contingency and instability of these medical 'systems' and, by extension, to suggest the constructed and agonistic nature of most representations of culture, both foreign and domestic. I hope that, once these broad contours of change have been charted, they will provide a context for other, more archive-driven studies of the history of medicine in China.

What Is Western? What Is Chinese?

'Western medicine' is used here as a label, or place-holder, for a changing assemblage of theories, technologies, and practices that defies easy definition. Some writers prefer to emphasize its eclectic origins by labelling it 'cosmopolitan' medicine, and, among anthropologists, the term 'biomedicine' is often substituted, to emphasize modern medicine's grounding in biological sciences and to de-emphasize its geographical origins.

The term 'biomedicine' is meant to signal a universal, scientific system of knowledge about the body in health and disease. However, even in the West, many other forms of medicine and healing remain available. In fact, as Arthur Kleinman notes, 'Because of its long development under the powerful regimen of industrial capitalism, biomedicine is the most institutionalized of the forms of medicine.'[10] Biomedicine today exists within a bureaucracy that controls the institutional settings and the terms of the encounter between patient and practitioner. Powerful professions regulate the practice of modern medicine, ostensibly to guarantee the quality of care, by splitting practice into many discrete specialties and monitoring the qualifications and permissible interventions of care-givers. Dominik Wujastyk suggests that the term 'modern establishment medicine' would avoid the use of other adjectives ('modern,' 'Western,' 'scientific') that make dubious status claims.[11]

Until at least the second decade of the twentieth century, however, medicine in Europe and North America was certainly not as institution-alized or as professionally consistent as these labels suggest. Theories and practices, therapies, and medical education all changed at an accelerating pace from the mid-nineteenth century onwards. This period saw the introduction of major abdominal surgery; the discovery of anaesthetics; the contested rise of germ theory; a new focus on physiology and laboratory medicine; and the start of new specialties (e.g., nursing and psychiatry) and new therapies (e.g., serum therapy against diphtheria and antibiotic drugs such as penicillin). Even the clinical trial, supposedly the gold standard of scientific medicine, was not required in the United States until, in the 1970s, the Food and Drug Administration insisted on 'adequate and well-controlled clinical investigations' for all new claims for drugs.[12]

Thus the medicine of the West changed dramatically in the course of the nineteenth and early twentieth centuries. The medicine taught in London in the 1830s to Benjamin Hobson, Britain's first Protestant missionary-physician to China, was very different from that taught to Chinese medical students in Japan around 1900. By 1921, when the Peking Union Medical College was reopened under the auspices of the American Rockefeller Foundation following the model of the United

States' leading medical school, Johns Hopkins, the theories, practices, drugs, and underlying world views of medical sciences in 1920s America were recognizably different from those of both mid-nineteenth-century Britain and turn-of-the-century Japan.[13] At each stage in this history, therefore, we need to consider what attributes constituted the 'Western,' or 'modern,' or 'scientific' medicine under discussion.

Whatever the content, Chinese sources remained fairly consistent in referring to *xiyi* 西醫 (Western medicine) in contrast to *zhongyi* 中醫 (Chinese medicine). Sometimes, *xiyi* was replaced with *yangyi* 洋醫 (foreign medicine), usually a derogatory term, or the more laudable *xiandai yixue* 現代醫學 (modern medicine). Similarly, Chinese medicine was sometimes referred to dismissively as *jiuyi* 舊醫 (old medicine), or patriotically as *guoyi* 國醫 (national medicine). Geographical origins were important, a fact that Chinese publications made clear when referring to Western medicine from Japan as *dongxiyi* 東西醫 (literally, 'eastern Western medicine'). This book adopts the same usage as the historical sources, with the result that the terms 'modern medicine,' 'national medicine,' 'Chinese medicine,' and 'Western medicine' appear frequently. None of these terms had a fixed meaning apart from the implied contrast with its civilizational other, but their rhetorical content was unmistakable.

Before the nineteenth century, Chinese people did not need to specify whether medicine was Western or Chinese. All medicine and healing was *yi* 醫. *Yi* was both a noun, referring to healers, and a transitive verb, 'to cure, to heal (someone or something).' A healer might be honoured with the title of 'imperial physician' (*tai yi* 太醫) or be a member of the literati class, a 'Confucian physician' (*ru yi* 儒醫). He, or (rarely) she, might be an itinerant peddler of medicines, a 'bell doctor' (*ling yi* 鈴醫), or, if female, a 'drugs woman' (*yao po* 藥婆), or be referred to as a 'quack' or 'vulgar physician' (*yong yi* 庸醫). Women were only rarely referred to as *yi*, although they were important in health care as midwives (*chan po* 產婆 or *wen po* 穩婆) and might also work as shaman healers (*shi po* 師婆). The word *po* here means 'old woman' or 'granny,' and it was used of women who made a living outside the home, which was generally frowned on under Confucian moral norms. So, no matter what service the *yi po* 醫婆 (medical grannies) provided to women and children in the sequestered inner quarters of well-to-do households, their name carried derogatory connotations.[14]

In its original sense, *yi* referred to an extensive sphere of human activity. The word for ailment, *bing* 病, could also mean any flaw or failing, so that to *yi* a *bing* might refer to the correction of flaws in a piece of craftsmanship or in an administrative policy as well as to the specific activity of healing illness. The word 'to treat' (which is not the same as 'to heal'), *zhi* 治, has a semantic range that extends from dealing with disease to administering a bureaucracy, 'to put in order, to govern.' There is a long history of metaphorical equivalence between the management of the human body and the management of the political realm. For instance, the foundational medical-cosmological text *The Yellow Emperor's Inner Canon* (*Huangdi nei jing* 黃帝內經) contains the famous observation: 'The Sagely Man treats incipient disease rather than existing disease, and incipient [political] disorder rather than existing disorder.'[15] Indeed, the educated elites of late Imperial China considered it part of their duty as good Confucians to study the literature of classical medicine, primarily in order to manage the health care of their families but also to demonstrate their virtue and competence as potential stewards and administrators of the empire. Fan Zhongyan (范仲淹, 989-1052), a leading politician and educator in the Northern Song dynasty, is supposed to have said: 'If high office is unattainable, none can fulfill so well as a good doctor the desire to save people and benefit the world.'[16]

In the course of the nineteenth- and twentieth-century encounter with the West, the word *yi* lost these associations with Neo-Confucian piety; instead, it became an example of a contested 'super-sign' in the sense analyzed by Lydia Liu. That is, it became a signifier that mediates between two or more languages, in the process changing its original semantic range while creating an illusion of intercultural equivalence. As Liu puts it: 'The super-sign is good at camouflaging the foreignness and internal split of a verbal unit by adopting the unchanging face of an indigenous word, be it in written or phonetic form, and projecting an illusion of homogeneity.'[17] During the course of the late nineteenth and early twentieth centuries, *yi* no longer referred to the whole of the cultural field of healing. It became ambiguous, requiring the modifiers we have seen – *xiyi, zhongyi, xinyi, jiuyi, guoyi,* and *yangyi.* To refer to the field of medicine, it became necessary to say *yixue* 醫學, a word that had originally meant 'school of medicine' but that had been adapted by seventeenth-century Jesuits to mean 'learned medicine,' a new usage that Protestant missionary translators revived in the nineteenth century to refer to 'scientific' medicine.[18] The act of splitting and renaming what had previously been merely aspects of *yi* emphasized newly contrasting epistemologies of health and disease. Today, it is easy to take these separate categories as natural and to forget that they are artificial derivatives of what was once a single, complex field of activity. The concept of a *Chinese* medicine did not exist until Chinese physicians found themselves forced to define their field in order to distinguish it from the medicine of the West.[19]

'Scientific medicine' was of little interest to most Chinese in the nineteenth century, and when Chinese people *did* adopt it, it was rarely for its therapeutic efficacy. Instead, they turned to modern medicine for a range of non-medical reasons: to bolster the position of the Chinese government vis-à-vis the imperial powers; to make the case for the overthrow of the last imperial dynasty; to provide new kinds of jobs for women as a route to female emancipation; or as a new route to individual positions of wealth or power. These and other motives for the adoption of the new medicine deflate our confident assumptions about the objectivity of science or the efficacy of medical therapies and point towards other values. If there is a common denominator in the motives of Chinese who adopted Western medicine, it is that medicine became symbolic of a shared striving towards the ideals of modernity. More surprising, perhaps, is that this striving for modernity was also shared by many supporters and reformers of Chinese medicine. The 'cultural conservatives' who fought to preserve a place for Chinese medicine in modern China were just as committed to modernization as were those who strove to abolish traditional medicine in the name of medical modernity. Chinese medicine was radically reconfigured in the process of the struggle to assert that it was both an essential part of Chinese culture and a praiseworthy example of 'folk science' that could be appreciated and validated by moderns.[20] As a result of this process, Chinese medicine today is neither traditional nor even purely Chinese.

Thus medicine carried with it many meanings that were only tangentially related to what sociologists call 'health-seeking behaviour.' Through the history of medicine we can follow the ongoing integration of China into the global economy of goods and ideas. Through medicine, we can interpret what modernity and science meant to both supply-side and demand-side actors. We can begin to understand why becoming modern and scientific was so important not only to the reforming elites but also to their more conservative opponents.

One of this study's most interesting findings is that the values associated with modernity (including science, democracy, linear time, and the commitment to progress in human history) came to be equally important in Chinese medicine. In this, Chinese medicine was part of a larger cultural undertaking. The indigenization of the values of modernity also led to the reformulation of many other 'traditional' spheres of knowledge and culture. The centrality of Confucianism in Chinese society was fundamentally undermined when the Imperial civil service examinations were abolished in 1905 and civil service appointments were filled instead by holders of degrees in the new sciences (such as engineering, geology, and international law).[21] After the First World War, when, in 1919, the victorious Allies refused to restore Germany's Chinese territories to Chinese sovereignty, a whole generation of Chinese blamed their culture and its inward-looking focus for China's weakness on the international stage. For this generation, who increasingly looked abroad for validation, the literary language of official communications seemed anachronistic; instead, they advocated for the use of vernacular Chinese even in written documents. In addition to importing many new words from the West, modern vernacular Chinese also adopted grammatical forms from European languages.[22] At the same time, the new Chinese literature was drawing many of its forms from Western literature;[23] Buddhism, Daoism, and Confucianism were all reformed to more closely resemble Western ideas of religion;[24] exposure to Western Enlightenment ideas of individual liberty and equality led to changes in family structure, particularly with respect to the status of women, and to a new legal code based on the principle of individual rights;[25] and it is hardly necessary to point out that the concepts of republicanism and communism are not indigenous to China.

In each of these areas, the encounter with Western forms led to the creation of a new technical lexicon, the mapping of new concepts onto pre-existing elements of Chinese culture, and the selective deployment of aspects of foreign disciplines by different people for divergent purposes. In the process, Chinese culture was repackaged into ontological categories defined against their Western counterparts, and these re-defined 'traditional' elements went on to shape Chinese culture for both Chinese and Westerners through the rest of the twentieth century and into the twenty-first.

In describing how Chinese people used medicine as an instrument of cultural and political self-fashioning, I examine negotiations of the meanings and contents of 'Western' and 'Chinese.' In twentieth-century China, science was an ideal trope, deployed to help correct some of the perceived failings of Chinese culture – just as, in the West today, 'holistic' Chinese medicine is often represented as a corrective to the mechanistic reductionism of modern clinical medicine. This analogy may make it easier to see that the flow and counterflow of science and culture consist of selective appropriations, of politically charged interpretations and reinscriptions of meaning. There are no pure cultural forms.[26]

The next chapter briefly outlines the diversity of healing in nineteenth-century China across the range of social class, nationalities, and gender. This spectrum of medical practices provides the substrate onto which idealized notions of 'Western' and 'Chinese,' 'modern' and 'traditional,' were to be imposed in subsequent decades. Chapter 3 examines the missionary medicine deliberately exported to China in the hope that the power of healing would open Chinese hearts and minds to Christianity more effectively than evangelism alone. As representatives of modern scientific medicine, missionaries were partially displaced after the end of the Sino-Japanese War in 1895 by Chinese enthusiasm for Japanese interpretations of science.[27] One overlooked aspect of Japanese influence in modern China is the way it served as a model for the reform of traditional culture as well as for the appropriation of modern science: this is the focus of Chapter 4. Chapter 5 explores the value of public health for the Chinese government, while Chapter 6 examines the political uses of medicine in the lives of influential Chinese. Chapter 7 describes the institutions created to support the new professions of medicine, and Chapter 8 highlights the effects of these cultural and institutional changes on the practice of Chinese medicine. The concluding chapter brings us full circle – to the new spectrum of medical practice of mid-twentieth-century China.

The Historical Context: Revolutionaries and Imperialists in China, 1839-1949

This overview is intended primarily for readers who may be unfamiliar with Chinese political history. Others may wish to skip this section and go directly to the next chapter.

The century preceding the founding of the People's Republic of China by the Chinese Communist Party (CCP) in 1949 was extraordinary in terms of its military, social, and cultural disruption. It is often called China's 'century of revolution.' From 1839 to 1842 and again from 1856 to 1860, military engagement with the British over trading rights (the 'Opium Wars') led to China's being forced to open coastal and inland port cities to foreign trade and to lease substantial territorial concessions to Britain and then to other imperialist nations, including France, the United States, Germany, Italy, Russia, and (after 1895) Japan. These cities, in which foreigners were allowed to live and trade, were known as the 'treaty ports,' and the succession of treaties that gave them these rights were known as the 'unequal treaties.' The treaty ports, together with their foreign and Chinese residents, were declared to be beyond the purview of the Chinese legal system. This extraterritoriality meant that foreigners were protected from Chinese prosecution unless a Chinese plaintiff could sue them in one of the foreign-run treaty port courts. The treaties also allowed for large reparations to foreigners from the Chinese government if their persons or property were unlawfully harmed even when outside the foreign concession areas. The treaty ports quickly became attractive refuges for dissident or fugitive Chinese avoiding prosecution, and regaining sovereignty over these key port cities was one of the priorities of the Chinese government during the Republican Era (1912-49).

From the mid-nineteenth century on, the stability of the Qing (Manchu) imperial dynasty was further threatened by devastating internal rebellions. In particular, the Taiping Rebellion of 1851-64 resulted in millions of deaths from fighting, displacement, and starvation. Southern China was laid waste not only in terms of its agriculture but also in terms of its cultural infrastructure and the ability of the population to contribute tax revenue. Close on the heels of the Taiping Rebellion came the Nian Rebellion in northern China, which reached its height in the period between 1853 and 1855, when the Yellow River broke its banks and switched course from the south of the Shandong Peninsula to the north, flooding thousands of hectares of arable land and displacing millions of farmers. Other, smaller rebellions erupted in Guangzhou (Canton) in the south and in the Muslim areas in the northwest and southwest.

The period from 1860 to 1895 is often referred to as the period of the 'Self-Strengthening Movement' (*ziqiang yundong* 自強運動) or the 'Foreign Affairs Movement' (*yangwu yundong* 洋務運動). When the Taiping rebels, who held the City of Nanjing and much of central and southern China by the early 1860s, advanced on the foreign treaty port of Shanghai they were effectively repulsed by British marines and artillery in 1860, and by British and French forces together with American mercenaries in 1862. The foreign artillery so impressed the Chinese generals and provincial governors Zeng Guofan and Li Hongzhang that, by 1863, they had created three small arsenals to provide themselves with similar modern weaponry. The year 1860 also saw the signing of the final Treaty of Tianjin between Britain and China and the establishment of the *Zongli yamen,* or Office for Foreign Affairs, the first institution in Chinese history to deal with foreign countries as equal sovereign states rather than as tribute-bearing satellites. It was quickly followed by the *Tongwen guan* 同文舘, or School of Foreign Languages, for training Chinese diplomats in Beijing. The function of the school soon expanded to include training in Western sciences, for which foreign teachers were employed. Later, similar schools were established at Fuzhou and Shanghai.[28]

Funding for these military and diplomatic projects was largely provided by revenue collected by the new Imperial Maritime Customs Service. This government office evolved from the Inspectorate of Customs, formed in Shanghai in 1854 when British, French, and American consuls offered to collect import duties on behalf of the

Chinese government during disruptions to normal trade caused by the Taiping Rebellion and the occupation of Shanghai by Triad (illegal secret society) rebels. Headed by a succession of British inspectors-general, this internationally staffed service became the Chinese government's main source of foreign currency and an important guarantor of China's international loans. Its steady income was also repeatedly mortgaged to foreign powers to pay for the various indemnities they imposed on China over the next half-century. Its revenues were also used to fund modernizing activities such as the new military arsenals and schools described above, and also the Plague Prevention Service set up in Manchuria in the wake of the plague epidemic of 1910 (see Chapter 5).

China lost control of the Southeast Asian peninsula in the Sino-French War of 1883-85. In the Sino-Japanese War of 1894-95, China and Japan used their new navies to contest their respective influence in Korea, and Japan won. The victorious Japanese imposed a burdensome war indemnity of US$200 million, payable in gold. Japan's victory surprised European observers and spurred many Chinese to advocate for the radical modernization of their military and civilian government.

Finally, in 1899, a group known to history as the Boxers because of their characteristic calisthenic exercises began a rebellion under the slogan of 'destroy the Qing and restore the Ming.' This was a reference to the Manchu ethnicity of the Qing ruling class, who had overthrown the last ethnically Han Chinese empire, the Ming, in 1644. When the Boxer rebels murdered two German missionaries, Germany's harsh military retaliation refocused the insurrection on the goal of driving European foreigners out of China. Conservative Manchu officials decided to support the Boxers, hoping that a combination of imperial troops and rebel forces would succeed in defeating the foreign forces in China. Empress Dowager Cixi declared war on all foreign powers in June 1900 and ordered provincial governors to send troops to Beijing. To the provincial governors, it was clear that the motley combined forces of untrained Boxer rebels and imperial recruits were no match for foreign armies, so they resisted the call to arms and made their own arrangements with the foreign consuls. The Boxers' two-month siege of the foreign embassies in Beijing ('the Siege of Peking') was routed in August by a combined foreign force. The foreign allies exacted a crippling indemnity on China: US$333 million to be paid over forty years, mainly from Customs Service revenues. Jack Gray estimates that the combined indemnity payments at the end of the nineteenth century consumed fully 44 percent of the Chinese government's annual revenue.[29]

By the turn of the twentieth century, it was clear to almost all Chinese that foreign powers were a threat to China. The consensus among the foreigners themselves was that their trading interests were best served by propping up the Qing imperial regime, but many Chinese were convinced that China's chances of survival as an independent state under the Manchu government were precarious. Eventually the Qing court, which had previously resisted attempts at structural reforms, embarked on a series of modernizations – the 'New Policies' (*xinzheng* 新政) – in the period from 1901 to the Chinese Revolution in late 1911. China was being forced to engage with foreign powers on terms that were set by the Westerners and that underlined China's subordination. To this day, Mainland Chinese historians refer to the period between 1895 and the founding of the People's Republic of China in 1949 as *guochi* 國恥 – [the period of] national humiliation.

The New Policies of 1901-11 aimed to create a constitutional monarchy and set a date for local elections in 1912-14, to be followed by elections for a national assembly. The proposals, modelled on the constitutional monarchies of the West, restricted the electorate to educated, propertied men and so would have won the support of many of China's elite. The measures also included reform of the educational system to include study of 'Western learning': science, international law, and foreign languages. The original intention was to gradually phase out the old-style civil service examinations based on expositions of classical texts. However, Japan's victory in the 1905 Russo-Japanese War, which seemed to represent the triumph of a newly created constitutional monarchy (Meiji Japan) over imperial autocracy (czarist Russia), persuaded the new Chinese Ministry of Education to prioritize educational reform. Thus, China abruptly abolished the entire civil service examination system as of 1906. Ironically, this act may have hastened the end of the Qing since, at one stroke, it alienated the thousands of local gentry who had spent many years of their lives studying in the hope of being able to advance through the examination system.

Among the many Chinese who were working for the overthrow of the Qing was Sun Yat-sen (Sun Wen 孫文, styled Zhongshan 中山, or Yat-sen in Cantonese pronounciation, 1866-1925), a Cantonese convert to Christianity who came from a farming family and who spent some time studying in Hawai'i before becoming one of the first students at the Hong Kong College of Medicine, run by two respected British physicians, Patrick Manson and James Cantlie. Sun graduated in 1892, but the British Medical Association did not recognize the qualifications of the Hong Kong graduates. Soon after, he turned to politics, organizing revolutionary secret societies, sponsoring anti-Qing propaganda, and travelling between China, Hong Kong, Japan, Hawaii, the United States, and England. Although the uprisings organized by his followers were initially unsuccessful, Sun's reputation was that of an inspiring leader and a committed republican whose success at raising funds from overseas supporters was considerable. In October 1911, the local government discovered a planned uprising in the inland city of Wuhan, thus forcing the rebels to mobilize quickly and to declare Wuhan independent of the central government. This triggered a series of similar declarations by most of·China's provinces, and a cascade of hastily formed provincial assemblies announced their support for a republic under Sun Yat-sen's leadership. Although the new Republic of China was declared on 1 January 1912, with Sun as its provisional first president, Sun's lack of military support persuaded him to cede the presidency to General Yuan Shikai 袁世凱, who commanded the most powerful Qing army. The first national elections were held in 1912, giving a majority of seats to Sun Yat-sen's newly formed Nationalist Party (the Guomindang 國民黨, or GMD [often rendered KMT, according to the Wade-Giles romanization as Kuo-min-tang]). Yuan Shikai, however, hoping to make himself the founder of a new imperial dynasty, outlawed the Nationalist Party in 1915. Even though Yuan died of kidney failure a few months later, his plans to re-establish a monarchy had already offended many regional leaders, who withdrew their support for the Republic and created their own local power bases, leading to the 'Warlord Period' of 1916-27. During

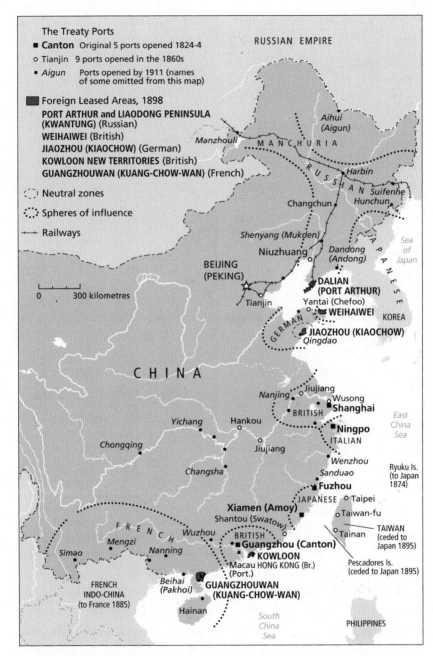

The Treaty Ports
- ■ **Canton** Original 5 ports opened 1824-4
- ○ Tianjin 9 ports opened in the 1860s
- • *Aigun* Ports opened by 1911 (names of some omitted from this map)

■ Foreign Leased Areas, 1898
PORT ARTHUR and LIAODONG PENINSULA (KWANTUNG) (Russian)
WEIHAIWEI (British)
JIAOZHOU (KIAOCHOW) (German)
KOWLOON NEW TERRITORIES (British)
GUANGZHOUWAN (KUANG-CHOW-WAN) (French)

⌣ Neutral zones
⫶ Spheres of influence
→ Railways

RUSSIAN EMPIRE

Aihui (Aigun)
Manzhouli MANCHURIA
RUSSIAN
Harbin
Changchun Suifenhe Hunchun
Shenyang (Mukden) Sea of Japan
Niuzhuang Dandong (Andong)
BEIJING (PEKING)
Tianjin DALIAN (PORT ARTHUR)
Yantai (Chefoo)
WEIHAIWEI KOREA
GERMAN JIAOZHOU (KIAOCHOW)
Qingdao

CHINA

Nanjing Jiujiang
Wusong
BRITISH Shanghai
Yichang Hankou Ningpo
ITALIAN East China Sea
Chongqing Jiujiang
Wenzhou Ryuku Is. (to Japan 1874)
Changsha Sanduao
Fuzhou
JAPANESE Taipei
Xiamen (Amoy) Taiwan-fu
Shantou (Swatow)
BRITISH Tainan TAIWAN (ceded to Japan 1895)
Mengzi Wuzhou Guangzhou (Canton)
Simao Nanning KOWLOON
Macau HONG KONG (Br.) Pescadores Is. (ceded to Japan 1895)
(Port.)
FRENCH INDO-CHINA (to France 1885)
Beihai (Pakhoi) GUANGZHOUWAN (KUANG-CHOW-WAN)
Hainan South China Sea PHILIPPINES

0 300 kilometres

Figure 1 Map of China showing treaty ports, circa 1920. *Source:* Map by Eric Leinberger. Based on the map "Imperialism in the 1890s" from *The Cambridge History of China: Volume 11: Late Ch'ing, 1800-1911* (Part 2. New York: Cambridge University Press, 1980).

this time, a series of short-lived governments was elected in Beijing, and these claimed control of tax and Customs Service revenue. The inability of these governments to extend their control into the provinces prolonged the political fragmentation, with Sun Yat-sen heading a rival government in Canton, and Western and Japanese authorities being in control of the many treaty ports.

Meanwhile, the First World War (1914-18) saw Japan joining the Allies and consolidating the territorial gains made after the 1894-95 Sino-Japanese War and the 1905 Russo-Japanese War. In 1915, Japan presented President Yuan Shikai with the Twenty-One Demands. In their original form these went far beyond recognizing and consolidating Japan's existing territorial concessions in Manchuria and the Shandong Peninsula, in effect making most of northeastern China into a Japanese protectorate while insisting that Japan be the only future beneficiary of any trading or territorial concessions in China. When the demands were leaked to the Western powers, Japan was forced to delete the most imperialistic clauses, but Yuan Shikai, whose ability to mount military resistance to Japan had been severely weakened by regional 'warlord' opposition, signed a 'Thirteen Demands' treaty with Japan in May 1915. This event caused great ill-will in China towards Japan and also raised Western powers' concerns about Japan's cavalier attitude towards international diplomacy. Meanwhile, China supported the Allied cause by sending about ninety-six thousand troops to serve on the Western Front, where they were not trusted to be combat forces but were used instead as front-line labourers, digging trenches and hauling artillery.

After the defeat of Germany, the Allies at the Paris Peace Conference shocked China by deciding *not* to restore the former German concessions to Chinese sovereignty, awarding them instead to Japan. Chinese public opinion exploded into outraged demonstrations in the cities. On 4 May 1919, a violently anti-Japanese, anti-imperialist demonstration of some three thousand students in central Beijing gave its name to a new movement dedicated to rescuing China from its international and domestic weaknesses. Many Chinese reformers and intellectuals in this May Fourth Movement blamed traditional Chinese culture for the defeat of republicanism and for China's vulnerability to foreign imperialism. Instead, they turned to two ideals of modernity, famously personified as 'Mr. Science' and 'Mr. Democracy' in the writings of Chen Duxiu 陳獨秀, the iconoclastic editor of the journal *New Youth (Xin Qingnian* 新青年) and co-founder of the Chinese Communist Party. To his generation, the concepts underlying Chinese medicine – *yin* and *yang*, the Five Phases, and belief in cosmic resonance between heaven, earth, and humankind – had to be expunged from the consciousness of modern Chinese citizens so that a new, strong nation could be created. In this, the leaders of the May Fourth Movement concurred with the New Culture Movement, which, a few years previously, had begun to increase political awareness among ordinary Chinese through emphasizing vernacular rather than classical literature and through attempting to reform the extreme hierarchies of the patriarchal Chinese family to allow for individual choice (e.g., in marriage), recognition of the individual rights of women, and engagement with modernist values. The modernism of this movement was expressed in a new orientation towards progress rather than towards an idealized Confucian past. It promoted science, democracy, and a commitment to racial improvement through eugenics and physical education in order to make Chinese people more evolutionarily 'fit' in an era of near-universal belief in the social-Darwinist concept of 'the survival of the fittest.'[30] Sports, physical education, and the banning of footbinding for women were thus the individualized, bodily expressions of a general concern to improve China's political and military position vis-à-vis that of the intruding foreign powers.[31]

Sun Yat-sen often appealed for Western and Japanese assistance, but only one country agreed to support the project of political reunification. In 1923, Soviet Russia, itself only six years old, said it would aid Sun's Nationalist Party if the Nationalists agreed to work together with the fledgling Chinese Communist Party, which had been formed in 1921. When Sun died in 1925, his reunification project passed to a young Moscow-trained military officer, Chiang Kai-shek 蔣介石 (1887-1975). With Soviet advisors on hand, the two organizations began their Northern Expedition to consolidate China's heartland under a single government in 1926. By March of 1927, a Communist advance contingent had succeeded in taking China's richest city, Shanghai, where it waited for the Nationalist army to bring reinforcements and organizational expertise. When Chiang Kai-shek's forces arrived, however, they moved to quickly disarm and round up the Communist forces, and then they slaughtered them. Thousands were killed on the mere suspicion of being Communist sympathizers, and surviving Communists were forced to flee or go underground, thus beginning an enmity that persists to this day.

Meanwhile, Chiang's forces continued to consolidate their positions, eventually uniting most of the provinces along the eastern seaboard and declaring Nanjing their capital city as political support was stronger there than around Beijing, where warlords Feng Yuxiang 馮玉祥 (1882-1948) and Yan Xishan 閻錫山 (1883-1960) still wielded considerable power. This period of Nationalist Party rule lasted from 1928 until the Japanese invasion in 1937 and is known as the 'Nanjing Decade.' It was a period of remarkable state-building activity, with the establishment of a modern banking system, unification and stabilization of the currency, energetic road- and rail-building projects, the creation of a new legal code, and – at least in the cities – substantial efforts to improve public health and sanitation and to expand the educational system. In 1930, the Nationalist government regained control over the trade tariffs that had previously been set by the imperial powers. The League of Nations provided technical expertise for state-planned industrialization projects, for example, sending engineers to help rebuild the Yangzi River flood control systems after a devastating flood in 1931.

Chiang Kai-shek continued to wage war against the Communists, many of whom had gathered in a rural area on the Jiangxi/Fujian border, where they proclaimed a Chinese Soviet republic in 1931. The Communists successfully used guerrilla tactics to repel several of Chiang's military expeditions but were finally encircled by Nationalist troops in October 1934. During the ensuing military retreat, constantly threatened by Chiang's forces, the Communists marched about nine thousand kilometres, taking a full year until they were finally able to establish a secure base in Yan'an in northern Shaanxi Province in late 1935. Mao Zedong's 毛澤東 (1893-1976) leadership during this famous 'Long March' consolidated his position at the head of the CCP, and Yan'an became the centre of Chinese Communist resistance during the War of Resistance against Japan (1937-45).

Support for the CCP was drawn mainly from the farmers, who benefited from land reforms and rural health and literacy programs. This
reliance on the peasantry to fuel the revolution was in contrast to Russia's
insistence on the vital role of an urban proletariat. The Communists
experimented with representative government. Under Mao's leadership
they also became expert at guerrilla warfare against both the Japanese
and Chiang Kai-shek's Nationalist army.

In China, the Second World War was almost synonymous with the
Second Sino-Japanese War, which lasted from the Japanese invasion in
1937 until 1945. The Nationalist government was forced to retreat from
Nanjing, first to Wuhan and then, in late 1938, to Chongqing, which
became the wartime capital, referred to by the Western media of the
day as 'Chungking, capital of Free China.'

This relocation of urban professionals and officials to the far more
rural hinterland forced many of them to experiment with local, small-
scale policy initiatives in contrast to their previous reliance on top-down
state-building activities. With no central government to back them up
and no certainty about the outcome of the war, doctors, educators, and
other professionals refocused their attention on local, realizable initiatives. The vibrant improvisation of the chaotic wartime years has been
all but ignored by historians of medicine, who have been overwhelmingly concerned with the narrative of China as a nation-state.[32] Kim
Taylor's work shows clearly that, by 1944, in the Communist headquarters in Yan'an, Mao Zedong was responding to the exigencies of isolation
and a largely peasant support base by advocating a 'united front' between
useful elements of traditional culture and modern, scientific behaviour.
In Mao's original formulation, old medicine and old-style doctors could
be made more scientific by uniting with new medicine, a process that
would involve discarding the feudal aspects of Chinese medicine, represented by 'illiteracy, superstition, and unhygienic habits.'[33]

As we shall see, the commitment to medical modernization was not
only a concern of politicians. For many Chinese in the early twentieth
century, hygiene and medical technologies were synonymous with
modernity and civilization.[34] Doctors of Chinese medicine also shared
these convictions and struggled to create their own version of a hygienic,

civilized medical practice. On many levels, medicine became a metaphor for the social and political health of the nation. It is hard to imagine a better topic through which to explore the creation of a Chinese modernity.

The Spectrum of Chinese Healing Practices

2

Even a quick glance at the state of medicine in China during the Republican period (1912-49) should be enough to convince us that the path to modernization includes stages during which 'the modern' coexists with 'the traditional.' At the 'Westernmost' end of the spectrum stood the American Rockefeller Foundation's state-of-the-art Peking Union Medical College (北京協和醫院). From 1921 on, the new college employed prominent Western physicians, was equipped with the best available technology, and trained elite Chinese students to be the future leaders of the medical profession in China.[1] Other institutions of Western medicine included smaller missionary-run hospitals and clinics as well as multi-denominational 'union medical colleges' that pooled missionary resources in order to provide more modern and expensive Western-style facilities. There were also the military hospitals of the Chinese, Japanese, and Russian armies; foreign-run medical facilities in the colonial treaty ports; Chinese Customs Service quarantine stations; and a growing number of private for-profit hospitals alongside a few run by regional and national governments. Medical practitioners in pharmacies and drugstores might prescribe Chinese-style or Western-style drugs or both. Western-trained physicians found private practice in major cities, as did others who claimed an education in Western medicine but – since licensing regulations were seldom enforced – could just as easily have acquired their knowledge from books or from working as hospital porters.

At what we may loosely refer to as the 'Chinese medicine' side of the spectrum, there were scholarly physicians who had inherited their knowledge from family members or through apprenticeships and who practised in their own clinics or in the homes of their patients. They included graduates of the new colleges of Chinese medicine as well as the famous Bamboo Grove monks (who specialized in gynecology) and martial artists (who were experts in orthopedic manipulation).[2] Add to the mix the specialists in minor surgery, acupuncturists, travelling peddlers of Chinese drugs, people who gave medical advice in temples, and massage therapists (many of whom were blind). Finally, dentists would pull a troublesome tooth for a fee and toss it onto the mound that advertised their occupation. Along with these predominantly male practitioners of medicine, women healers were active as midwives, as specialists in pediatric care (using moxibustion and massage), and as smallpox variolation specialists.[3]

Illiterate healers are, by definition, unlikely to leave written accounts of their practices, so the writings of educated observers are essential for our understanding of popular and folk healing practices. Unfortunately, such observers were rarely sympathetic, reflecting their class and cultural differences. We will bear these prejudices in mind as we review two commentaries in order to assess the starting point for our examination of medical change in China. The first source, 'The Chinese Arts of Healing,' was written by John Dudgeon, who gained his MD and Master of Surgery from Glasgow University in Scotland in 1862, travelled to China in 1863, and lived there until his death in 1901. While in China, Dudgeon served as physician to the British Legation (embassy) in Beijing and was professor of anatomy and physiology at the *Tongwen guan* 同文館, variously translated as Office of Combined Learning, School of Foreign Languages, or (as in Dudgeon's *British Medical Journal* obituary), the Imperial College. The *Tongwen guan* trained Chinese in foreign languages and foreign affairs on behalf of the *Zongli yamen* 總理衙門 (the Chinese Foreign Office), and medicine was part of that agenda. While serving in Beijing, Dudgeon published prolifically in both English and Chinese, mostly on medical subjects but also on his observations of famines, diet, hygiene, bound feet, the opium trade, and the size of the Chinese population.[4] His observations on 'The Chinese Arts of Healing' were serialized in the *Chinese Recorder* in nine articles published between September 1869 and October 1870. They give an overview of healing practices in the Beijing area from the point of view of an enthusiast for Enlightenment rationality and Protestant evangelical Christianity.

Our second source for the spectrum of Chinese healing practices is an article by Qiu Jisheng 裘吉生 (whose legal name was Qiu Qingyuan 裘慶元, 1872-1947) titled 'Medical Customs of Shaoxing,' published in the *Shaoxing Journal of Medicine and Pharmacy* in 1915.[5] Qiu was a native of Shaoxing, Zhejiang Province. He became a member of the anti-Manchu Restoration Society on its founding in 1904 and was involved in several anti-Qing activities. Through his Shaoxing connections he grew acquainted with several famous revolutionaries, such as the female martyr Qiu Jin 秋瑾 and her cousin Xu Xilin 徐錫麟, the literary modernist Lu Xun 魯迅, and the Restoration Society founder Cai Yuanpei 蔡元培, who went on to become chancellor of Beijing University and a major May Fourth-era intellectual.

Qiu Jisheng supported a revolutionary purge in medicine as in politics, being an ardent supporter of the reform and modernization of Chinese medicine in order to ensure its continued existence as part of a modernized Chinese culture. He collected and republished old medical texts, lectured at the new schools and colleges of Chinese medicine, and was involved in several early Chinese medical journals, including the *Shaoxing Journal of Medicine and Pharmacy* from its inception in 1908.

Bear in mind that both John Dudgeon and Qiu Jisheng were assessing Chinese medical customs against a standard. In Dudgeon's case, it was the medicine of mid-nineteenth-century Scotland; in Qiu's, it was a combination of the secular medicine of the elite literary tradition (which was still relatively inaccessible to Dudgeon) and the discourse of what Ruth Rogaski terms 'hygienic modernity.'[6] Dudgeon lived in Beijing, in the north, whereas Qiu lived in Shaoxing, in the southern Lower Yangzi region. Dudgeon wrote before the culture shocks of the 1894-95 Sino-Japanese War and the 1900 Boxer Rebellion, whereas Qiu wrote in the early years of the Chinese Republic. Each man judged what he saw and found it wanting.

Dudgeon's 'Chinese Arts of Healing'

Dudgeon divided the 'Chinese arts of healing' into three broad fields: magic, charms, and gymnastics. Although he occasionally referred to classical literature such as the *Yellow Emperor's Inner Canon* (*Huangdi nei jing* 黃帝內經), the ideas contained within it fell squarely into his category of superstition and magic. Nonetheless, Dudgeon was fairly sympathetic to Chinese culture in general, noting similarities between Chinese and 'primitive' European thought, as in this early quote:

> We find the Chinese describing particular diseases according to particular planets, portioning out their relations to these heavenly bodies, to the five elements, colours, tastes, points of the compass, &c., &c.; and gravely assigning every disease to the predominance of one or other, and treating them accordingly. In this respect their pathology even to this day resembles Galen's which depended on the four elements, the four humors, the four qualities, and these in combination. Like him the Chinese are diligent observers of the phenomena of disease; and they might become first class physicians, if their predilections and reverence for the theories of their ancestors did not warp and bias their judgment.[7]

Dudgeon perceptively noted that many Chinese technical and religious texts were written in such a way as to be confusing or even unintelligible to outsiders. (One might note in passing that medical terminology in English is not exactly transparent either.) Because of this, he regarded even literate physicians as 'quacks and sorcerers,' claiming that all were charlatans out to make money from unsuspecting clients. Figure 2 shows an 'itinerant healer' photographed by missionaries in the 1860s as an embodiment of the 'quack' competition.

Other aspects of 'magic' included temple medicine. Here, Dudgeon found deities presiding over particular diseases, especially smallpox. The simplest appeal for a cure called for patients to rub the part of a temple statue that corresponded to the location of their own disease. In another method, patients or their family members would choose a numbered stick from a bamboo tube containing up to a hundred such sticks, then toss coins or other two-sided objects in order to divine whether the number on the stick was *yang* (correct) or *yin* (incorrect). Once confirmed, the patient consulted a numbered list of recipes, choosing the recipe that corresponded to the number on the stick.

Temple medicine was a recurrent concern for the Chinese government, which feared that charismatic healers could turn their followers into rebels. According to Dudgeon: 'It is deemed an offence against the state to assemble, especially for women and girls, at these temples for purposes of jugglery, burning incense, witchcraft and healing of disease.'[8] The Yellow Turban Rebellion, which occurred during the Han dynasty, had grown out of such heterodox healing, as had several more recent uprisings. In the eighteenth and nineteenth centuries, this resulted in imperial proclamations against the rebuilding of temples without court permission.[9]

Temple priests might also visit patients at home, where they offered food to appease the spirits responsible for the disease or placed mirrors to repel them. They would also chant 'formularies' (probably spells ordering the disease demons away), while ringing bells and beating gongs. Dudgeon considered these visits to constitute one of the ways that dangerous epidemics (such as diphtheria, typhus, cholera, and smallpox) were spread around the city.

Spirit-mediums might also be consulted, either to discover the cause of disease or, by use of a writing-brush, to elicit a prescription while the medium was in a trance state.[10] There was also a specifically Manchu form of shamanism called *tiao shen* (跳神 'jumping spirits'), in which the medium invited the spirits by playing a tambourine while jumping on one foot. Families might resort to an expert in one of several different varieties of fortune-telling, some based on astrology, some on divination using the *Book of Changes* (*Yijing* 易經).[11] Fortune-telling was often the occupation of blind people. According to Dudgeon:

> The number of tolerably well-dressed blind individuals with official hats, carrying gongs, cymbals or three-stringed guitars, has often struck the foreign resident in Peking. Those with musical instruments are employed generally at the theatres and places of amusement; the others are fortune-tellers who are supported in this superstitious

manner. They receive about a penny for their services, which are usually solicited by women.[12]

Turning to literate sources, Dudgeon notes the parallelism in the vocabulary of health and disease, on the one hand, and political orthodoxy and rebellion, on the other. He translates *xie qi* 邪氣, the pathological *qi* that is the opposite of healthy *qi*, as 'depraved air,' saying:

> Disease is caused by the exit of the Shenchi [*shen qi* 神氣, spirit *qi*] or animal spirits and the stealthy admission of depraved air. They often ascribe pain and disease to depraved air which has not been driven out and dispelled ... and this air getting into the natural blood and air ... causes confusion and strife – and this we call pain ...
>
> In Chinese medical works we read constantly of this disease-causing air and of devils and spirits in the same sense. Chêng-ch'i [*zhengqi* 正氣, upright or normal *qi*], or Yang-ch'i [*yang qi* 養氣], stands for shen [spirit, deity], and Hsieh-ch'i [*xie qi*], or Yin-ch'i [*yin qi* 陰氣], for Kwei [*gui* 鬼, ghosts/demons] ... They are not considered really devils or spirits by the literary classes (although the common people most frequently do so) but simply ideas or imaginings of the heart.[13]

As a result of these beliefs, ordinary people often placed great faith in the use of charms, Dudgeon's second art of healing. In the Yuan and Ming dynasties, healing by charms had been one of the thirteen departments of instruction at the Imperial Medical Academy.[14] By Dudgeon's day, it had been prohibited as a heterodox practice; he reports how an old woman was imprisoned in 1870 for offering healing by charms outside one of Beijing's city gates. Nonetheless, healing by charms remained ubiquitous, was applied to all kinds of ailments, and was practised by laypersons as well as by various kinds of priests. Generally, the *fu* 符 (charm or talisman) was written on a piece of yellow paper, which was then burned, and the ashes were put into water, tea, or alcohol for ingestion by the patient. For some kinds of diseases, the ashes of charms were combined with particular herbal decoctions, a combination of ritual therapy and medication. Prayers would be said over the patient

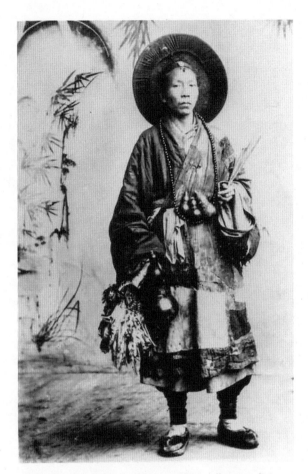

Figure 2   Photograph of Daoist priest selling medicines
and charms, late nineteenth century. *Source:* Manly Papers,
Courtesy of Special Collections, Yale Divinity School Library.

while he or she drank the medicine. In other cases, the patient would
lie down while the practitioner would mutter the prayer or incantation,
write the character of the charm in water or oil around the affected part,
and then apply the ashes of the burnt charm to the patient's skin. Alterna-
tively, the intact charm could be carried on the person in a little bag or
pasted onto his/her bedpost or door. The written characters used as
charms were not regular Chinese characters but, rather, imaginary com-
posites, often containing within them the character *gui* for ghost or

demon, one or other of the Five Phases (as appropriate) for the ailment concerned, and words relating to imperial orders, such as *shang* 尚 (to be in charge of) or *ling* 令 (an order). The accompanying prayers or incantations were an essential part of this kind of therapy. Dudgeon was sympathetic to this for, as he notes, alluding to Christ: 'Physicians have been told by one of themselves, that if they desire and hope for cures, they must with true faith call on God and teach their patients to do the same. Some sorts of devils are not cast out but by fasting and prayer.'[15]

Dudgeon provides several examples of prayers that were used while applying charms, all of which invoke a version of Chinese cosmology that includes demons as well as more benign but powerful spirits and deities, such as Laozi, or the spirits of various stars, or 'heavenly doctors.' Although Dudgeon refers to this as 'silly and nonsensical,' he was clearly alert to what we now call the placebo effect, attributing curative success to 'the great faith in the method demanded in both doctor and patient' and noting, as a comparison, that 'bread pills are often success-fully used at home.'[16]

In the *Chinese Recorder*, Dudgeon had originally intended to discuss gymnastics as his third observed mode of healing. However, his observa-tions on this subject did not appear until 1895, when he published a translation of a Ming dynasty treatise, the *Yan ling pian* 延齡篇 (*Treatise on Extending Life*), calling it 'Kung-Fu or Tauist Medical Gymnastics' in the *Journal of the Peking Oriental Society*. It contains various calisthenic and therapeutic exercises, often combined with recipes for medicinal decoctions. In contrast to his attitude towards other healing practices, Dudgeon has only high praise for 'Kung-fu,' which he says is 'founded on principles originally pure and free of all the superstition with which it is today surrounded,' arguing that it 'has all the characteristics of an ancient scientific method.'[17] Probably the rise of sport culture in Britain in the second half of the nineteenth century influenced Dudgeon's relatively favourable opinion of Chinese traditions of therapeutic exer-cise.[18] His classification of 'Kung-fu' exercises as a 'Chinese healing art' reminds us that comparing 'medicine' across cultures is far from self-explanatory. It also underscores the fact that, for the most part, Dudgeon was recording what foreign visitors to Beijing could observe while out on the streets. The forms of healing that went on within households, including the visits of learned Confucian scholar-physicians, were not easily accessible to the foreign observer.

Qiu Jisheng's 1915 Account of the 'Medical Customs of Shaoxing'

Household healing practices, by contrast, are the starting point for our Chinese observer of the medical marketplace, Qiu Jisheng. Qiu notes that it was common for householders to act as their own family's doctor, often resorting to a wide variety of dubious practices.[19] Qiu saw local Zhejiang culture as particularly superstitious, so we cannot assume that all the forms of folk practice that he describes were universal in China. But he argues that, since doctors everywhere have to compete with folk customs and unorthodox practitioners, it is essential to understand their role in society. Obviously, such a view presupposes that the reader is a member of the rational, literate elite who would be interested in such customs in order to counteract and discredit them. The following summary omits many of his deprecating remarks about the needless suffering caused by healers whom he generally regarded as inferior and about patients whom he regarded as dangerously ignorant. Qiu's account is valuable for its careful description of healing occupations and behaviour according to sex and class, and for its estimates of how much the different practitioners were able to charge for their services.

Qiu clearly disapproves of all the home healing methods he describes, including both those that regard disease as the invasion of a pathological entity to be removed and those based on the idea that changes in behaviour and temperament involve soul loss. Among the former, the technique of 'absorption by Earth' imagines disease to be the result of noxious *qi* in the body – something that could be removed by covering a bowl containing rice and a single iron nail and waving it in front of the body of the sick family member while chanting a spell that begs the deities of the Earth to absorb noxious *qi*. In the latter category, delirious speech and talking while asleep were ascribed to loss of the *hun* 魂 (soul), which had to be retrieved. To do this, members of the family would go to the local Earth God temple, taking an umbrella, broom, lantern, and some of the patient's clothing. At the temple, they would request that the soul of the patient be released and then dress the broom in her/his clothes and walk home, holding the umbrella over the patient's effigy.

While walking, the person bearing the lantern would murmur, 'Come home _____,' while the person holding the effigy would murmur, 'I'm coming home.' This would lead the patient's soul back. Apparently even quite wealthy people believed in this practice; Qiu knew of one successful doctor who even instructed patients in how to do it. Similarly, when children panicked or cried for long periods, this was called 'fright,' a symptom of the fact that the soul of infants was easily dislodged. So whenever a small child fell over, the parents would take a bit of dirt and rub it onto the tip of the child's nose, then cover her or his ears with their hands while reciting a preventive rhyme. Jean Ewen describes this custom in the late 1930s: 'If a child fell off a donkey or a chair or just fell, his mother or another adult quickly picked up a handful of earth, smeared his head with it, and muttered, "*Ohme two fu.*" [The name of the Amitabha Buddha in Chinese.] This was done three times to make sure his soul was still with him – a sort of "God bless you.""[20] According to Qiu, if a child cried at night, 'rather than investigating the cause of the ailment,' the parents might just write a charm on a piece of yellow paper and paste it on an outside wall overlooking the street to encourage the 'Night-crying Man' to stay away.

Infections were seen as numinous forces that could be bribed or persuaded to move on, which led to the custom of 'selling colds.' When someone caught a cold they would write 'cold for sale' on an envelope in which a penny was placed and then put the envelope in the street, the idea being that anyone who picked up the money would acquire the cold from the sufferer along with the money. Similarly, children's sprains and other minor injuries could be blamed on demonic forces, such as 'wind-arrows,' which could be drawn out by the mother's chanting a spell while pinching the injured part.

Qiu's discussion of home healing methods clearly demonstrates that his agenda was to illustrate how badly Chinese medical customs were in need of modernization. He completely omits any mention of helpful home healing practices, such as dietary modification or physical exercise.[21] Even when describing treatment with herbal remedies, he disparages the custom of cooking up the prescription at the bedside because it was done in compliance with a superstitious belief that carrying the medicine through a doorway would cause it to lose its efficacy.

Other behaviours Qiu targets include people's 'deluded belief' (*mixin* 迷信) in spirits. Some of the most popular healing methods of this time involved asking the spirits to write medical prescriptions. Every town and village had altars for divining, at which people who asked for medical help would petition the spirits with a detailed written description of the sickness. Two diviners would hold a plate filled with sand and, after turning it this way and that, would see traces of characters that they would write down one by one to make up a 'planchette prescription' (*jifang* 乩方). If the prescription did not work, it was just considered to be the patient's bad fortune. Since the procedure cost only incense and candles, no one had any grounds for complaint.

Petitioners could also visit Shaoxing temples devoted to Hua Tuo 華陀 (a semi-mythical doctor of the late Han/Three Kingdoms period) or King Yan 閻王 (Yama, king of the Buddhist Underworld), where rows of herbal prescriptions were printed on a board and arranged by numbers. After burning incense and prostrating her/himself in prayer, the patient would shake a container of strips of bamboo (*qian* 籤) until one fell out. The number written on this stick would indicate the number of the printed prescription that, for a small fee, the patient would be given. The prescription might call for the patient to take incense stick ash, divine cinnabar (*xian dan* 仙丹), regular herbs like *fuzi* 附子 (aconite) and *dahuang* 大黃 (rhubarb root), or housedust (which was ingested as a drug). This use of 'stick prescriptions' (*qian fang* 籤方) is similar to what Dudgeon describes. Its ubiquity even led to a saying: 'If anything happens, ask the *qian*-sticks' (*you shiqing qiu qian* 有事情求籤).[22] This practice persists in Taiwan and has also recently been revived in Mainland China. I observed it in the Nanputuo Temple in Xiamen and in other smaller temples in Fujian Province in the 1980s and 1990s, and Adam Chau describes it as recently as 1998 in northern Shaanxi Province.[23]

In the towns, divination (*wen bu* 問卜) was often performed by blind men, called 'blind masters.' When sick people asked them for prognoses, the blind masters would use numerology to divine various methods of averting disaster. People followed their instructions to the letter, and Qiu notes with some bitterness that even patients who were happy to tamper with a doctor's herbal prescription regarded the blind masters' pronouncements as sacrosanct.

Sometimes the sick preferred to consult the spirits more directly. 'Ghost-seers' (*guiyan* 鬼眼) would charge several hundred copper coins (the standard value of a copper coin was one-thousandth of a silver tael) to come to the patient's room, look all around, spend a long time talking and gesticulating to the empty air, and then announcing that there were so many male, female, large, or small ghosts present. The sick person would ask the ghost-seer to identify the ghost and would then be told that it was a particular relative. Then the patient would ask the ghost how to avert disaster. The ghost-seer, often assuming the voice of the ghost, would tell her or him what to do. Similarly, 'enlightened grannies' (*wupo* 悟婆) were possessed by female immortals or gods. Asked about a patient's illness, the 'grannie' would give a big yawn, showing that she had entered a trance state and was in communication with the spirit world before pronouncing, for instance, that the person had angered someone who was seeking redress.

Qiu, like Dudgeon, regarded these interventions as dangerous quackery and as obstacles to medical modernization. By contrast, psychiatrist Arthur Kleinman's 1980 study of shamanic healing in Taiwan credits shamans with a potentially valuable role in mediating family relations and managing mental and psychological distress. He reminds us that, in shamanic healing, the patient-healer relationship is sacred, deriving much of its potential efficacy from its folk-religious character.[24]

Other behaviours aimed to protect a family member from the baleful influence of spirits. Having tried the previous solutions, family members might stand outside a sick person's door and mumble a rhyming spell that told the spirits of disease that this was a poor household, asking them if they would please take some food and consider visiting other, richer, families instead. Or, should a patient became delirious, her or his random speech would be interpreted as a conversation with nearby ghosts, and carers would cover the body in a fishing net in the belief that doing so would ward off ghostly influence.

People envisioned disease-causing spirits as operating in a hierarchical society much like their own, so some patients would invoke greater spiritual authorities to control the trouble-making spirits of disease. Popular among these authorities was Jiang Taigong 姜太公, a famous military strategist who had advised the kings of Zhou in their efforts to overthrow the Shang dynasty in the eleventh-century BCE. Jiang was venerated as a commander, and, in writing, patients would invoke his authority on a slip of bamboo, which they would then wear in their hair to repel the forces of disease. There was a similar rationale for the habit of wearing a copy of the official calendar around one's neck when venturing out to see a doctor (*gua liriben* 掛曆日本). Because the calendar described the movements of the stars and constellations, wearing it lent the patient some of the supernatural power of the heavenly bodies and helped her or him to ward off evil spirits.

Female sufferers of 'hysteria' (here Qiu uses *xuesidili* 雪司地里, a transliteration of the Western word), or what was locally referred to as seizures or palpitations, often rejected medication and, instead, sought supernatural protection at local temples. Mothers took their daughters, sisters-in-law accompanied wives; even so, Qiu accused the monks of taking advantage: 'More than avaricious, their behaviour is an offence to public decency.'

Adding to these local resources for the treatment of disease were the various kinds of travelling healers and itinerant doctors (river-and-lake doctors, *jiang hu yi* 江湖醫), who came either on market days or (if from more distant locations) just once or twice a year. Street healers (*guo lu langzhong* 過路郎中), who had a rattle made of a round hollow iron tube with balls inside, would shake these as they called out their various kinds of expertise. Some would first needle people and then use hollowed-out ox-horns to create a vacuum and draw blood, like the 'Japanese cupping method for treating stagnant blood.'[25] Others came in groups of three or four to set up a stall at a busy marketplace, where they laid out exotic objects like animal bones and snakeskins to attract attention. Claiming to have cured famous people, they would sell poultices and plasters and treat people with acupuncture. A few times a year, a martial artist (*daquantou* 打拳頭) would attract attention by practising martial arts moves and, once a crowd had gathered, start selling drug plasters. Usually they donated the first three products and charged a few copper coins after that. Sometimes they even took a stick and hit themselves, then applied one of their plasters to show how it would heal the injury immediately. Other specialists in physical ailments were the tiger-skin merchants (*hupi ke* 虎皮客). They carried a long stick covered with a real tiger's skin and sold various ox and horse bones, tendons, and organs. When people saw the tiger skin, they would buy the bones and tendons to use as cures for leg pain. (Tiger bones are famous for their ability to heal stiffness and joint pain.) The items varied in price up to several *yuan.*

These itinerant healers operated in the streets or at the marketplace, but some also visited clients in their homes. This was particularly true of women healers, such as the toothworm removers (*xiao yachong* 消牙蟲). Operating in small groups, they went to street corners, called out that they removed toothworms, then went to the side doors (the entrances to the women's quarters) to seek customers. They would first decide on an arbitrary price, anything from ten cents to a dollar or two, and then, no matter what the cause of the toothache, they would call for a bowl of water. Taking a bone needle and poking it into the afflicted part, they would tap the needle into the bowl, where a wriggling worm would appear. Qiu notes with disapproval that not only women but also some respectable gentlemen allowed themselves to be taken in.

He is less disapproving of drug peddlers (*caoyao dan* 草藥担), men who carried drugs in baskets on shoulder poles and called out the names of drugs while walking the streets. Buyers would describe their ailments, and the peddler would sell them one or two herbs for a few dimes. Often their strong remedies were quick and effective, but other times people got sick after taking them, apparently because, according to Qiu: 'drug peddlers know their drugs but don't really know diseases.'

The category *Jianghu yi* 江湖醫 (river-and-lake doctors), or travelling doctors, is now listed in Chinese dictionaries as 'old,' that is, as referring to pre-1949 society; however, in Hong Kong in 1954, the 'Society for the Study of National Medicine' (*Guoyi xue she* 國醫學社) published a book, *Transmitted Secrets of River and Lake Medicine* (*Jianghu yishu mizhuan* 江湖醫術秘傳), which gives a sense of the range of conditions treated and approaches used by this type of doctor in the mid-twentieth century. The first (and long) section addresses 'Chinese and Western secrets about venereal diseases,' and it is followed by chapters on acumoxa, charms, pediatric massage, treatment of *sha zheng/sha qi* 痧證/痧氣 (a disease category that overlaps with cholera), smallpox, measles, remedies for treating injuries, and, finally, horse medicine and cow medicine. In contrast to

Qiu's account, this book contains information about many herbal remedies as well as instructions for making plasters and using acupuncture, moxa, and massage. However, the herbal formulae often refer to just one or two drugs, which are used in large quantities and are expectated to have an immediate effect. The section on Western understandings of venereal diseases describes bacteria (microbes, *wei shengwu* 微生物), how to give injections of Compound 606 (the breakthrough 'magic bullet' against syphilis, formulated in 1910 and also marketed as 'Salvarsan') to fight syphilis, as well as the correct use of mercury and other Western drugs.[26] The category of 'river-and-lake,' or 'itinerant,' doctors is one that does not presuppose any particular regional, national, or theoretical viewpoint. It collectively describes people who peddle different kinds of healing remedies and expertise, and who travel in the course of their work. In this sense, the Christian missionaries who carried patent remedies to attract crowds at Chinese marketplaces, the better to have an audience to hear the gospel, also belonged to the category of 'river-and-lake doctors.'

Qiu's final categories are 'official doctors' (*guan yi* 官醫) and 'semi-official doctors' (*ban guan yi* 半官醫). The fallen Qing dynasty had used the term 'official doctors' to refer to local medical officials employed to attend to prisoners. Rather cynically, Qiu describes their main duty as writing prescriptions for prisoners on the verge of death so that the prison records would indicate that they had died of illness rather than of malnourishment or some other form of maltreatment. They received salaries of three or four *yuan* a month. After the fall of the Qing, these positions were abolished, but several similar uses of official funds remained, including:

- Military doctors (*junyi* 軍醫). At the troop garrison headquarters in Shaoxing the medical officer was a medical graduate of one of the new technical colleges, and he or she prescribed only Western drugs.
- Office doctors (*ju yi* 局醫). The city Office of Opium Prohibition had employed a Chinese-medical doctor whose job was to investigate and treat cravings. The post carried a monthly salary of twenty *yuan,* and the doctor attended every afternoon. The office was closed in 1915.

- School doctors (*xiao yi* 校醫). Both the teacher-training college and the middle school paid a doctor of the Japanese style of modern medicine forty *yuan* a month to visit twice a week. For the most part, they prescribed Japanese drugs.
- Orphanage doctors (*yingtang yi* 嬰堂醫). The foundling hospital/ orphanage manager appointed two Chinese-medical specialists in pediatrics (who alternated attendance) as well as a specialist in 'external medicine' (*waike* 外科, a specialty that included skin conditions and minor surgery). The orphanage had its own drug dispensary that dealt exclusively with Chinese herbal medicines, which were dispensed free of charge.
- Welfare agency doctors (*shantang yi* 善堂醫). The United Welfare Agency (*tongshantang* 同善堂) paid for a Chinese-medical doctor and his or her assistants to vaccinate against smallpox during the forty days after Chinese New Year. They vaccinated at least three thousand people annually.
- Red Cross doctors (*hui yi* 會醫). The Shaoxing branch of the Red Cross had established a city hospital, and in 1914 it appointed a Chinese doctor trained in Western medicine and a Chinese-medical doctor. Patients of the Western-style doctor were examined and given drugs, while patients of the Chinese-style doctor were only given prescriptions. It was necessary for Western-style doctors to dispense drugs because Western-style pharmaceuticals were hard to come by. Between them, they saw thirty to forty patients on a slow day and up to two hundred on a busy day. The fee to see the Chinese-medical doctor was eleven *cash* (1.1 cents) or ten cents for an emergency appointment. A regular consultation with the Western-style doctor cost ten cents, nearly ten times as much as the fee to see the Chinese-medical doctor. The Red Cross also kept a subscription book, which enabled Red Cross members to recommend patients to various doctors in the city. Participating doctors hung a red cross sign outside their clinics.

In addition to these official posts there were charity dispensaries that were organized by wealthy local philanthropists. One had been set up in 1915 and employed four Chinese-medical doctors: a gynecologist, a generalist, a specialist in epidemics (*shanghan* 傷寒), and a vaccinator. Both the doctors and the drugs were free, at considerable expense to the single benefactor. All drugs were of Chinese origin, and the doctors attended to over five hundred patients a day. There were other, smaller dispensaries in the rural areas, most of which did not donate medicines but also employed Chinese-medical doctors.

Qiu also describes the various kinds of Western-style medical practice in and around Shaoxing. There were already several Western-style hospitals in Shaoxing city, each organized by one or two Chinese graduates of Western medicine. Their fees were ten cents for morning clinics, one *yuan* for afternoon clinics, and three *yuan* for home visits, plus travelling expenses of about one *yuan* for every two Chinese miles (*li* 里). All the hospitals had inpatient rooms, and daily room prices varied from fifty cents to two *yuan*. The majority of their patients were surgical cases.

The rural areas around Shaoxing also had a couple of Western-style doctors who worked in clinics and dispensed drugs, two female doctors who specialized in Western-style obstetrics, and two Western-style dentists.

Qiu has a separate category for the practice of doctors trained in modern medicine in Japan: *dongyi* 東醫 (eastern medicine). This reflects differences both in political origin and in the kind of medicine practised as, at the beginning of the twentieth century, Japan's medicine was modelled on Germany's. In Germany, state medical officers wielded a great deal of political power and clinical medicine emphasized the role of laboratory science much more than was the case in Anglo-American medical practice. The single Japanese-style modern doctor in the Shaoxing region charged the huge consultation fee of twenty cents, in addition to fees for drugs, in spite of the fact that the one-person clinic did not have any inpatient beds or much in the way of medical facilities.

Finally, Qiu turns his attention to *zhongyi* 中醫 (Chinese-style doctors). It is interesting to notice that he identifies this as a category that is quite distinct from that of popular healers, whom he disparages. Chinese-style doctors are mainly identified by their specialties, such as wound treatment, eye diseases, throat diseases, pox, childbirth, children's medicine, acupuncture, external medicine/surgery, and internal medicine. It is sometimes difficult to understand Qiu's criteria for elevating some kinds of healer to the category of *zhongyi*. For example, it is clear from his description of their market stalls and sales practices that he disapproves of itinerant sellers of plasters for limb injuries, but he also describes wound medicine (*shangke* 傷科) as a Chinese-medical specialty. Expertise in this form of medicine was generally transmitted orally, and it was often practised by monks at temples. The most effective treatments were plasters, but wound doctors would also prescribe myrrh (a dried plant resin) for internal administration, and some also made up herbal decoctions.

Similarly, treatment of the eye (*yanke* 眼科), such as couching for cataract, is well attested as a lower-class occupation. Early Western missionaries tended to specialize in cataract surgery because it was one kind of intervention with which their patients were familiar and that they would request once they had been convinced of the surgeon's skill. In Shaoxing, there were several families of Chinese eye doctors who claimed lineages of more than twenty generations. Their drugs generally consisted of secret formulae and were externally applied. Qiu acknowledges that they were both quick and effective.

Pox medicine (*douke* 痘科) was not threatened by the arrival of Western methods. Even in 1915, there were still many people who believed in variolation (inoculating smallpox by blowing dried scabs up the noses of children) to induce the disease in what it was hoped would be a mild form. In the mountainous rural areas, some farmers became part-time variolators each spring. They charged one *yuan* for every male child and twenty cents for every girl. Inoculators competed with each other by advertising their survival rates, and in recent years some had switched to using cowpox vaccine, with excellent results.

Specialists in throat medicine (*houke* 喉科) were under threat not so much from Western medicine as from the newly virulent epidemics of diphtheria.[27] Two established family lineages had had their remedies prove ineffectual during recent outbreaks. In addition to their secret prescriptions, they used coarse iron scalpels to cut open the pharyngeal membrane, but with little effect.

Shaoxing also had a clan of hereditary childbirth experts (*chanke* 產科). Seven or eight of them had their clinics side by side. Some

Chinese-medical internists would also attend women in labour, but most patients preferred the hereditary specialists or the monks of the famous Bamboo Grove Monastery.[28] The clinic fee varied between ten and twenty cents, while home visits cost one *yuan* plus transport and mileage fees. All told, these healers were about half as expensive as a Western-style physician. Additionally, there were two Western-style women obstetricians, though not many people knew of them, and many ordinary midwives (*wenpo* 穩婆), who were politely referred to as 'birth-attending mothers-in-law' (*shousheng waipo* 收生外婆).

Children's medicine (*erke* 兒科) was a separate discipline, and there were a few local hereditary experts who cultivated the air of being literate Confucian pediatric physicians. Some internists also treated children, and some had also begun to provide cowpox vaccination. Their fees were similar to those of childbirth specialists. Additionally, some children's doctors specialized in treating acute and chronic 'fright' (*jingke* 警科), mainly with acupuncture and massage. *Jing* 警 (fright) is a culture-bound syndrome in which children who are perceived to be behaving abnormally (e.g., becoming listless or crying a lot) are thought to be in danger of losing their souls. Their parents take them to be ritually treated by a specialist who is able to call back their souls.[29] The fees of these specialists started at ten cents and went up from there. Qiu maintains that, generally, the upper classes did not believe in soul loss, although Christopher Cullen's study of medicine in late Imperial China suggests that there may well have been exceptions.[30]

Sha 痧 was another disease that is hard to capture with modern medical terminology. It was an acute seasonal syndrome, characterized by a granular rash, vomiting, and/or diarrhea. Sometimes translated as 'Asiatic cholera' (which, however, is a relatively new disease that was first documented in China in 1822), it must also have encompassed other biomedical diagnoses (such as gastroenteritis and sunstroke), and all internists were familiar with treating it. There were a couple of hereditary specialists in this disease who were quite successful. And then there were what Qiu refers to as 'the shaven-headed charlatans,' monks who took payments to serve as proxies for the actual sufferers, receiving acupuncture and skin-scraping treatments on their client's behalf, with the paying client believing that the treatment given the proxy would effect her or his own cure at a distance. Qiu notes that merchants were especially likely to believe in this 'preposterous' treatment method.

Even though acupuncture (*zhenke* 針科) is described in the classic medical texts, elites of Qiu's time no longer practised it. However, it was still practised at monasteries and nunneries, where many people went for treatment. Qiu notes that a few modern acupuncture clinics, presided over by famous experts, were beginning to appear in Chinese cities. I return to the revival of acupuncture in Chapter 8. For the most part, however, acupuncture and minor surgery were closely related, low-status occupations. The Chinese word for minor surgery and dermatology is *waike* 外科 (external specialty). Similar to the 'sores doctors' (*yang yi* 瘍醫) of ancient times, specialists were skilled in the use of knives and scalpels, plasters and decoctions. During his investigations in Shaoxing, Qiu found that many patients who had been treated unsuccessfully by Western-style doctors had finally been cured by Chinese-style surgeons. However, the Chinese surgeons took advantage of their reputation for excellence by doubling their fees in urgent cases, and this made people reluctant to visit them. Qiu also notes, with disapproval, that some surgeons took old, used dressings and displayed them as advertisements of their trade, hanging them as shop-signs outside their clinics (rather like the striped poles of old-style European barber-surgeons), thereby 'allowing germs to spread.'

'Experts in internal medicine' (*neike* 內科) constitutes by far the largest category of Chinese-style doctors. In the entire Shaoxing territory Qiu counted over 280. Some of them also had other specialties, such as surgery, women's and children's medicine, and moxibustion, and some even used Western methods and drugs. Some had independent clinics, others set up shop inside drugstores. There were over 190 drugstores, and most of them had annual turnovers of several tens of thousands of *yuan*, mainly as a result of prescriptions written by internists. City pharmacies often provided free prescriptions to the poor, but rural pharmacies were more likely to assess how rich their clients were and to charge accordingly.

Finally, Qiu notes the presence of venereal disease specialists (*xiati bing ke* 下體病科) in Shaoxing. There were a few of these, all of whom displayed signs advertising their ability to treat syphilis, sores and chancres, and sexual infections.

Qiu's account is valuable for several reasons. First, it corroborates many of Dudgeon's observations, while providing them with greater context. More important, it allows us to see how attitudes towards disease management varied by income level, education, and geographical location. Qiu suggests, for example, that the local elites were less likely to consult acupuncturists or to take their children to experts in 'fright' disorders. He is suspicious of healing monks, referring to them as 'shaven-headed charlatans' for offering – for a fee – to endure medical treatments in the place of their actual patients, and as 'an offence to public decency' for the way they took advantage of women suffering from hysteria. At the same time, he acknowledges the primacy of the Bamboo Grove monks when it came to obstetric medicine. He also admits that even elites were likely to believe that tooth cavities were caused by toothworms and to conduct some form of divination to determine what had caused their disease and how to go about treating it.

In her recent book on women's medicine in late Imperial China, Yi-Li Wu discusses how Qiu Jisheng originally dismissed traditional obstetrical manuals as useless and as full of superstition. He changed his mind, however, after friends told him of their wives' experiences of labour. The first friend's wife died in childbirth under the care of a doctor of Western medicine, while the second friend's wife survived a difficult labour (which ended in a stillbirth) under the care of a traditional-style doctor who prescribed a herbal formula. These incidents persuaded him to include the source of that herbal formula, an obstetrical text by Qing dynasty doctor Shan Nanshan (單南山), in his *Hundred Masters of National Medicine* (*Guoyi bai jia* 國醫百家), a compilation of praiseworthy texts of Chinese medicine that he published serially between 1918 and 1921.[31]

Henrietta Harrison's exploration of the diary of Liu Dapeng (1857-1942), a rural *juren* 舉人 (degree-holder) from Shanxi Province in north China, shows how members of the Confucianist elite viewed disease as a disruption of the moral order of the universe and were likely to blame illnesses on their own or their families' moral transgressions. The twentieth-century example of Liu Dapeng illustrates how the concept of retributory illness persisted even as people adopted a more secular approach to medical treatment. This meant that, even though people like Qiu viewed them with suspicion, priests retained an important role as mediators between the macrocosmic order and the social environment.[32]

Many local communities across China maintained temples to the 'King of Medicine' (*yaowang* 藥王), Sun Simiao (孫思邈, lived seventh century CE). Sun and other famous, deified physicians whose statues were honoured in these temples were important patrons of a folk medicine of religious healing, and drug peddlers and fortune-tellers could often be found looking for business at these temples.[33] Starting with the late Qing New Policies reforms of 1901-11, and again during the Nanjing Decade of 1928-37, the government ordered that temples devoted to 'superstitious' religious practice be commandeered to house modern schools. Even so, in the first half of the twentieth century there are many accounts of how Daoist and Buddhist monks conducted ceremonies in order to request divine intercession during epidemic outbreaks and of how communities continued to organize anti-epidemic festivals.[34]

Qiu's classification of healers attempts to draw a clear distinction between Chinese-style doctors (*zhongyi*), on the one hand, and spirit doctors (*shen yi*) and river-and-lake doctors (*jianghu yi*), on the other. This is in line with his objective, which was to create a reformed, modern Chinese medicine that would be able to resist the imperialism of Western medicine just as the regaining of Chinese national sovereignty would be able to resist imperialist encroachment. This theme – the creation and maintenance of a boundary between a respectable, modernizing Chinese medicine and all other healing practices – is explored more fully in later chapters.

Omitted from Qiu's account is self-medication through patent remedies that were available in every drugstore. Since at least the Ming dynasty, Chinese pharmacies had been turning classic prescriptions and secret remedies into convenient pills and powders, which were sold in small porcelain bottles adorned with slogans and marketing images.[35] By the early twentieth century, these had been replaced by glass bottles and modern advertising. But there was no equivalent of the US Pure Food and Drug Act (1906), so manufacturers were not required to list their ingredients – something that benefited unscrupulous Western companies just as much as it did Chinese companies. In China there was a burgeoning trade in medications of deliberately ambiguous origin, such as the famous Tiger Balm, T.C. Yales' Brain Tonic, Five Continents Drugstore's Manmade Blood, and the infamous Canadian product Dr. Williams' Pink Pills for Pale People. This lack of scruples on the part of Western drug manufacturers may explain why Qiu omitted patent remedies from his critical survey.[36]

In this rich, lower Yangzi municipality, Qiu's account also demonstrates the substantial penetration of modern medicine: by 1915, there were already several private hospitals of modern medicine, two private clinics run by solitary physicians, a small hospital run by a Japanese-trained doctor, and a couple of modern obstetricians. A Japanese-educated doctor was employed by the city as the school doctor, and the military barracks also had a Western-style doctor trained in one of the new technical colleges of medicine. So both local and national government organizations were employing doctors of modern medicine, whereas the recent Qing government had hired doctors of Chinese medicine for the Opium Bureau. Further to this, 'semi-official' posts, such as attendant doctors for the city orphanage or the United Welfare agency, were still staffed by doctors of Chinese medicine.

Interestingly, we also see that the local Red Cross Association employed *both* a Western-style *and* a Chinese-style physician to work in its hospital. Patients were free to choose either doctor, though the fee to see the Western-style doctor was much higher. Elizabeth Sinn describes a similar situation with regard to the Tung Wah Hospital in Hong Kong in the late nineteenth century. Caroline Reeves's study of the Chinese Red Cross shows how the organization grew out of existing welfare agencies (*shan tang* 善堂) and indicates that it was common for Red Cross hospitals to employ both Western-style and Chinese-style doctors. Access to modern medicine was necessary to preserve the internationalism that the Red Cross represented, but it was expensive, in scarce supply, and unfamiliar to most of the association's clientele.[37] If *shan tang* clinics and Red Cross hospitals were routinely employing both kinds of doctor, the famous battles between Western and Chinese in medicine may well have been exaggerated. Certainly the Chinese-medical literature of the Republican era enthusiastically encourages people to utilize the best of both traditions. And, as we see in the next chapter, medical missionaries frequently borrowed from Chinese medicine to make their practices more attractive to their patients and potential converts. The headline battles over political patronage and legitimacy have served to obscure an extremly messy process of medical modernization, one in which medical pluralism and combined therapies were much more common than adherence to idealized pure types.

Yu Xinzhong has recently published a study of Qing dynasty medical customs in the lower Yangzi region for which his principal sources are local gazetteers, the guides produced from a collaboration between local dignitaries and representatives of the imperial government. Inevitably, the gazetteers reflect the outlook of the elite, who tend to look down on many of the same practices that Qiu and Dudgeon found unacceptable. In the Qing, however, the line between reason and superstition was not so rigidly policed. Yu notes that Xu Dachun, a famous eighteenth-century Confucian physician, argued that even though most prescriptions obtained by divination and other supernatural means were vulgar and heterodox, sometimes they turned out to be as effective as the great classical prescriptions. Xu explained this by arguing that appeals for guidance from the spirit world were sometimes answered by the spirits of medically knowledgeable men who had died before their time. Because of their early deaths, their spirits lingered awhile between heaven and earth and, when asked, would prescribe good medicines. Thus even the scholarly elite believed in the continuing influence of the dead on the living.[38]

Why did ordinary people continue to engage in healing practices that, in the eighteenth century, already looked foolish to Chinese elites? Yu suggests several ways of making sense of these behaviours: first, because the fees for literate doctors were much higher than most could afford, there were not many doctors available in some areas and/or they would not make home visits, so it was important to have home remedies available. Second, it was important for the sick to feel cared for and for family members to express their filial devotion by searching for cures.

For poor patients and their families, the healing options might be restricted to inexpensive offerings to deities or to picking up a temple prescription or charm to burn and take with wine. Such treatments were efficacious as expressions of concern, if not as medical care. Finally, social interventions (such as advice given by spirit-mediums in trance, often in front of several family members as well as the patient) were psychologically efficacious. A shaman's advice was the equivalent of a modern biomedical doctor's diagnosis: even if the disease was serious, it was reassuring to have it identified and explained in familiar terms.

Anthropologist Judith Farquhar noted this effect in the 1990s when observing a Chinese-medical doctor, Dr. Zhao, who supplemented his diagnoses with divination. Every year, month, day, and hour in the Chinese calendar has an association with one of the Five Phases of Chinese cosmology (Wood, Fire, Earth, Metal, and Water); therefore, after calculating the patient's Phase strengths and weaknesses from her or his birthdate, the doctor would alter his prescription to address these aspects of the patient's problem as well as their obvious medical symptoms. Farquhar notes that patients found it immensely reassuring to discuss how their treatment was to be tailored to their precise astrological constitution: 'By mapping an Eight Character birthdate over a Five Phases understanding of physiology, he not only fills time with significant content for the client, he rationally structures an intervention on the basis of that significance.'[39]

Many of the 'superstitious' practices that are not acceptable in today's 'traditional Chinese medicine,' and that were looked down on by elites in the late nineteenth and early twentieth centuries, survived in Taiwan and Hong Kong as well as in other Chinese communities, and, since the 1980s, they have re-emerged in Mainland China. It is not difficult to find restored medical temples in which one can consult the *qian* sticks for a prescription, and sets of *qian* sticks and prescriptions corresponding to each number are openly for sale in stores, along with almanacs that list lucky and unlucky activities as well as the locations of various spirits around the house for each hour of every day. This is important information: if you tread on the location of the foetus spirit when you are pregnant, for instance, you are likely to suffer a miscarriage. *Qigong* 气功 teachers can now be found and, for a fee, will instruct you in the mysteries of healthful breathing. (*Qigong*, or *'chi gung'* is a practice of aligning breath, movement, and awareness for exercise, healing, and meditation.) Some of them have adapted their skills to modern concerns: for example, *jianfei qigong* 减肥气功 (fat-reducing qigong) will help you lose weight.

Numerous competing healing methods, along with a multiplicity of healers, resulted in an early twentieth-century cacophony that was an embarrassment to medical and Confucian elites alike. For some, the answer seemed to lie in the wholesale adaptation of modern/Western medicine. Others wanted to winnow away the chaff of superstitious practices to obtain a kernel of rational Chinese medicine. The case for rational Chinese medicine had to be made simultaneously against Western medicine, on the one hand, and against superstition, on the other. As we see in the following chapters, Chinese-medical doctors were helped by the fact that the case for 'Western' medicine was also far from unified.

Missionary Medicine from the West **3**

To make Zhang Zhongjing's famous Cinnamon Twig Decoction, use cinnamon twig, peony root, fresh ginger root, dried jujube dates, and dried licorice root.[1] Each ingredient has its function according to the principles of combining Chinese herbal formulae. Cinnamon twig as the ruler (*jun* 君) expresses the therapeutic aim, which is to release wind-cold from the body's exterior layers of skin and flesh to the outside. The minister (*chen* 臣), peony root, supports the ruler cinnamon by providing supplementary benefit to the *yin* (interior) of the body's *yin-yang* economy. Ginger root and the jujube dates are the assistants (*zuo* 佐), which modify the main drugs or moderate side effects. Licorice root is the envoy (*shi* 使), directing the formula to the body's centre.[2]

Lest it seem that these categories are the imaginings of the ignorant itinerant herbalists about whom Qiu complained in the last chapter, here is W. Hale White on how to compose prescriptions, from the first edition (1892) of his popular textbook on *materia medica*, used in updated versions in American and British medical schools until the 1930s:

> The more complex prescriptions consist of
> The Basis, or principal active ingredient *(curare).*
> The Adjuvans, or that which assists its action *(cito).*
> The Corrigens, or that which corrects its operation *(tuto).*

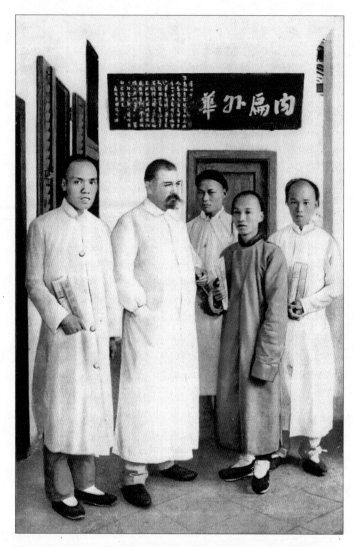

Figure 3   Postcard labelled "Ein Missionsarzt in China mit seinen Schülern" (A missionary doctor in China with his students), depicting a missionary of the Swiss Basler Mission. The placard above the door would have been a gift from a grateful patient; its headline reads "In internal [medicine as good as] Bian [Qüe], in surgery, [the equal of] Hua [Tuo]," referring to the skills of two legendary ancient physicians. Produced late nineteenth or first decade of the twentieth century.

Source: Author's collection, gift from Cyrus Veeser.

The Constituens, vehicle, or excipient, which imparts an agreeable form (*jucunde*).

... For example, in Pilula Rhei Composita [a purgative] the rhubarb is the basis, the aloes and myrrh form the adjuvans, and the peppermint is the corrigens to prevent the griping. In Mistura Cretae the cinnamon water is the vehicle.[3]

Even the nineteenth edition (1927) repeated this text, having only dropped the Latin parentheses and with a different formula as the example.

In fact, the principles of drug combination used by Chinese and Western-trained physicians throughout the nineteenth and early twentieth centuries were remarkably similar, something that is often forgotten today. Medical students of that time, East and West, learned about *materia medica* in categories that were defined according to therapeutic action, such as reducing a fever, functioning as an emetic, causing blisters, inducing purging, and so on. They were also expected to learn how to identify plants and medically relevant chemicals and animals. Radical change to Western pharmaceutical practice did not begin until the second half of the nineteenth century, when chemists started to subject herbal drugs to laboratory analysis, in the process isolating compounds like morphine, codeine, and quinine. For the most part, doctors East and West were compounding medicines from the raw *materia medica* and according to the same basic principles.[4]

Thus when Peter Parker, the first Protestant missionary physician in China, came to live, work, and spread the twin gospels of scientific medicine and Protestant Christianity, parts of his medical practice bore amazing similarities to Chinese practice. For example, in Figure 3 we see a placard in Chinese comparing the foreign doctor to the legendary physicians of Chinese antiquity, while his students are carrying Chinese-language texts and wearing gowns that combine European and Chinese tailoring. Having seen the range of Chinese healing practices, these similarities come as a bit of a surprise. After all, the history of missionary physicians in China has been examined and retold primarily as part of the spread of Western influence, being interpreted variously as a marker of progress towards modernization or as evidence of the reach of

Western imperialism into Chinese culture and into the lives and bodies of individual Chinese. Indeed, as we noted in the introduction, some missionaries were so successful at attuning their practice to local Chinese sensibilities that, by the early twentieth century, their clinics were acknowledged to be less modern and scientific than those established by the Chinese themselves.

If the gulf separating 'Western' medicine as practised by missionaries and 'Chinese' medicine was smaller than has previously been thought, we are left with the question of how much influence medical missionaries actually had in China. How many Chinese regarded them as the bearers of science and progress? Were they simply visible reminders of China's weakness on the international stage? Given that they represented a new model of health management, what influences did medical missionaries exert on Chinese efforts to create a modern nation?

Two themes recur in this examination: commensurability and accommodation. Commensurability (the similarity, in practice, between nineteenth-century Western medicine and Chinese medicine) is exemplified in Zhang Zhongjing's Cinnamon Twig Decoction, while accommodation (the willingness to adapt and downplay differences in order to appeal to Chinese patients) may be seen in comments made by Harold Balme, president and former dean of medicine at Shandong Christian University, in 1921. Balme noted the recent shifts in the objectives and methodology of missionary medicine:

> Twenty years ago it was almost utopian to think in terms of modern science in relation to mission hospitals. At that time the great objective was the winning of patients' confidence and friendship and in that endeavor it was inevitable for medical missions to be established and carried on under conditions which were frankly opposed to every idea of hygiene and good nursing, or of scientific methods of diagnosis and treatment.
>
> But to-day ... [there is] a growing demand on the part of many of the Chinese themselves for a higher level of hospital efficiency – a demand to which medical missionaries all over China are giving considerable attention.[5]

Balme's analysis suggests that early missionaries made considerable accommodations in order to meet Chinese expectations, at least in the early years, and that their focus on adapting to local conditions may eventually have impaired their credibility as purveyors of 'scientific medicine.'

The history of missionary medicine in China is a large topic, worthy of a far more in-depth treatment than is possible here. It is certainly true that missionary medicine was an essential element in Christianity's penetration of nineteenth- and early twentieth-century China, and it provided models that were selectively adapted by both Chinese doctors and political administrations. Here, however, I focus on how missionary medicine turned out to be not so much a marker of cultural difference as a tool for reducing the perception of alterity.

Commensurability is most readily seen in the use that Western medical missionaries made of drugs. For early medical missionaries in China, particularly those who established themselves inland, maintaining an adequate supply of drugs was a problem, with the result that local substitutes were in high demand. The *Chinese Recorder* often carried short articles in which physicians shared their discoveries about the Chinese names, and relative strength and purity, of local drugs. This is not surprising since many herbal and mineral drugs available in China – such as 'rhubarb, camphor, opium, sulphate of soda, nitrate of potassa [sic], liquorice, anise-seed, cinnamon, musk, asafoetida, etc.'[6] – were common to the pharmacopeia of both traditions. In 1871, F. Porter Smith published a guide to Chinese drugs, with the telling title of *Contributions toward the Materia Medica and Natural History of China, for the Use of Medical Missionaries and Native Medical Students*. In addition to identifying drugs by their Latin, Chinese (characters and pronunciation), and common English names, Smith gave instructions on how to apply Chinese drugs to Western pharmaceutical preparations. Smith's guide was of sufficient value for G.A. Stuart to revise and republish it in 1911 as *Chinese Materia Medica: Vegetable Kingdom*.

Similar investigations focused on Chinese mineral drugs. In 1889, Dr. J.B. Neal published chemical analyses of locally purchased samples of sixteen substances, including carbonates of lead, zinc, iron, copper, and sodium; sodium sulphate; calomel; alum; gypsum; vermilion; sulphide of arsenic; nitre [KNO_3]; and ferrous sulphate. In 1891, he supplemented these with a further list, which included analyses of local kaolinite, mercury, cinnabar, mica, pumice stone, ammonium chloride, and several others. Bernard Read, working with Chinese colleagues at the Peking Union Medical College in 1925, published a comparison of the market prices and relative purity of several locally available inorganic drugs in order to help foreign-trained doctors buy local supplies as sagaciously and as cheaply as possible.[7]

The search for local drug substitutes could lead to creativity or to conflict. For example, as late as 1923, a Dr. Patterson wrote to the *China Medical Journal* about her difficulty obtaining the constituents of one formula, Cataplasma kaolini USP, which was useful as a hot poultice in mild local infections. The standard formula was a mixture of kaolin (a kind of clay), glycerin, boric acid, methyl salicylate, thymol, and oil of peppermint. Dr. Patterson had experimented with various locally available substitutions for kaolin, glycerin, boric acid, and methyl salicylate, and she recommended 'Native peanut oil [instead of glycerin], native talc or soapstone, [instead of kaolin and boric acid], thymol, oil of peppermint, oil of eucalyptus.' In the next issue of the journal, Read agreed that peanut oil was a good substitute for glycerin but pointedly reminded Patterson that 'Kaolin exists in China in great abundance, hence ... there is no reason why there should be any departure from the original formula for kaolin poultice.'[8]

At other times, on encountering patients who had been successfully treated with local preparations, missionaries decided to investigate further. For example, Dr. Butchart, working in Taiwan, reported to the 1907 Conference of the Medical Missionary Association that

> he saw an epidemic of malaria last Fall in which there were many who could not have used *quinine*, but who got better, and their prescription from the native doctors showed that cinnamon had been given. Is this a parasiticide? It would be well to investigate and see what native drugs are parasiticides.[9]

These frequent attempts to understand and to operate in the Chinese pharmaceutical world suggest that the missionaries were not as dismissive of Chinese pharmacy as they were of Chinese medical theory. Given

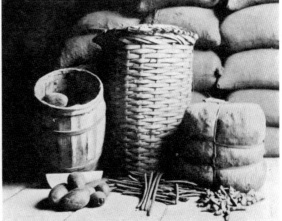

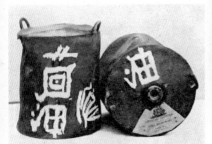

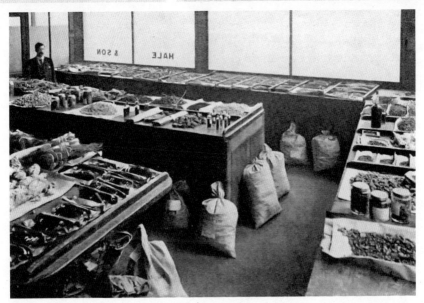

Figures 4, 5, and 6 Photographs from the fourth (1924) edition of a common medical textbook, Greenish's *Materia Medica*, first published in 1899, showing raw drugs of Chinese origin shipped for sale in Europe and the Americas. *Source:* Author's collection.

that even Western pharmacists obtained many of their products (e.g., kaolin, rhubarb, and camphor) from East Asia, this is perhaps not surprising. Figures 4 to 6 feature reproductions from the fourth (1924) edition of a common medical textbook, Greenish's *Materia Medica*, first published in 1899, showing drugs of Chinese origin.[10]

As pharmacy became more of a laboratory science in the late nineteenth and early twentieth centuries, many Chinese herbal drugs were analyzed for their pharmaceutically active constituents. Studies were undertaken in Japan as early as the 1880s, and, by the 1920s, Chinese university laboratories were also publishing in this new field. More famously, the drug *mahuang* 麻黃 yielded the stimulant ephedrine, first isolated by the Japanese chemist Nagai Nagayoshi 長井長義 (1844-1929) in 1885 and successfully developed as a drug to treat asthma by Peking Union Medical College researchers K.K. Chen and Carl F. Schmidt in 1924.[11] In another example, research into the Chinese herb *danggui* 當歸 resulted in an extract that was marketed in Europe as a new commercial emmenagogue (menstruation-promoting drug), 'Eumenol,' as early as 1898.[12] In a process now known as 'bioprospecting,' many drugs were analyzed for active principles that, once isolated, could be repackaged and sold as modern (i.e., Western-medical) drugs.[13]

Most doctors saw patented drugs as a great improvement in pharmacy because of their standardized preparation and, therefore, predictable strength. This standardization was a marker of modernity and one of the reasons for the presumed superiority of modern medicine, as demonstrated by this 1892 *New York Times* article, ironically titled 'Progress in China':

> The missionaries are doing much to dispel the mysticism and reverent awe which the Chinaman holds for the concoctions of snakes, toads, lizards, etc., prepared by the native doctors. They recommend standard remedies which have long been favorably known in America and Europe, such as Dr. Pierce's Golden Medical Discovery, a remedy for all cases of *blood-taints* or *humors*, which has had years of uninterrupted success in the United States, and numbers its cures by the tens of thousands.[14]

Dr. Pierce's Golden Medical Discovery was, in fact, an alcoholic herbal panacea containing unknown ingredients for which the main competitor in the United States was Lydia E. Pinkham's Vegetable Compound.[15] The *New York Times'* enthusiasm for these nostrums was modified by the scandals that precipitated the US Pure Food and Drug Act, 1906.

Before that date, drug manufacturers were not required to state the ingredients of their preparations, and the inclusion of narcotics such as opium and stimulants such as cocaine was common practice. After all, opium will reliably dull pain and cocaine will give most patients a lift!

To identify the appropriate local *materia medica* to use in their formulae, missionaries had to become better linguists. This was just one of the accommodations they made. In addition to such basic skills as learning to speak some Chinese, they also needed to be able to observe proper etiquette when dealing with officials, patients, and patients' families. Many physicians felt this to be a considerable burden as it took valuable time away from clinical work.

A lack of sensitivity to Chinese cultural norms could do more than merely alienate potential patient-converts: it could endanger both doctors and patients. One example of this involves the nineteenth-century physicians' habit of pickling excised body parts and keeping them in glass jars. Chinese reverence for the body as a sacred gift from one's parents presented grave obstacles to medical missionaries when they proposed surgery and amputations, but the display of body parts could lead to actual violence: 'We now notice the troubles which arise from the medical work ... [It is] generally believed that the riot in 1868 which occurred in Yangchow [Yangzhou] was hastened by a physician, who put a human foetus in a bottle and allowed it to be seen by the Chinese.'[16]

Missionaries also noticed early on that Chinese patients rarely displayed pain as to do so would have caused them to lose face. They would also have been anxious to avoid causing the doctor embarrassment by indicating the suffering he or she was inflicting. Unfortunately, this stoic behaviour led many Westerners to infer that Chinese actually experienced less pain than Caucasians: 'There is a very general impression among foreigners that the pain sense of the Asiatic, particularly the mongolian races, is not nearly so highly developed as in other races.'[17] As a result, many decided that it was not necessary to use chloroform when operating on Chinese. The suggestion that impassivity in the face of pain might rather be the result of self-control had been made as early as 1877 by John Dudgeon, who was, as we have seen, unusually culturally sensitive, but the prejudice remained, and it caused a great deal of unnecessary suffering to Chinese patients.[18] However easy it is in hindsight to label this misconception as racial prejudice, in the mid-nineteenth century most Westerners agreed that race was responsible for many 'physiological' differences that we now ascribe to culture. In effect, not using anaesthetics was a decision based on apparently sound empirical evidence: to many missionaries, this was not only reasonable but also scientific.

Other accommodations involved adapting the clinical encounter to the cultural sensitivity of Chinese patients. Soon after his arrival in China in 1904, Edward Hume of the Yale-in-China mission observed that patients might leave his clinic in scorn if he failed to take the pulses at both wrists in the Chinese style. In Chinese medical theory, the condition of different internal organs is detectable at different points on the wrists: heart and liver on the left, for example, and lungs and digestive system on the right. So for the doctor to feel the pulse at only one wrist was, to most Chinese patients, a sure sign of ignorance and incompetence.[19]

Another common Chinese expectation was that a competent doctor would adjust the contents of a medical prescription according to the stage of disease and recovery. As one Chinese MD advised his Caucasian colleagues: 'Continued administration of the same drug for a length of time is sure to induce the patient to dispense with your services. When it is necessary, as in cases of the iodides for syphilis, the doctor ought from time to time to alter the taste, odour, or colour of the preparation.'[20] This suggests that the Western idea of a disease as a fixed taxonomic entity was slow to be accepted in China, where the expectation was that treatment would be continually adjusted to match the dynamic between the disease and the natural recuperative powers of the human body. In this instance, too, the Chinese idea of disease as a dynamic process recalls the humoral Western medicine of the immediately preceding past. Because of this conviction that local conditions influenced the manifestations of diseases, James Henderson, in his influential *Shanghai Hygiene* of 1863, discusses such factors as temperature, humidity, geology, drainage and cultivation, the proximity of the sea and of rivers, elevation, positions of mountains, prevalent winds, and trees and vegetation. He also analyzes the diet, drink, exercise, clothing, bathing, and perspiration of Westerners in Shanghai. The Imperial Maritime Customs medical officers, who were often also medical missionaries, adopted this multiple local-factor approach in their medical reports for the rest of the nineteenth century.[21]

The ways in which patients behaved in foreign hospitals also necessitated multiple accommodations. Not only were hospitals built to reflect indigenous architectural styles, but men and women were physically separated and consulting rooms and even operating rooms were visible to other patients in order to allay Chinese suspicions that foreigners might experiment on Chinese bodies.[22] Most hospitals abandoned the rule that patients must be bathed on admission because so many Chinese considered this a danger to their health, especially when the weather was cold and they were already sick. In general, Chinese also resisted the bland, overcooked food that Westerners considered suitable hospital fare, instead bringing in friends or relatives to cook for them on-site. Medical missionaries allowed this because they had neither the funds nor the nursing staff to provide alternatives. The fact that the cooking and nursing were handled by the patients' families gave early hospitals a chaotic atmosphere. To some missionaries, this was one of their advantages: 'The hospital is far more homey and far more human than eleven-tenths [sic] of our rule-trodden institutions in the dear homeland, and it suits the Chinese patients very well indeed.'[23]

Accommodation was not always just a way for medical missionaries to get along with their Chinese patients: it could also lead them to revise their medical beliefs. For example, we are now accustomed to thinking of epidemic diseases as being caused by the spread of infectious germs, usually either viruses or bacteria. For most of the nineteenth century, however, diseases – particularly epidemic diseases – were thought to be spread either by exposure to infectious miasmas or by direct contact with an afflicted person or with their clothes or bedding. This 'spread by direct contact' is the narrow meaning of the word 'contagious,' just as the word 'malaria,' from the Latin for 'bad air,' expresses the conviction that foul odours could cause disease. Before the advent of the germ theory of disease causation and the elucidation (ca. the 1880s) of the lifecycles of particular disease-causing organisms, debates on whether particular diseases such as cholera and plague were infectious (spread in air or water) or merely contagious (spread by direct contact from person to person) raged within the international community, and there was little consensus on how best to prevent their spread. Malaria, for example, was not considered contagious, and, before the discovery in 1897 that it was transmited through mosquito bites, nobody was able to prevent it. Compounding the problem, Western medicine's most effective remedy, quinine, was expensive and in short supply. For example, when Edinburgh University's first Chinese graduate, Dr. Wong Fun, was employed as a medical missionary by the London Missionary Society in Canton in 1857, he did not have enough quinine to meet the demand for treatment of intermittent fevers, even though the doses given to Chinese were 'much smaller than might be required by a European.'[24] International sanitary conferences were convened as early as 1851 to discuss how to contain the spread of cholera, smallpox, and plague, but it was not until the seventh such conference, held in Venice in 1892, that the first limited agreements were reached between nations regarding treatment and quarantine measures for dealing with ships found to be harbouring cholera. In 1893, ten nations signed an agreement regulating ship quarantine measures and pledging urgent mutual notification of any cholera outbreaks.[25] However, there was still a consensus that foul air, or 'miasma,' was injurious to health. For this reason the sanitation movement of the mid-nineteenth century was concerned with the provision of clean piped water, the construction of underground sewerage systems in towns, and building programs that allowed for adequate ventilation and light. None of these measures was based on the idea that bacteria or viruses were the main agents of disease; rather, diseases were thought to be caused by miasmas given off from decaying matter or, in particularly unhealthy areas, emitted from the soil.[26] In fact, as late as 1907, in London medical schools bacteriology was still an elective course and not part of basic medical education.[27]

The first therapeutic application of germ theory in China involved Koch's tuberculin, which was available in Hong Kong and Shanghai in 1891. Originally touted as a cure for tuberculosis, it turned out to be a dismal failure. Doctors continued to use it as a diagnostic tool because it produced a rapid and easily identifiable skin reaction in infected patients. Later in the 1890s, von Behring's and Kitasato's serum therapy for diphtheria helped save many lives, but serum therapy proved difficult to reproduce for other infectious diseases, and there was often strong popular opposition to inoculation.[28] Moreover, most physicians in China during this period had had no training in bacteriology or laboratory methods, did not own microscopes, and had likely never seen a microbe for themselves. In 1910, Jefferys and Maxwell noted that the last conference of the China Medical Missionary Association had resolved

> that boards require their medical mission candidates to show evidence that they have made *a special study of tropical diseases*. Preferably that they have taken a practical course in tropical medicine or at the very least have attended a course of lectures on the subject and have been thoroughly trained in practical bacteriology and microscopic methods.[29]

This confirms the general impression that most medical missionaries – like their metropolitan counterparts – had not been trained in bacteriology before this date.

Additionally, medical missionaries in China generally lacked both the funds and the authority to undertake public health measures, whether informed by the old (miasma) or new (germ) theories. For several reasons, they were also less interested in preventive medicine than in curative medicine. In 1932, a survey of the medical missionary community revealed that its members considered prevention less demonstrative of goodwill than cure. Furthermore, the survey indicated that preventive medicine was thought to yield no monetary returns, a consideration especially important during the worldwide depression of the 1930s, when missions were urged to be self-supporting. Medical missionaries also argued that large-scale preventive work was a function of government, that their own training had been in curative medicine, that 'any large success in death prevention would but aggravate the ominous problem of overpopulation,' and that preventive medicine did not lend itself to evangelistic efforts as well as did the personal contact between patient and doctor.[30]

More surprisingly, the writings of some nineteenth-century medical missionaries indicate that most of them considered Western-style sanitary measures unnecessary or superfluous in Chinese towns. Dr. James Henderson, who was instrumental in planning the sanitation measures in Shanghai's International Settlement, wrote in 1864: 'I have often been asked to explain how it is that comparatively there are so few epidemics of low fever among the Chinese? Shut up as they are in cities, in narrow crowded streets, and in low, damp houses, with city, streets, houses and people filthy in the extreme.'[31] In 1877, Dr. John Dudgeon went further, using his years of observations of life in China to cast doubts on the assumptions of Western 'sanitary science':

> If we bear in mind the utter absence of all sanitary science ... the narrow streets, pent-up houses, dense populations, want of ventilation, earthen floors, absence of cellars, sewers and other channels for under-ground purification, stagnant pools and pits of putrefaction in all directions, with a high atmospheric heat for half the year, it is astonishing that the country is not swept incessantly by fearful epidemics, and ere long depopulated ... Now if all this be true – and no one who knows China will fail to admit the truth of the description – we may well ask, is their general freedom from disease, and especially acute disease, and the general health, vitality and activity they exhibit not altogether very remarkable?[32]

This doubt concerning the relevance of their Western medical knowledge to Chinese conditions was repeated in the reports of the mainly British physicians who served as medical officers in the Chinese Imperial Maritime Customs Medical Service: 'The sanitary legislation of Western cities is based on the one idea that disagreeable and offensive odours are necessarily deleterious to health. The condition and mortality of Peking would seem rather to explode this belief.'[33] When these officers attempted to convince their European colleagues back home of the good health that prevailed in China in spite of the abominable sanitary conditions, their observations were met with scathing disregard. For instance, when John Dudgeon, in his role of customs medical officer for Beijing, read a paper to the Glasgow MedicoChirurgical Society to this effect, the *Lancet* responded:

It may well be that Dr. Dudgeon has acquired a sort of affection for
China, which makes him:
'to her virtues very kind,
And to her faults a little blind.'[34]

Medical missionaries, then, were overwhelmingly concerned with
clinical practice, partly because they lacked the necessary authority to
implement sanitary measures but also because their concerns were to
make contact with individual Chinese and to undertake the healing of
existing ailments, healing being, for them, 'the divinely appointed substitute for miracles.'[35] Activities aimed at disease prevention lacked the
proselytizing potential provided by clinical medicine. Further to this,
attempts at large-scale sanitary policing, such as that enforced by the
Hong Kong government during the outbreak of bubonic plague in 1894,
aroused such resentment in the population that, should missionaries
have attempted anything similar, they would have endangered both
their lives and their mission.

When Western representatives did undertake public health functions,
however, elements of accommodation were often apparent. In treaty port
settlements such as Shanghai and Tianjin, municipal councils of foreign
residents established institutions that were responsibile for maintaining
public health functions of a standard comparable – and in some cases
superior – to those of contemporary European cities. In Shanghai, in
particular, in the second half of the nineteenth century the Municipal
Council of the International Settlement undertook extensive programs
to provide roads, drains, sewerage systems, and clean water, but these
services were not extended to the Chinese parts of the city.[36] Foreign
control of these treaty ports provided missionaries with an opportunity
to attempt to control epidemics through the use of new understandings
derived from germ theory and research into the lifecycles of disease-
causing parasites. In 1913, Dr. W.W. Peter of the American YMCA in
China founded the Joint Council on Public Health Education in
Shanghai. He was deeply conscious of the fact that this was a departure
for missionary medical work. His 1917 appeal to members of the China
Medical Missionary Association for financial support not only stressed

the urgent need but also indicated that their support of public health work would show 'that interest in this work is general among medical missionaries.'[37]

The Joint Council on Public Health Education's activities show how attempts to make medical education effective in China entailed cultural hybridization. Public events such as exhibits, lectures illustrated with lantern slides, and, most of all, 'moving picture shows' such as 'War on Mosquito' and 'Fly' had the greatest impact. In this the council borrowed from Chinese popular tradition, according to which communities responded to outbreaks of epidemic disease by collectively organizing processions and ceremonies to frighten off plague demons or to appease offended gods. Local gentry might also band together to provide charity dispensaries and clinics during epidemics, employing local doctors and paying for medicines either for the duration of the outbreak or even, as during the spring epidemic season, on a regular basis.[38]

The YMCA in China went further, cooperating with city officials, local churches, and city chambers of commerce to organize public health festivals that were remarkably similar to traditional anti-epidemic processions, complete with local musicians with trumpets, cymbals, and drums, along with large banners and floats bearing huge models of flies to illustrate the importance of keeping flies off food in order to prevent the spread of cholera and typhoid.[39] Historian Peter Buck recalls hearing of a Chinese observer who, at one such procession, remarked that it was no wonder foreigners made such a fuss about flies if flies were so large in foreign lands![40] In 1920, by contrast, the *China Medical Journal* reported the apparent congruence between Chinese and Western ideas of disease causation:

> A missionary physician relates that one day the servants on his mission compound were given an address on sanitation. Many of them had been in contact with the church for several years. At the close of the address, a Chinese, who had listened attentively, remarked that the foreigners seemed to be just as much worried about bacteria as the Chinese were about demons, and in his opinion there was not much to choose between these different enemies of mankind.[41]

That both the invisible disease-demons of Chinese folk tradition and invisible germs required attentive ritual behaviours to contain and control them is further illustrated by the autobiography of a young Chinese student, who recalled his mother's death from tuberculosis in the 1920s. In Chinese translation this disease is conflated with the traditional concept of lung wasting (*feilao* 肺癆). The faces of those who died of lung wasting were traditionally covered with a white cloth to stop the worms of consumption from leaving the corpse in search of another victim: 'Mother lay on a long, narrow, wooden bench, her face covered with a sheet of paper, soaked in alcohol. The faces of people who die of tuberculosis are always covered in this way. There is a superstition that the germs that caused the infection fly out through the nostrils.'[42] With the advent of germ theory, white paper replaced the white cloth, and alcohol, a germicide, helped keep it in place. Accommodation and adaptation thus led to apparent commensurability even in the 1920s.

By the 1920s, however, missionary success at accommodating local conditions had become a liability. The Republican government realized that, in its fight to regain national sovereignty, it had to demonstrate that it could provide internationally acceptable standards, be they with regard to military medicine, port quarantine facilities, or public health administration. As, in the early twentieth century, pharmacy became more of a laboratory science, use of raw *materia medica* declined in favour of chemical extracts and commercial preparations.[43] This increased emphasis on the laboratory made missionary clinics and hospitals start to look old-fashioned to the increasing numbers of Chinese who were studying in the West and in Japan. At the same time, allowing family nursing and cooking in mission-run hospitals, while eminently sensible from a therapeutic perspective, failed to meet the standards of scientific hospital care of the 1920s and thus became another example of the backwardness of missionary medicine.

Seen in this light, the 'scientific' medicine brought by the nineteenth-century West seems scarcely distinguishable from the Chinese 'idolatrous superstitions' it was intended to replace. We cannot blame missionary physicians for their convictions of medical superiority: in some areas, such as surgery, they certainly excelled. They were also sincere in their

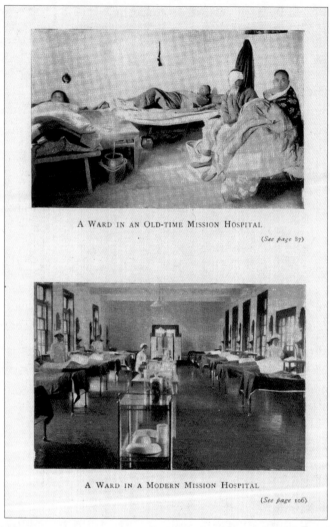

A WARD IN AN OLD-TIME MISSION HOSPITAL

(See page 87)

A WARD IN A MODERN MISSION HOSPITAL

(See page 106)

Figure 7 Photographs of old and new missionary hospital wards.
Source: China and Modern Medicine: A Study in Medical Missionary Development
by Harold Balme (London: United Council for Missionary Education, 1921),
plate facing page 97. Author's collection.

desire to heal their Chinese patients. But their rhetoric of science and medical progress did not match the reality of their situation. China, the modernizing state, now required modern medicine. Paradoxically, it would find significant support in this quest from a triumphant foe – Japan.

The Significance of Medical Reforms in Japan

4

One of the 'fathers of modern Chinese literature,' Lu Xun 鲁迅 (1881-1936), wrote about his early enthusiasm for Western medicine in the preface to his best-known collection of short stories, *Call to Arms* (*Nahan* 呐喊):

> Recalling the talk and prescriptions of physicians I had known and comparing them with what I now knew, I came to the conclusion that those [Chinese] physicians must be either unwitting or deliberate charlatans ... From translated histories I also learned that the Japanese Reformation had originated, to a great extent, with the introduction of Western medical science to Japan.
>
> These inklings took me to a provincial medical college in Japan. I dreamed a beautiful dream that on my return to China I would cure patients like my father, who had been wrongly treated, while if war broke out I would serve as an army doctor, at the same time strengthening my countrymen's faith in reformation.[1]

Other Chinese shared Lu's 'beautiful dream' and looked to Japan to provide an example for China's modernization. Perhaps surprisingly, given reactions like Lu Xun's to practitioners of traditional Chinese medicine, Japan's experience provided support both for advocates of

Western medicine and for those who valued more traditional approaches. To understand how this came about, we need to appreciate the Japanese path to modernization.

After Japan defeated China in the war of 1894-95, Chinese intellectuals and bureaucrats constantly invoked the Japanese reforms of the Meiji Restoration (1868-1911) as the model for China to follow with regard to military modernization, constitutional reform, education, and the teaching and regulation of science and medicine. Admiration for the rapid assimilation of the technologies of modernity was reinforced by Japan's alliance with the Western powers during the Boxer Rebellion of 1900. When Japan consolidated its status by defeating Russia in the 1905 Russo-Japanese War, Chinese students rushed to study the Japanese model of East Asian modernity. In doing so, they were reversing a long history in which Japanese scholars had looked to China for guidance.

Japan had been importing Chinese models of government institutions and laws, Chinese translations of Buddhist sutras, and Chinese medical books and practices since the seventh century. Over the course of the following centuries, Japanese elites continued to import, read, and comment on Chinese medical works. By the beginning of the Tokugawa period (1616-1867 CE), the most important currents of medical thought in Japan were those that followed the works of the first-century physician Zhang Ji, author of the *Treatise on Cold Damage* (*Shanghan lun* in Chinese, these same characters are pronounced as *Shinkanron* in Japanese), and the teachings of the Chinese 'four great physicians of the Jin and Yuan dynasties' (1115-1368 CE).[2]

Western medicine first arrived with Portuguese Jesuit missionaries in the middle of the sixteenth century. This link between foreign religion and medicine was reinforced after 1590 by Franciscan missionaries, who built leper hospitals as extensions of their new convents.[3]

This kind of foreign medicine was termed 'southern barbarians' medicine' (*namban igaku* 南蛮医学) or 'red-hair medicine' (*kōmō igaku* 红毛医学), and it was based on the Galenic humoral pathology of the period. Humoral pathology, like Chinese medicine, defined health as a state of being in balance with cosmic forces. The four elements of air, water, fire, and earth corresponded to one of four bodily humours:

blood, phlegm, yellow bile, and black bile, respectively. The preponderance of a particular humour determined a person's constitution: blood correlated with a sanguine temperament, phlegm with a phlegmatic temperament, yellow bile with a choleric temperament, and black bile with a melancholic temperament. Heat and cold, moisture and dryness expressed two further axes of this correlative system: fire/yellow bile was hot and dry, earth/black bile was dry and cold, water/phlegm was cold and moist, and air/blood was moist and hot. This system provided a way of understanding the influence of the environment on the body's health.[4]

Around this time, Christianity came under attack in Japan, culminating in the 1641 series of edicts from shōgun Tokugawa Iemitsu calling for *sakoku* (closed country) in order to prevent further evangelism from the West. No Japanese ships were to sail for a foreign port without a licence, no Japanese could leave the country without a permit, and any Japanese who attempted to return from abroad risked execution. By this date, all foreign traders but the Dutch – who were viewed as simple merchants without religious motives – had been banished entirely, and even they were soon moved to the tiny human-made island of Deshima in Nagasaki Bay. The self-imposed isolation of the *sakoku* period was not absolute. In spite of a 1630 ban on the importation of European books, there was a large trade in European medical wares such as 'saffron, saltpeter, borax, corrosive sublimate, alum, gums, catechu, liquid storax.'[5] One leading official called these medicines 'the only essential items' of trade with the West. Still, for the next two centuries, all official trade with foreign countries was conducted through Nagasaki.[6]

Most Chinese physicians who visited Japan during this period were also confined to Nagasaki. Although contact and trade with China was not as rigorously proscribed as that with Western nations, exchange of medical ideas certainly slowed. This can be seen in the fact that the Chinese medical developments of the Qing dynasty (1644-1911) attracted little attention in Japan. Examples include the new theories of 'warm disorders' concerning the etiology and treatment of epidemic fevers that flourished in China during the seventeenth and eighteenth centuries but that attracted little attention in Japan,[7] and variolation, a technique invented in the second half of the sixteenth century in China. Variolation had spread to Korea, Russia, and Western Europe by the end of the Ming dynasty (1644) but was not seen in Japan (i.e., in Nagasaki) until 1744.[8]

After 1671, the Japanese interpreters in the Dutch warehouses were given formal instruction in reading and writing Dutch, and (later) they were also granted special permission to observe the practices of the Dutch physicians. Four of the leading Japanese families of interpreters at Deshima were able to use the information they gained from the Dutch physicians to establish their own medical lineages. These interpreters were also responsible for some of the first books about Western medicine to be published in Japan.[9] These and the handful of other Japanese writings on Western medicine published before 1774 were not direct translations; rather, techniques from abroad were discussed and selectively assimilated into Japanese medical practice.

The first direct medical translation was published in 1774, laying the foundation of what was to become *Rangaku* 蘭学 (literally, 'Dutch studies'). It was a translation of a simple anatomical atlas, originally published in German as *Anatomische Tabellen* by Johann Adam Kulmus in Danzig in 1722 and translated into Japanese (using Chinese characters) from a 1734 Dutch translation. The principal translators, Maeno Ryōtaku 前野良沢 and Sugita Gempaku 杉田玄白, had been inspired by attending the dismemberment and rough dissection of a female criminal at an execution ground, where they determined that their newly acquired German-Dutch anatomical tables offered a much closer representation of what they saw than anything then available in the Sino-Japanese medical tradition. In 1773 they published a trial extract of their translation, calling it *A Short Atlas of Anatomy* (*Kaitai yakuzu* 解体約図), which consisted of only three pages of plates and a short report. They wanted to test the waters of official opinion because they knew of at least one other Dutch translation that had been confiscated and had its plates destroyed by the police because its illustrations contained some letters of the Roman alphabet.[10] Their plates and introductory text show that Japanese interest in anatomy was mainly concerned with correcting the tenets of Chinese medicine. There were no descriptions of the characteristic Renaissance-style muscle anatomy in these new Japanese medical works, indicating that Western accounts of the musculature were not of prime importance to the Japanese. On the other hand, demonstrations that the body does not contain exactly 365 bones (one for each day of the year), or that the lung is not composed of 'six lobes and two ears' (as described in the Sino-Japanese medical tradition), were of much greater relevance to the Japanese physicians.

The effect of this work owed more to its graphic style than to the novelty of its message. Yamawaki Tōyō 山脇東洋 (1705-62) had compared Dutch and Chinese anatomical drawings over a decade earlier, endorsing Dutch anatomy in his *Record of the Internal Organs* (*Zōshi* 臓誌) in 1759. The crucial difference between Yamawaki's work and Maeno and Sugita's translation was that Yamawaki had employed traditional Japanese artists to make the illustrations. Even though his book discussed and endorsed the Western body-image, it was still a Japanese medical work. Maeno and Sugita's book, on the other hand, was a new genre, a straight translation, with illustrations painstakingly copied from the Dutch copper plates. The realism of these illustrations made a dramatic impression on readers as they were graphic representations of a system of medicine based on a very different conceptualization of the body.[11]

Maeno and Sugita's valiant translation also demonstrated the possibility of creating specialized scientific vocabularies in Japanese. In its wake, in 1783, the *Rangaku* scholar Otsuki Gentaku published a beginner's textbook of the Dutch language and, in 1786, founded a school of Dutch studies in Edo. By the 1840s, Dutch studies were being taught in several public institutions, including government schools.[12]

It is important to understand that 'Dutch' – and by association all foreign learning – was not studied merely because it was in accord with the new value being placed on graphical realism in Japan. The applied sciences transmitted by Dutch East India Company surgeons through their interpreters were particularly relevant to Neo-Confucian scholars who valued 'practical learning' as opposed to the 'empty learning' of Buddhism and Daoism. Practical learning was useful in governance and was applicable to the welfare of society. Thus the eighth Tokugawa shōgun, Yoshimune (ruled 1716-45), endorsed the study of new Chinese astronomical texts even though they had been produced by Christian converts. He also allowed the translation of navigational and medical texts brought by the Dutch. Slowly, *Rangaku* was losing its association with undesirable Christian proselytizing and was beginning to be seen as a source of useful new information.[13]

Along with this eighteenth-century relaxation of attitudes towards foreign knowledge came an enthusiasm for Western things that mirrored the crazes for chinoiserie and japonaiserie in Europe. During this 'Hollandomania' *(ranpeki)* new translations of medical works had a ready readership, even finding their way into the collections of rural doctors, who used them to supplement their ongoing research.[14] A stellar example of this kind of influence appears in the work of the Japanese doctor Hanaoka Seishū 華岡 青洲 (1760-1835) from Wakayama Prefecture, near Osaka. Hanaoka was fascinated by the legend of Hua Tuo, the great surgeon of Chinese antiquity famed for using a special powder that rendered patients insensible. Hanaoka also read Western works on surgery and used his knowledge of Chinese *materia medica* to develop the world's first general anaesthetic in 1805. His formula, developed by experimenting on animals and on his own wife, consisted of six plant drugs from the Chinese pharmacopeia, including aconite and datura. With this innovation, Hanaoka was able to build a reputation for major surgery, particularly the excision of breast tumours. He saw himself as combining Chinese-style internal medicine with 'Dutch' surgery, and his procedures became known as the 'Hanaoka method,' which his many students made famous throughout Japan.[15]

Several Western physicians who came to Nagasaki as employees of the Dutch East India Company became influential early teachers of Western medicine. During the 1820s, the German medical doctor Philip Franz von Siebold was employed by the Dutch in Deshima and was permitted by the Japanese to establish a private medical school in Nagasaki. He taught chemistry, geology, mineralogy, and physics as well as the medical sciences of the period.[16] The Dutch army surgeon Johannes Pompe van Meerdervoort arrived in Nagasaki in 1857, and the Japanese government quickly asked him to tutor twelve Japanese medical students. Van Meerdervoort also succeeded in receiving permission to dissect the bodies of several executed criminals in order to teach his students practical anatomy.[17] By the time he left Japan after five years, he had given medical diplomas to 61 students, taught a total of 150, and seen a 120-bed Western-medical hospital erected in Nagasaki at government expense, to which new medical school buildings were attached.[18]

Information about Western learning was most effectively propagated in the private schools of the *Rangakusha* (Dutch scholars). The most famous of these was Ogata Kōan 緒方洪庵 (1810-63), who started his school in Osaka in 1838. He taught Western medicine to three thousand students between 1838 and 1862.[19] In the years between the publication of Sugita's *New Atlas of Anatomy* in 1774 and the Meiji Restoration of 1868, at least twelve private schools of Western medicine were founded in Edo (modern Tokyo), Kyoto, Osaka, and Nagasaki, compared with the twenty-seven schools of Sino-Japanese medicine established during the same period by *daimyō* (feudal lords).[20] Of the forty-nine recorded medical schools run in the provinces under *daimyō* administration during the last years of the Tokugawa regime (i.e., before the Meiji Restoration of 1868), at least seven taught Dutch medicine.[21] In her study of several early nineteenth-century physicians, Ann Jannetta concludes that *Ranpō* 蘭方 (Dutch medicine) could function as a route to social mobility for its students, who created far-flung social and intellectual support networks for each other. These scholars' networks and their knowledge of the West primed them for leadership positions when, after 1868, the Japanese government adopted European models of modernization.[22]

In 1854, as a result of US naval officer Commodore Perry's successful intimidation of the Japanese government, new ports were opened to international trade. In 1855, Japan's treaty with Russia gave Russians the right to trade as well as extra-territorial rights. This concession was followed up by American negotiators who succeeded in obtaining extra-territoriality for American citizens in 1857, along with permission for them to establish permanent residence in the cities of Shimoda and Hakodate. Through 'most-favoured nation' clauses, the Japanese government was pressured into extending these concessions to other Western nations, engendering much popular resentment among its own people. Renegotiation of these 'unequal treaties' was a high priority in Japanese foreign policy for the rest of the century and was finally achieved after Japan demonstrated its military might by defeating China in the 1894-95 Sino-Japanese War.

The Tokugawa government's capitulation to these foreign demands during the late 1850s and 1860s was a major catalyst for the downfall of the shōgunate and the restoration carried out in the name of the Meiji Emperor, who assumed the throne in 1867 (aged fifteen) and whose faction had consolidated power by the following year. From the start, the restoration took as its slogan the establishment of 'a rich country and a strong army,' and it looked to Western technologies to achieve this. A strong army required healthy soldiers and citizens, necessitating an army medical service. So in early 1874, the Meiji government established the Department of [Western] Medicine in the Ministry of Culture. Its first director was Nagayo Sensai 長与専斎 (1838-1902), a graduate of Pompe van Meerdervoort's medical school in Nagasaki who had recently returned from the Iwakura mission, a year-long inspection tour of Europe and the United States. By the end of the year, Nagayo had formulated a new medical act, requiring that all medical practitioners be licensed. Physicians who had been in practice before February 1875 were granted a licence without examination, but thereafter all doctors had to pass an examination in six Western-medical subjects. This edict was first carried out in Tokyo, Kyoto, and Osaka; by 1884 it was in force across the entire country. Although the 'grandfathering in' of established physicians was intended to minimize opposition to the new regulations on the part of the physicians of Sino-Japanese medicine *(kanpō)* and their supporters, the edict aimed to replace *kanpō* with Western medicine within one generation.[23]

According to figures for 1875, there were 22,527 physicians of *kanpō* and 5,123 physicians of Western (Dutch) medicine in Japan, a ratio of more than 4:1. The government decided to train more doctors of Western medicine as quickly as possible, and, by 1897, just twenty-two years later, there were 39,390 licensed physicians in Japan. Of these, over fifteen thousand were doctors of Western medicine who had passed the licensing examinations since 1875. Only forty-six of these men had qualified abroad, which indicates Japan's success in setting up a domestic system of training in Western medicine. Another forty-nine hundred physicians were doctors of Western medicine who, in 1875, had been granted licences without examination. The total number of *kanpō* physicians had shrunk to about nineteen thousand, already less than half of the total number of licensed medical practitioners in Japan.[24]

Kanpō advocates launched initiatives to defend their status. In 1879 *kanpō* physicians organized conferences, founded a society, and petitioned the government for the inclusion of a medical licensing examination specifically in *kanpō* medicine. The society had seven hundred members at its peak and petitioned the government three times – all unsuccessfully – before its closure owing to financial difficulties in 1886.[25] The next major attempt to regain official status for *kanpō* medicine started in 1890, when Dr. Asai Atsutarō 浅井厚田朗 founded the Imperial Sino-Japanese Medical Association. This association reached a membership of three thousand *kanpō* physicians, with support from another 100,000 non-medics.[26] The new Japanese Constitution had been promulgated in 1889, and 1890 was the year of the first elections for the new two-chambered Diet. This change of constitution, with legislative powers passing to an elected body, gave supporters of Sino-Japanese medicine a new source of authority to petition. In 1891, Asai's Medical Association petitioned the Imperial Diet to exempt traditional doctors from the medical licensing examinations. They succeeded in persuading a group of twelve Diet members to bring a motion in their support, which was read in 1892. Their case remained undecided, however, because of the early dissolution of the Diet later that year.[27]

These attempts to relegitimize Sino-Japanese medicine in Japan brought a strong response from a prominent physician of Western medicine, Surgeon-General Ishiguro Tadanori 石黒忠悳 (1845-1941), who mounted a campaign to prevent the licensing of *kanpō* practitioners. He argued that, even though scholars of the old medical books were to be admired, most *kanpō* doctors were quacks. The persistence of such low-calibre doctors would encourage mediocre doctors from abroad (he was referring to China and Korea) to earn their living in Japan, thus draining the country's resources. He further maintained that a modern medical system must meet particular hygienic, legal, and military requirements, among which were public health, epidemic prevention (including international quarantine measures), autopsies to determine the cause of death, and field surgery. Sino-Japanese medicine delivered none of these. If Japan were to encourage the practice of *kanpō,* the status of Japanese medicine as a whole would suffer in the eyes of the international community. Instead, Japan should build on its successes, such as its admission to the International Red Cross Society in 1887 – an accolade denied China until 1904. (Ishiguro himself was later to be intimately involved in the administration of the Japanese Red Cross during the Sino-Japanese War of 1894-95, for which he would be awarded samurai status and the rank of baron.) In 1892, in addition to giving public lectures denouncing *kanpō,* he published his broadsides as *A Comparison of Eastern and Western Medical Arts.* The arguments he employed in favour of Western medicine were very explicit in assessing it as an essential part of the machinery of modern state-building. Ishiguro's complaints about quack *kanpō* physicians were not couched in terms of the harm they might cause their patients but, rather, in terms of the potential damage they might do to the prestige and finances of the Japanese state.[28]

In 1894, the supporters of *kanpō* resubmitted their bill to the Diet and succeeded in getting it passed at the first reading, in spite of Ishiguro's campaign. However, in this year the Sino-Japanese War broke out. By the time the petitioned amendments to the licensing laws were read before the eighth session of the Imperial Diet in 1895, opinion had hardened towards everything Chinese and the amendments were defeated. In 1898, the *kanpō* society folded. Its founder, Asai, wrote an epigraph for himself in 1900: 'For ten generations we have continued our fathers' profession, but now we face the end of the line. Heavy-hearted, worried and distressed, I do not know how to proceed.'[29]

The future of *kanpō* medicine in Japan did indeed look bleak at this time. Between 1894 and 1909 the leaders of the licensing movement died. In the fifty-eight years from the start of the Meiji Restoration in 1868 until the start of the revival movement in 1926 (the start of the Shōwa emperor's reign), only thirty-two *kanpō* books were published in Japan. There were no publications at all in the decade between 1898 and 1907, and only eleven for the entire period between the Sino-Japanese War (1894-95) and 1926.[30]

Kanpō's resurgence had an unlikely source – a licensed practitioner of Western medicine. In 1910, Wada Keijūrō 和田啓十郎 (1872-1916)

published the first edition of his *Iron Spear of the Medical World* (*Ikai no tettsui,* 医界之鉄椎).[31] This book was republished four times between 1910 and 1922 and was also translated into Chinese and Korean. In it, Wada praised the clinical effectiveness of *kanpō* medicine and explicitly castigated pro-Western theorists who had condemned it without any experience of its practical efficacy. He claimed that, although Western medicine might provide precise diagnoses, it was unable to deliver the corresponding therapies. One of Wada's principal targets was the same Ishiguro Tadanori who had been leading the offensive against *kanpō* medicine. In his extended 1915 edition, Wada published a point-by-point repudiation of Ishiguro's arguments against Sino-Japanese medicine and then related how he had called on the baron to ask him to contribute a preface. In Wada's own account, Baron Ishiguro angrily replied that he had yet to find anything of practical value in all his extensive readings of the classical medical works. Wada, in turn, insisted that *kanpō* medicine was indeed practical and asked whether Ishiguro had had any experience of it. Ishiguro readily admitted that he had not. Wada then argued that no one could be expected to understand Sino-Japanese medical concepts using only the theories of Western medicine and that practical experience provided the best evidence of *kanpō*'s benefits.[32] The consequences of the outbreak of the First World War in 1914 and the severing of the drug supply from the West were to bear him out since, after the war, even Ishiguro retracted his earlier extreme position:

> When I think of how, in the past, I exerted myself to the utmost to realise the goal of the abolition of *kanpō*, and insisted on [Western-medical] drugs of only the finest quality, always taking German drug quality as the standard; now I look back, and it seems that 49 of the last 50 years have been mistaken.[33]

Wada's book spurred a growth of interest in *kanpō* medicine among Western-trained physicians in Japan, many of whom claimed to have had experiences like Wada's, in which chronic illnesses had been cured through *kanpō* treatment after Western medicine had proved ineffectual.[34]

However, it was not until the late 1920s that Sino-Japanese physicians started to organize themselves into any kind of renewed political force. Zhao Hongjun claims that this movement in Japan was inspired by the successes of the supporters of Chinese medicine in China, who effectively repulsed attempts to establish Japanese-style restrictive licensing legislation in 1929. Yu Yunxiu, who had received his Western-medical training in Japan and, at the time, was virulent in his opposition to Chinese medicine, states the opposite, insisting that the formation of the Sino-Japanese Medical Association in late 1929 was a great inspiration to the Chinese-medical community in China.[35] While it is clear that there was an enormous traffic in ideas and medical information between China and Japan in this period, the *kanpō* revival movement seems to have started slightly earlier. In 1926, the pharmacist Asahina Yasuhiko 根本曽代子 (1880-1975) read a paper to the Japanese Medical Association's Seventh Congress titled 'Research into Unprocessed Sino-Japanese [herbal] Drugs.'[36]

This was a time of increasing nationalism, which would eventually lead to the Japanese invasion of Manchuria in 1931. Japan had proved itself as a world military power during the First World War and, in return, had been awarded Germany's rights and concessions in Shandong Province, causing widespread outrage in China. In 1921, at the Washington Conference, Japan had signed a naval treaty with Great Britain and the United States to limit relative battleship tonnage ratios to 3:5:5, respectively, thus quantifying Japan's status as a maritime power.[37] With this status and the proven ability to rapidly modernize, the Japanese clearly felt that scientific explorations of native *materia medica* were much less threatening to their national pride than they had been in the 1890s.

Suddenly, books and articles describing the modern uses of *kanpō* burgeoned, and by 1938 at least six national organizations were promoting Sino-Japanese medicine, and each was publishing its own journal. Five new motions requesting the legal recognition of *kanpō* as a medical specialty were presented to the Imperial Diet between 1929 and 1940. One such resolution – for the government to establish a research institute for *kanpō* medicine – was passed by both houses in 1930 but was never implemented.[38]

Although the *kanpō* revival movement ground to a halt during the Second World War, it achieved more than just a succession of enthusiastic publications. Most significant was the pharmacological research into such Chinese drugs as ginseng, ephedra, pilose deer antler, cow-bezoar, and monkshood root. These investigations set the scene for what was to become Japan's main interest in *kanpō* – the discovery of new active principles in the traditional pharmacopeia. It was not until the 1970s, when Japanese national pride had recovered from the setbacks of the Second World War and the consequent American occupation (1945-52), and after Japan had gained admittance to the United Nations (1956) and embarked on the modern 'economic miracle,' that schools and research institutes devoted to the new Sino-Japanese medicine began to be founded in Japan.[39]

This is the background to the situation Chinese students encountered when they studied in Japan. On arrival, they could find evidence both for Western medicine (as an aid to building the state) and for a 'scientized' traditional medicine with Chinese roots (as a way of maintaining cultural identity). Japanese influence appeared along a broad spectrum of Chinese political beliefs. The communist revolutionary Guo Moruo 郭沫若 (1892-1978) studied medicine in Japan, as did the late Qing revolutionaries Qiu Jin 秋瑾 and Chen Yuan 陈垣, whose views we consider further in Chapter 6. Although Sun Yat-sen, provisional first president of the Republic of China, studied medicine with the British in Guangzhou and Hong Kong, he enjoyed much support from the Japanese and, in turn, supported the establishment of Western medicine as the state-sponsored medical system.[40] The more conservative Ding Fubao 丁福保 spent twenty years translating Japanese textbooks of modern medicine into Chinese, dominating the considerable market for this kind of information for the whole of the first two decades of the Republic of China.

Many of the prominent politicians of the early Republic had been trained abroad, several of them in Western medicine. So when the Guomindang (Nationalist Party) under Jiang Jieshi (Chiang Kai-shek 蔣介石) assumed control in 1928, and its Nanjing government convened its first Health Commission in February 1929, it seemed entirely natural that the eighteen members of the commission should all have been trained only in Western medicine. In fact, at least ten were graduates of foreign medical schools in Europe, the United States, or Japan.[41.]

One of the members of the 1929 Health Commission was Yu Yan 余巖 (styled Yunxiu 云岫, 1879-1954). Yu was one of the first generation of students sent to study in Japan in the last years of the Qing. In 1908, he enrolled in Osaka Medical University's premedical program, and he graduated with a medical degree in 1916. He interrupted his studies for just over a year, starting in November 1911, a month after the Chinese Revolution, to join a group of fellow Chinese medical students in Japan who organized themselves into a Red Cross medical team and returned to volunteer.[42] This patriotism re-emerged in Yu's offensive against Chinese medicine, which commenced the year after his return to Shanghai with the 1917 publication of his *Straight Talk about the Spiritual [Pivot] and the Plain [Questions]* (*Ling, Su shangdui* 靈素商兌). It consisted of a wholesale attack on the theoretical foundations of Chinese medicine, as found in the *Yellow Emperor's Inner Canon* (*Huangdi neijing*). Starting by demolishing 'superstitious' beliefs in such notions as *yin*, *yang*, and the Five Phases, Yu continued by explicating the inadequacies of Chinese-medical ideas regarding the structure and function of the internal organs, blood vessels, and acupuncture tracts, and disease causation. Yu insisted that he was not ridiculing China's ancient learning per se, and he emphasized that much of the Western-medical knowledge on which he drew was very new. The real targets of Yu's broadside were the medical practitioners of the day, who insisted on blindly clinging to their outdated medical traditions, flagrantly disregarding modern proofs both of their own inadequacies and of the efficacy of more modern (Western) methods.[43]

Yu Yunxiu's offensive drew little response until 1922, when a prominent Chinese-medical practitioner and classical scholar, Yun Tieqiao 惲鐵樵 (1878-1935), published a rebuttal in his *Record of Wisdom Observed in the [medical] Classics* (*Qunjing jianzhi lu* 群經見智錄). Thereafter, articles rebutting Yu's arguments appeared frequently in the Chinese-medical press.[44]

By the time the Nanjing government's Health Commission first met in 1929, Yu was fighting to eliminate Chinese medicine altogether. The commission considered four proposals that dealt with medical registration and policies towards Chinese medicine. Of these four, Yu's proposal was considered last and was by far the most radical. Called 'Proposal to Abolish Old [Chinese] Medicine in Order to Remove Obstacles to Medicine and Hygiene,' it recommended that all Chinese-medical practitioners be required to register with the government before the end of 1930 in order to be issued with a licence to practise. All except those who were over fifty and who had been practising for over twenty years would be required to take classes in modern medicine and hygiene, the course to be completed by the end of 1933. Schools of Chinese medicine, Chinese-medical reports in periodicals, and advertising for anything other than 'scientific medicine' were to be outlawed.[45]

Yu was explicit about his intention to abolish Chinese medicine as quickly as possible. He wrote in the introduction to his motion: 'For every day that old medicine is not abolished, the people's ideas will not change, the cause of modern medicine will not be able to progress, and sanitary measures will not be able to advance.'[46] Yu's strategy was thus much more confrontational than that so carefully implemented by Nagayo Sensai in Japan in the early 1870s. Nagayo had not required established physicians to take classes, and he had allowed all Sino-Japanese practitioners who had been in practice for only five years to continue unhindered. He had also seen no need to attempt to censor the Sino-Japanese medical community. As we have seen, public opinion was already very favourably inclined towards Western medicine in Japan in the 1870s, and, by 1897, more than half of all licensed doctors in Japan had been trained in Western medicine. By 1922, Japan had a ratio of qualified Western-medical doctors to the population of approximately 1:1000.[47]

The situation in China in 1929 was very different. Even after the three associations that supported doctors of Western medicine had amalgamated in 1932, their total membership was still only 794. This was a great increase over the thirty-six founding members of the Chinese Medical Association in 1915, but it still only represented one Western-medical doctor for every 500,000 inhabitants. Moreover, almost all of these doctors lived and worked in the big cities.[48] Given the relative dearth and inaccessibility of Western-medical care, it is no wonder that Chinese public opinion was much less convinced of the wisdom of wholesale conversion to Western medicine than was Japanese public opinion. Even among the government elite, Yu had clearly underestimated the sympathy for Chinese medicine, as the response to his motion was to show.

According to Yu Yunxiu's own account, he encouraged the commission members to discuss his motion in detail, but they were tired and declined. Notwithstanding, the motion was carried, with only two or three members expressing any doubts.[49] This outraged the Chinese-medical community, which called a national congress in Shanghai to protest the motion, repeatedly petitioned the government, sent telegrams, and lobbied furiously. Acrimonious debates in the press over the proper role of traditional medicine in the new Republic had been commonplace for some time, so the battle lines had already been drawn. Moreover, immediately prior to the convening of the Health Commission, the government had published its 'Basic Principles of the National Health Administration,' establishing the commission as an exclusively Western-medical government department. The government also published provisional regulations governing pharmaceutical practice, which required all pharmacists to be licensed and to be qualified in Western pharmacy.[50] Yu Yunxiu thus became a target for the Chinese-style doctors' fury and frustration.

The Chinese-medical community's lobbying was effective enough to change several commissioners' minds, so much so that, when Minister of Health Xue Dubi 薛篤弼 (1892-1973) returned from a visit to a disaster area in the northwest (which had necessitated his absence from the original meeting), he came out in opposition to the motion. This left Yu Yunxiu unprotected – he said he felt as though people wanted to hack him into tiny pieces – and, although he tried to carry his argument into the newspapers, only two agreed to print his letters, and one of these responded with an editorial that was critical of him.[51]

Yu's confrontational approach meant that he alienated even those reform-minded Chinese physicians who were later successfully integrated into a less threatening modernization program. Indeed, one supporter of the reform – but not the abolition – of Chinese medicine wrote in

1932 that Yu's motion was the event that had made the debate public knowledge and was the main reason that enough support was found to establish the Institute of National (i.e., Chinese) Medicine the following year.[52] The late 1920s were a period of rising nationalism and opposition to foreign imperialism in China, sentiments that the Chinese-medical community used to great advantage.

Yu continued his anti-Chinese medicine polemics into the mid-1930s by criticizing Chinese enthusiasm for Japanese attempts to modernize Sino-Japanese medicine. However, after the state funded the Institute of National Medicine in 1930, he turned his attention to the study of old Chinese medical works in the hope of informing such pharmacological research as the analytical pharmacognosy pioneered in Japan. It was this new-found enthusiasm for Japan's 'scientization' of traditional *kanpō* medicine that other Chinese visitors would also bring back to China.

Well before the Japanese established their Imperial Sino-Japanese Medicine Association in 1929, the Chinese-medical scholarly community felt the influence of Japan. For instance, the Japanese conversion to Western medicine in the early years of the Meiji Restoration meant that there was less demand in Japan for Chinese-medical books, which were discarded and sold very cheaply. Several Chinese scholars built valuable collections of rare Chinese works by buying copies suddenly available in Japan. They discovered titles that had been thought lost as well as several rare editions of classical texts. Thus, the Cantonese scholar Han Moyuan was able to purchase a 1307 edition of Sun Simiao's *Supplementary Prescriptions Worth a Thousand in Gold* (*Qianjin yi fang* 千金翼方, written in the seventh century CE) and a 1640 edition of Wang Tao's *Arcane Essentials from the Imperial Library* (*Waitai biyao fang* 外台必要方, eighth century), both editions having been unknown in China. Han reprinted them in 1874. The diplomat and bibliophile Yang Shoujing 楊守敬 (1839-1915) also brought back several hundred rare Japanese editions of Chinese books in the late nineteenth century. In 1884, he published a collection of thirteen of these, followed by a rare Song dynasty (960-1279 CE) edition of Zhang Ji's first-century classic, the *Shanghan Zabing Lun* (*Treatise on Cold-Damage and Miscellaneous Disorders*), in 1902.[53]

Since the late eighteenth century, the Chinese intellectual current of 'evidential research' (*kaozheng xuepai* 考證學派) had become popular in Japanese medical scholarship, inspiring publication in Japan of several critical editions of the Chinese-medical classics as well as reference works and compilations. When, in the late 1920s, the champions of the Chinese-medical cause started to publish their own collections of important medical works with the intention of making classical Chinese medicine more accessible and demonstrating the value of the Chinese-medical tradition, many of them repaid the favour by including Japanese works of the Sino-Japanese tradition in their collections. For example, in 1923, Qiu Jisheng, whose description of popular medical practices we encountered in Chapter 2, included eight Japanese titles in his collection of ninety-nine less accessible medical works, *Double Three Medical Collection* (*San san yi shu* 三三醫書). In 1931, He Bingyuan 何炳元 (styled Lianchen 廉臣, 1861-1921), included three Japanese titles in his collection, *Mr He's Medical Collection* (*Heshi yixue congshu* 何氏醫學叢書). Both Qiu and He were eminent in the Chinese-medical world, running study societies and publishing medical journals. He Bingyuan and Yun Tieqiao made frequent reference to Japanese editions and commentaries in their own studies of Zhang Ji's *Treatise on Cold Damage*, but they were far surpassed in their enthusiasm for Japanese scholarship by the Shanghai physician Lu Pengnian 陸彭年 (styled Yuanlei 淵雷, 1894-1955). Lu Yuanlei made a total of 674 references to forty different Japanese authors in his 1931 *Modern Exposition of the Treatise on Cold Damage* (*Shanghan lun jin shi* 傷寒論今釋). Lu and Yun were two of the most respected spokesmen for Chinese medicine in the Republican period. Their teaching positions at accredited schools of Chinese medicine indicate a widespread regard for Japanese medical scholarship of the 1920s.[54]

This appreciation of Sino-Japanese medical publications continued even after the commencement of aggressive Japanese imperialism in China in 1931. In 1936, the World Press (*Shijie, shuju* 世界書局) in Shanghai published a collection of seventy-two Japanese medical works, the *Sino-Japanese Medical Collection* (*Huanghan yixue congshu* 皇漢醫學叢書), edited by Chen Cunren 陳存仁 (1908-90), who was working under the auspices of the Institute of National Medicine. Half of this collection was devoted to books representing the recent revival of *kanpō* medicine in Japan and half to old books that were rarely available in China. Chen indicated that the distinguishing features of *kanpō* medicine included the preservation of skills now lost on the mainland (such as bone-setting and abdominal diagnosis), certain obstetrical operations, and the relocation of acupuncture points and tracts. He further argued that scholars and scientists in the 'advanced nations' of Japan and Germany had endorsed the validity and usefulness of Chinese medicine. They had also started to translate Sino-Japanese medical books and use scientific methods to investigate the merits of Chinese medicine.[55]

The application of scientific methods, both in the investigation of Chinese medicine and in its redrafting by 'traditional' physicians for their new medical schools, became the major innovation in the Chinese medicine of the 1920s and 1930s. In 1932, Wang Shenxuan 王慎軒 (1900-84) collected a large selection of essays that he deemed to represent the best of what was new in Chinese medicine. Thirty of these were by Japanese authors. The whole collection represented concerted attempts to assimilate and accommodate Western ideas of cellular anatomy, pathological anatomy, physiology, and pathology.[56]

The influence in China of Japanese efforts to reconcile *kanpō* with modern science is difficult to quantify, particularly since one result of Japanese imperialism in China is that many Chinese were and are reluctant to acknowledge Japanese influence. Thus, Zhu Weiju 朱味菊 (1884-1951), having spent over a year in Japan at the invitation of his Japanese teacher of (Western) medicine, published a compilation of his lecture notes on pathology, *Pathology Elucidated* (*Bingli fahui* 病理發揮), in 1931. This was a bold attempt to reconcile germ theory and cellular pathology with the concepts of Chinese medicine. Even though Zhu rejected the Chinese medical and cosmological concepts of the Five Movements and Six Qi (*wu yun liu qi* 五運六氣) as so much unscientific superstition, expressing ideas very similar to those published earlier by Wada Keijūrō, he nowhere mentions his debt to Japanese scholarship. Significantly, the title-page calligraphy to Zhu's book was contributed by Yu Youren 于右任 (1879-1964), a member of the Guomindang Central Executive Committee and chief of police. Yu was a supporter of cooperation between the Guomindang and the Communists in a united front against Japanese aggression. In an age when Chinese medicine was being sold to the public as part of a unique Chinese cultural heritage, proposals for its modernization were unlikely to gain adherents by admitting to having been inspired by Japanese imperialists.[57]

Such factors make it difficult to decisively determine the order of Chinese and Japanese influence on each country's respective medical modernization. What is important to note about this complex of alternating influence and parallel change is that, in each country, both modern medicine and traditional medicine emerged with renewed strength. Previous cultural exchanges, dating back centuries, meant that each of the modern rivals had preserved the other's medical culture in written collections of classic works. Thus, Chinese visitors to Japan could find Chinese medical treasures as well as new Western techniques and methods for modernizing traditional medicine. At some point, all of these elements – cultural uniqueness, Western influence, and innovative hybridization – would contribute to China's effort at state-building, a subject to which we now turn.

Public Health and State-Building   5

Without the provision of adequate machinery and facilities for the
prevention and treatment of disease, easily accessible to the public,
no Government can be considered modern or complete.

-LEANG-LI T'ANG, *RECONSTRUCTION IN CHINA: A RECORD OF
PROGRESS AND ACHIEVEMENT IN FACTS AND FIGURES*

Public health as a Western concept was created in the mid-nineteenth
century in Britain, France, and Germany as a direct result of the political
economy of utilitarianism. Since an unprecedented accumulation of
labour was needed to service the factories and workshops of the newly
industrialized urban centres, frequent illnesses among the labour force
were expensive. Throughout most of the nineteenth century, people
thought that infectious diseases were caused by the foul air, or miasma,
given off by dirt, excrement, and stagnant water. Thus, the nineteenth-
century campaigners for sanitary reform, such as Edwin Chadwick in
Britain, assumed that by eliminating the sources of foul air and noxious
odours, they would be eliminating the cause of many of the most serious
diseases. Although a few private employers applied these principles
directly, such as, famously, the Cadbury family in the late-nineteenth-
century construction of their workers' town at Bournville, the sanitary

movement as a whole addressed itself to the state. This was the first time that the health of poor people was considered economically (as opposed to morally) relevant to the governing classes. So our current understanding of the term 'public health' grew out of a concern for national economic efficiency, and, thus, public health activities became the legitimate and proper concerns of the state.[1]

Any examination of the concept of public health in nineteenth-century China, however, has to acknowledge another meaning of the term. Activities that Westerners might normally label as related to 'public health,' such as the building of drains and the issuing of medicines during epidemic disease episodes, were classified quite differently in pre-twentieth-century China. Similarly, the concept of public health that developed in China differed from the concept that developed in the West. To see the evolution of both concept and activity, we need to turn to premodern times.

Historians have found various kinds of 'health-seeking behaviour' that predate a state-centred concept of public health in China. For example, as mentioned earlier, the *Yellow Emperor's Inner Canon (Huangdi neijing)* states: 'The Sagely Man treats incipient disease rather than existing disease, and incipient [political] disorder rather than existing disorder.' The same word, *zhi* 治, is used both for disease treatment and for political rule or control.[2] Many early Chinese texts contain admonitions for the proper siting and care of wells and irrigation channels, the disposal of human waste, personal hygiene, and the correct disposal of the dead. And, although it is difficult to draw conclusions about actual practice from these admonitions, it is clear that they were all matters of common concern.[3] What is more certain is that great care was taken to build urban water supply and drainage networks, for example in Beijing at the beginning of the Qing dynasty (1644). Chinese motivations for building urban waterways included the provision of fresh drinking water and drainage, but they also included the desire to assist the transportation of goods, to prevent large-scale fires, to control flooding, to provide a line of defence, and to supply the lakes and ponds that were built both for aesthetic reasons and for the cultivation of water plants.[4] The Chinese practice of variolation was also considered effective enough to be adopted in most European countries during the course of the eighteenth century. Moreover, as Angela Leung argues, it was not unknown in China for the imperial authorities to explicitly support measures that we in the West would normally associate with public health. These included the publication and distribution of efficacious prescriptions under the Tang dynasty (608-906 CE), the construction of infirmaries in major cities to segregate the seriously ill during the Song dynasty (960-1279 CE), and the establishment of charity pharmacies that gave out free medicines, especially during epidemic outbreaks, also first recorded under the Song.[5]

These activities were part of 'emergency (or calamity) relief,' *jiuhuang* 救荒 or *jiuzai* 救災, terms also applied to efforts employed in the face of natural calamities such as epidemics, famine, drought, flood, and storm damage.[6] Some of these measures might resemble Western public health activities; however, in the West the idea of public health referred to an ongoing agenda of disease-preventative activities, while in China calamity relief was, by definition, only offered after a calamity had already occurred (which is not to ignore the considerable efforts that often went into contingency preparations such as the civilian granary system).

Starting in the sixteenth century, official responses to epidemics were usually in the form of ad hoc distributions of medicines or money with which to buy them. An exception was the founding of special quarantine villages about forty *li* (about twenty-five kilometres) from the Beijing city wall during the early years of the Qing (Manchu) dynasty (1644-1911). These villages were used to house smallpox cases. This unusual measure was adopted because the Manchus, coming from the sparsely populated north, had not been exposed to smallpox, and, on occupying Beijing, their mortality from the disease was very high. Both the Shunzi emperor (1638-61) and the Tongzhi emperor (1856-75) died of smallpox, and high nobles and even members of the Imperial clan were not permitted to enter the palace until they had survived the disease.[7]

Compensating for the relative absence of government-funded health care provision in late Imperial China, local associations of gentry scholars or merchants founded charity dispensaries and clinics, particularly in the Lower Yangzi region. By the late Qing (mid- to late nineteenth century) such privately funded initiatives had arisen all over China. Clinics and dispensaries were typically run by a society of respectable

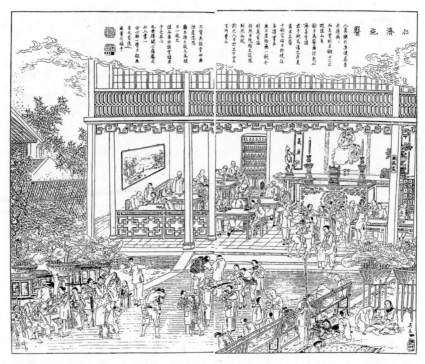

Figure 8　Illustrated newspaper article praising the members of the Renji Charitable Society in Shanghai, who paid ten reputable local physicians to provide free treatment to the poor for a day. *Source: Dianshizhai Huabao* 點石齋畫報 [Lithographic pictorial] no. 48, 1885. Courtesy of Cambridge University Library.

local individuals, each paying subscriptions in order to fund the activities, although these projects could also be undertaken and funded by a single individual or family. These groups would employ local doctors in rotation or for a particular season (typically the 'epidemic' season – spring and summer). Some limited themselves to prescribing and dispensing medicines; others also maintained a sick room for those too ill or poor to be returned home for care. Some also provided coffins for the dead. Carol Benedict notes that the local gentry also funded processions and ceremonies to frighten off plague demons or to appease offended gods.[8] Figure 8 illustrates a dispensary in which, on a particular day in Shanghai in 1885, the members of a philanthropic society have temporarily employed ten physicians to provide free medicine for the poor.

The pursuit of elite status in their community motivated local gentry to establish and fund charitable health work. As Leung indicates:

> The decline of the state's role and the rise of organized private initia-
> tive in public health was important in China more for social than
> for health reasons. It marked an avenue for local elites to assert their
> leadership and influence in an area where the state had left a vacuum.
> In the more complexly stratified, competitive society emerging after
> the late Ming, this opportunity was especially useful to merchants
> and other local rich men who lacked official status.[9]

It was especially gratifying for a family without official bureaucratic or scholarly status to earn recognition in a local official gazette through meritorious philanthropy. The Qing government actively encouraged these initiatives, most famously in a 1731 edict from the Yongzheng emperor: 'I exhort every wealthy household to be constantly vigilant, even in peacetime, in dispensing relief and aid to the poor.'[10] Thus, while local levels of investment in charitable health activities were extremely variable, it is clear that the support of a local charitable pharmacy or dispensary was an expression of the donor's importance and social standing.

In China, delegating responsibility for the welfare of the poor to local notables was part of what Susan Mann, following Max Weber, calls 'liturgical governance.' The leaders of local communities 'were to assume collective liability for the welfare of members, in exchange for and in affirmation of their privileged monopoly on wealth and power.'[11] As Mann notes, later in the dynasty the pressures of urbanization resulted in the transfer of these liturgical responsibilities to tradesmen's associations and occupational guilds. This local provision of charitable medical aid runs counter to the modern idea of public health as one of the prime functions of the state.

We have seen in our earlier discussion how the Western missionary presence in China did not substantially change Chinese orientation towards the concept of public health. Indeed, the first appeals for China's adoption of Western-style sanitation and public health works came from political reformers rather than from doctors, echoing the role of utilitarianism in the birth of the sanitary movement in Britain. However, the Chinese drive for greater attention to matters of health, hygiene, and sanitation (the various translations of the Sino-Japanese term *weisheng* 衛生) was not inspired by a concern to increase industrial labour efficiency. For the Chinese, the most compelling argument came from studying the works of Charles Darwin, T.H. Huxley, and Herbert Spencer in translation. As Frank Dikötter notes, in China, evolution and natural selection were interpreted as operating on racial groups rather than on individuals. Dikötter identifies the period from around 1903 until 1915 as the time when Chinese identified 'racial evolution' in terms of a struggle for survival among nations.[12]

Beginning around 1908, contributors to the medical periodical press frequently couched their appeals for the promotion of medical studies and the introduction of sanitary measures and legislation in terms of promoting national and racial survival in the face of Western imperialist expansion. Here is an example, closely patterned on the opening passage of the canonical Confucian text *The Great Learning* (*Daxue* 大學):

> Alas! The China of today is a sick nation weakened by injury and oppressed by noxious influences. How can we find someone to treat the nation, to eradicate the roots of the ailment and turn weakness into strength? Although we may wish to strengthen the nation, it is first necessary to strengthen the race. To strengthen the race it is first necessary to pay attention to hygiene/*weisheng*. To do this, we must first understand physiology, and if we wish to understand physiology, we must first promote medicine.[13]

As Ruth Rogaski shows, the Chinese term *weisheng* was originally used to indicate a wide range of private, culturally sanctioned activities intended to 'guard or protect life,' such as modifying the diet according to age, life stage, and state of health, or practising calisthenic exercises or breath training. Because of the increasing popularity of scientific and medical translations of Japanese works in the early twentieth century, the meaning of the word *weisheng* came increasingly to stand for activities associated with the state management of the health of public spaces and citizens' bodies: meanings rendered in English on a spectrum from 'hygiene' to 'sanitation' to 'public health.'[14] Similar arguments urging the government to assume responsibility for these functions are found throughout the Republican period, both in Chinese-medical and Western-medical journals. In 1916, the *Shaoxing Journal of Medicine and Pharmacy*, run by practitioners of Chinese medicine who advocated its reform along scientific lines, reported on the importance of a recent international sanitary conference by linking the health of individuals, the health of the nation, and the struggle for existence:

> A person's spirit/mind (*jingshen* 精神) lives in the body. The 'original *qi*' (*yuanqi* 原氣) of a nation exists in the bodies of its people. There is a saying in Western philosophy: 'A healthy mind lives in a healthy body.' If we extrapolate from this, then 'a healthy nation resides in a healthy population.' The protection of health is the role of hygiene/public health (*weisheng*). Now, in the world of living things, the struggle for existence does not abate for an instant.[15]

The author of an article titled 'Medical War' claimed that the First World War was an example of what occurred when nations followed T.H. Huxley's slogan 'survival of the fittest.'[16] A proponent of greater state support for Western medicine argued that China should follow the example of the United States and Europe and invest in public health and preventive medicine because the protection of the health of the people was the secret behind the strength of Western nations.[17]

These are just a few of the ways in which notions of social evolutionism (or social Darwinism) were interpreted in racial and nationalist terms, framing the 'struggle for existence' for China. Advocates of greater state involvement in public health activities frequently referred to China as 'the sick old man of Asia' – a term originally coined to indicate the political and economic bankruptcy of the last years of the Qing dynasty – and argued that China was perceived in this way because so many of its people were unhealthy. To be sure, this notion of dangerous degeneracy was not a purely Chinese phenomenon. The powerful concepts of progress and evolution were matched by an equally powerful debate about the extent and causes of degeneracy in European and American society.[18] To many Chinese commentators, however, the only way to improve the evolutionary 'fitness' of the Chinese nation/race was to improve the health and physical fitness of its people. This was the thinking that led to the construction of large drill yards in educational establishments all over China and the imposition of the compulsory exercise drills that have persisted in schools in China to this day. Those attending lectures at the *Tongji* Medical School of modern medicine in Shanghai in 1911 heard the case in unequivocal terms:

> The twentieth century is the autumn of the competition for existence among races. It is also the extreme of the violent war between man and microbes. If man is victorious in war then his race is strong and the nation is prosperous. If man is defeated in war then his race is weak and the nation is wiped out. The vastness of China's territory is more than twice that of other strong nations; the population is the largest in the world. But the political administration becomes more corrupt, and national power and influence are reduced by the day. Although the reasons for this are very complex, the principal cause is inattention to public health. If one were to examine the rural population, the numbers of aged, handicapped and sick would amount to 30 or 40 percent, and the numbers of weak constitutions and consumptives would be 60 or 70 percent. With such a sick nation compared with the strong tiger-like, wolf-like enemies at our borders, how can we avoid being crushed like dead leaves? Alas! The main cause of China's poverty and weakness is inattention to public health.[19]

Preventing Plague and Containing Imperialism: Manchuria in 1910

Of course, it is one thing to talk about building a strong nation through public health and another thing to implement the measures necessary. Plague germs, the threat of foreign aggression, and imperialist nations' concerns about diluting their access to Chinese wealth gave the Chinese government its chance. China learned both the necessity and the advantages of using public health as a tool of government when a virulent epidemic of pneumonic plague broke out in Manchuria in 1910.[20] Back in 1905, at the end of the Russo-Japanese War (fought in Manchuria over control of the Liaodong Peninsula), the victorious Japanese had taken control of both the Russian trade concessions in Manchuria and the

South Manchurian Railway as far north as Changchun. The Russians retained control of the Chinese Eastern Railway, which forms a loop with the Trans-Siberian Railway, passing through Harbin on its way east to Vladivostok. Both the Russians and the Japanese stationed troops along their railways as these were vital logistical and trade arteries. In addition, the Japanese South Manchuria Railway Company managed large swathes of land bordering the railway, including settlements of varying sizes.[21] Construction on these railways had started in the second half of the 1890s, so rapid access to this vast area, rich in mineral resources, was still relatively new (Figure 9).

In 1910, approximately 100,000 labourers migrated into Manchuria to take advantage of the opportunities the new railways offered. Some ten thousand of these were amateur trappers, keen to obtain skins and furs for the European market, including the fur of the tarabagan (a large marmot), which – as it turned out – harboured plague. Pneumonic plague first appeared in Manchouli, a remote northern settlement near the borders of Mongolia, Russia, and Manchuria, in October of 1910. From there it spread along the railway to the Chinese settlement then known as Fuchiatien (Fujiadian 傅家甸), geographically adjacent to the Russian-administered city of Harbin but under purely Chinese control. The settlement of Fuchiatien had grown up since the Boxer Rebellion of 1900 as a result of the large Russian subsidies that flowed into Harbin. As such, it was something of a shantytown, lacking even such basic facilities as hard roads. Harbin itself had a population of about sixty-five thousand, including fifteen thousand Chinese, most of the rest being Russian.

At this time, the United States was pursuing its 'Open Door' policy with regard to the annexation of territory in China. It argued that any further annexation of Chinese territory beyond the 'spheres of influence' already established by the turn of the century would be to the disadvantage of all the imperial powers since the potentially lucrative Chinese market would be fragmented. Germany and Britain agreed with the American position. Thus several powers were apprehensive that the outbreak of plague would give Russia or Japan a pretext to expand their territorial control in Manchuria. The United States minister to China, W.J. Calhoun, approached the Chinese official responsible for

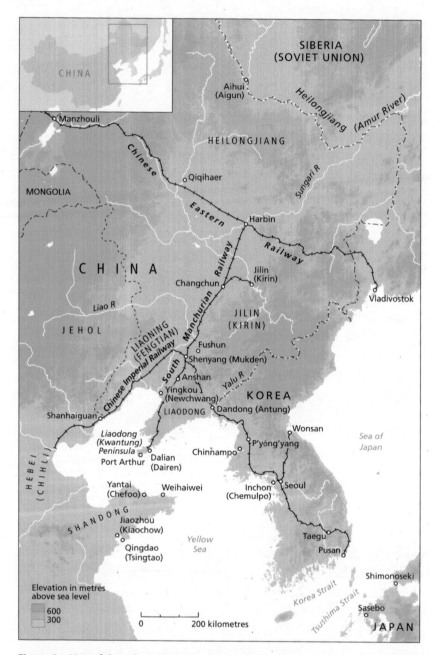

Figure 9   Map of the railway system in China in 1910. *Source:* Map by Eric Leinberger. Based on the map "Railway building, late Ch'ing," from *The Cambridge History of China: Volume 11: Late Ch'ing, 1800-1911,* Part 2. New York: Cambridge University Press, 1980.

managing the outbreak, a Cornell graduate and second vice-president of the Board of Foreign Affairs, Sao-ke Alfred Sze (Shi Zhaoji 施肇基), urging,

> ... the necessity for active and effective work upon the part of the Chinese, in order to prevent any excuse for interference by either Russia or Japan, or both, under plea of necessity for the protection of their respective local interests, or for the prevention of the spread of the plague to Korea or Siberia. He [Sze] promised that neither money nor effort would be spared.[22]

In fact, the Russian administrators of the Chinese Eastern Railway had already instigated quarantine regulations that prevented any Chinese from boarding the train at Manchouli unless they had first spent five days in supervised quarantine. Other nationals were not subjected to this control. When it was seen that this measure and the closure of all infected houses were still insufficient to halt the spread of the plague, the Russian railway authorities imported special railway cars and forced the entire Chinese population of Manchouli to live in them in quarantine for five days. In the meantime, Russian troops disinfected the Chinese residential areas and burned any property where there had been known cases of plague. These steps brought 'indignant protests' from the Chinese, but 'owing to the easy methods of the Russian police in enforcing their orders,' there was little active opposition to them.[23] They were also effective, and Manchouli was declared free of plague within a few days of these draconian measures. However, the epidemic continued to spread in Harbin. Although the Russian authorities established an isolation hospital to hold up to two thousand 'suspects' (invariably lower-class Chinese) and instituted checkpoints on the roads in order to stop the free movement of Chinese between Fuchiatien and Harbin, the daily death toll reached over a hundred by the end of the year. At about this time, the Russians started to complain of Chinese lack of cooperation, while Chinese expressed their resentment at what they saw as Russian interference. The Chinese authorities in Fuchiatien also declined medical assistance from the Russians, thus fuelling Russian fears.[24]

Sze's response to these twin threats of a widespread outbreak of plague and increased imperialist activity was to second the vice-director of the Imperial Army Medical College in Tianjin, Dr. Wu Lien-teh (Wu Liande) to 'plague prevention' (in fact, containment) duties in Harbin and Fuchiatien. Wu was a Malay Chinese with British nationality who had obtained his medical degree from Emmanuel College, Cambridge. He had been instructed in the latest bacteriological techniques at both the Pasteur Institute in Paris (then headed by Roux and Metchnikoff) and Robert Koch's Institute of Infectious Diseases in Berlin. He knew Vice-President Sze personally.

Wu applied for, and was granted, the emperor's permission to carry out two culturally repugnant measures deemed necessary to bring the plague under control: conducting autopsies on unclaimed plague corpses and cremating plague victims' bodies in order to prevent re-infection (Figure 10). (Hundreds of corpses had simply been abandoned on the frozen ground outside Harbin.) Both of these actions would violate the Confucian values of non-mutilation of the body, alive or dead, and prevent families from affording their relatives a respectful burial and assuring themselves of good fortune through showing piety towards their ancestors. Over five hundred labourers, who had mostly been rendered unemployed as a result of the Russian authorities in Harbin's expulsion of poorer Chinese residents,[25] were put to work digging the necessary pits and cremating corpses. Wu was also empowered to commandeer the services of over seven hundred local policemen for sanitary policing and to recruit and train two hundred for more specialized duties. Over a thousand soldiers were employed in house-to-house searches, disinfecting dwellings, isolating the sick in hospitals and their contacts in camps, establishing military cordons along the transport routes, and closing schools and theatres. The anti-plague effort was directed by a medical team of twenty doctors of Western medicine and twenty-nine senior medical students who had volunteered their services from medical schools all over China. The effort cost the imperial government 150,000 taels.[26]

Despite their considerable public relations work, the members of Wu's team met noticeable resistance. A French Catholic priest, having

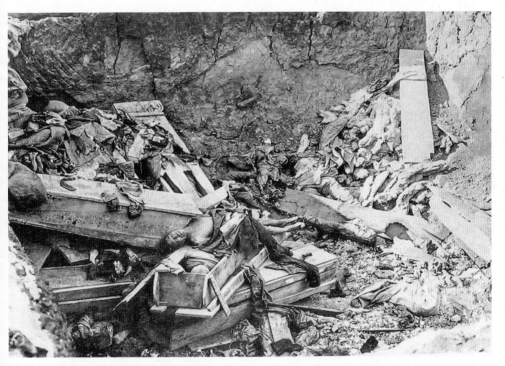

Figure 10   Photograph of corpses awaiting cremation during the outbreak of pneumonic plague, Mukden/Fengtian, early 1911. *Source:* North Manchurian Plague Prevention Service Reports, 1911-13. Courtesy of Countway Library of Harvard University.

allowed three hundred people to stay in his church compound, claimed the right to extraterritoriality and had the bodies of dead refugees secretly removed at night. Any businesses that had contact with a plague patient or someone suspected of having the plague were instantly closed down, so it is no surprise that the local population resented the authoritarian management of the epidemic. The Commercial Guild of Mukden (Fengtian in Chinese, the modern city of Shenyang) on the South Manchurian Railway route accused the sanitation department of incompetence, obstructed its house-to-house searches, and set up its own plague control measures. These included employing five hundred sanitary police and two traditional doctors as well as opening their own plague hospital.[27] The guild's doctors and most of their patients died of plague; then again, the plague hospitals run by Wu also had a mortality rate of very nearly 100 percent. The popular perception that no one suspected of having the plague ever escaped from the sanitary police alive was, therefore, close to the truth.

The Mongolian viceroy of Manchuria, Xiliang (Hsi-liang 錫良), in the preface to his report to the emperor on the plague outbreak, acknowledged the necessity of the strict policing measures employed by Wu Lien-teh in the name of Western medicine, but he complained of the prohibitions on public prayer and sacrifices and the censure that newspapers and disapproving officials directed at him personally:

> The new plague prevention regulations have the definite advantage of isolating relatives. Fearing calamity, [the sanitary police] carry infected persons to a hospital and isolate the remainder. The fate of life or death is decided between dawn and dusk. Blood relatives are not permitted to see [each other]; a gesture, a backward glance, they swallow their words and are separated for ever ...
>
> The new plague prevention regulations have a further advantage in their severing of communications, checking the stampede at once. Traders do not travel, but are restrained, complaining, in their lodgings. The depth of their resentment is indescribable ...
>
> The new plague prevention regulations have a further advantage in carrying out disinfection, thereby cutting off the remaining evil. Where death has already occurred, should [the family] want a burial, the ground is frozen solid and soldiers are unable to break it. Should they want to place it in a temporary site [i.e., above ground, awaiting burial], the pestilential *qi* will move freely and new outbreaks will continue to multiply. Inevitably everything is seized: their clothing and bedding, inner and outer coffins, and committed to the flames. Alas! What crime have our people committed that having already died of plague, they suffer such redoubled oppression?[28]

Viceroy Xiliang clearly did not enjoy acting as the cultural broker for this first Chinese experiment in modern sanitary disease control. The measures had not been intended for his or his subjects' approval: they were carried out for reasons of international politics. This became even more apparent when the plague mortality figures began to drop, the last death in Harbin occurring on 1 March 1911. The Chinese government, quick to capitalize on its perceived success, called the first international scientific conference to be held in China: the International Plague Conference. This took place in April 1911, with delegates from eleven nations, including the United States, Britain, Russia, and Japan (with the famous bacteriologist Kitasato heading the delegation). Here, too, the Chinese were anxious not to allow either the Russians or the Japanese to dominate the proceedings; therefore, they invited the scientific delegation from the United States to arrive two months early and provided its members with experimental material in the form of corpses for autopsy, live tarbagans, and even plague patients with whom to try out intravenous injections (of vaccine, presumably). This facilitated substantial scientific contributions from the United States, which was seen as a non-predatory power, thereby depriving the other nations of any opportunity to dominate.[29]

In his opening address to the conference, Wu Lien-teh sketched the policies that China had implemented for dealing with the plague, including the autopsies and the incineration of plague corpses, measures that 'still conjure up in the native mind all that is repulsive and contrary to natural feelings.' These actions on the part of the Chinese government, he said, 'must prove to you that the Government is moved by the highest motives of humanity and is ready to lay aside age-long prejudices, to spend money unsparingly, and to possess itself of all that science can impart for the saving of life and the elimination of national perils.' In conclusion, he reminded the delegates that this was the first international medical conference ever held in China, and he looked forward to the 'beneficial results' their presence would have on 'the future progress of medical science in China.' The conference, he declared, neatly summing up the Chinese motivation for staging it, 'gives China a strong position among nations seeking the welfare of their people.'[30] As Mark Gamsa has argued, the entire containment effort in Harbin was an exercise in colonial control by both the Chinese and the Russian authorities, both of whose medical leaders had spent time at the Institut Pasteur in Paris. Andrew Cunningham's analysis reminds us that the Chinese internal colonialism depended on the authority of the laboratory as the defining justification for public health interventions.[31]

One outcome of the conference was a proposal to establish a plague prevention service for Manchuria, to be funded by Customs Service revenue from the Harbin customs circuit. Haines Wilson, a Briton who served as the Harbin circuit commissioner, and Wu Lien-teh compiled an application to the customs service (then run by another Briton) in May 1911 for Mexican $90,000 (sixty thousand 'customs taels': Mexican silver dollars were widely used as standard currency in the absence of a national mint). After being reviewed by the Ministry of Foreign Affairs and the diplomatic bodies of the Western powers in Beijing, the appropriation was approved.[32] The need for the support of foreign interests in China is clear from Wu's own account:

> The building of hospitals at Harbin, Manchouli, and Lahasusu was begun, for which various sums had already been voted. In October [1911] the revolution broke out, and the Manchurian Customs were hypothecated to the payment of the Loans and Boxer Indemnity. The Manchurian Customs Revenue thus passed into the control of the representatives of the [foreign] Powers in Peking who at first refused to continue this Service. Six months then passed, and now, as a result of representations from the Wai Chiao Pu [*Waijiao Bu* 外交部, Ministry of Foreign Affairs], a dispatch, dated September 19th, 1912, has been received from the Diplomatic Body, saying that the sum asked for, namely, Roubles 78,000, has been sanctioned, and work could commence at once.[33]

This new organization, the North Manchurian Plague Prevention Service, was China's first attempt at a public health service. As Carl Nathan observes: 'When epidemics swept Manchuria, Plague Prevention Service hospitals attended exclusively to infectious disease control. In the lulls between epidemics, however, the hospitals were thrown open as a free, general medical service for North Manchuria, representing the service's major extra-epidemic activity.'[34]

There is no doubt that Wu was hoping to expand the activities of the Plague Prevention Service into a public health service for the whole of China, preferably under his own leadership:

One of the most important objects of the Service is to utilise every means at its disposal with a view to giving an efficient training in preventive medicine to medical men who will, in future, carry their acquired knowledge to other portions of the country. This, in itself, is a cause worthy of energetic support, seeing that such work has been commenced in China only under the auspices of the North Manchurian Plague Prevention Service ... It is to be hoped that not only will the encouraging progress thus made in preventive medicine in China be allowed to continue, but that an impetus will be given to extend our sphere of activity.[35]

The Plague Prevention Service produced its own vaccines and sera for plague, cholera, rabies, typhoid, and scarlet fever, and it undertook epidemiological and bacteriological research on epidemic diseases in general. The reputation of the new and aspiringly modern Chinese state, as well as the interests of both the Chinese government and of Wu Lien-teh and the emerging profession of foreign-trained medical staff under his command, were well served by the recognition of their efforts at international medical and sanitary conferences and the publication of their research results in foreign journals.[36] For Wu Lien-teh, trained in the foremost medical research establishments of Europe and possessing an anglophile and anglophone background, these were genuine attempts to introduce Western medicine, along with Western concepts of public health and sanitation, in order to assist the development of China. For the Chinese government, however, support for Wu's public health activities and scientific legitimation for the Chinese public health effort were parts of an ongoing struggle to achieve credibility in the modern world order.

The Central Epidemic Prevention Bureau

When pneumonic plague broke out for the second time in China, this time in Shanxi Province in 1917, the Chinese government obtained a loan from foreign banks of US$1 million with which to combat it. The mortality in this outbreak was much lower than it was in the 1910 outbreak, totalling around sixteen thousand over seven months. The Chinese government decided to use the unused portion of the loan to establish the Central Epidemic Prevention Bureau in Beijing in 1919. Like the North Manchurian Service, the work of the Epidemic Prevention Bureau was funded by the Chinese Customs Service, to the tune of US$110,000 a year.[37] Here, again, we see a public health initiative that was dependent on the approval and support of the foreign community in China since all appropriations made by the customs for use in China needed the support of the diplomatic community.

This new public health initiative, modelled on Wu Lien-teh's service, came under heavy censure from some members of the medical profession in China. In particular, in 1924 the editor of the *Republican Medical Journal*, Hou Yuwen 侯毓汶, objected to the activities of the Central Epidemic Prevention Bureau on two grounds: first, that, in the wake of extensive flooding after heavy rains in the summer of 1924, members of the bureau staff had done nothing to prevent the inevitable epidemics in the area; rather, they had made only two visits to the area and produced one report. What use was this to the peasants?[38] Second, the bureau was in fact carrying out one of the activities that properly belonged under the remit of the hygiene department (*weisheng si* 衛生司), a division of the Ministry of Internal Affairs (*neiwu bu* 內務部), in the very unstable central government of the period. The bureau's actual activities were not in plague prevention but in infectious disease research. According to Hou, in order to avoid the expensive waste of scarce financial resources, the bureau should take over the laboratory research functions of the government hygiene department and, accordingly, should be renamed the Institute of Infectious Diseases (*chuanranbing yanjiusuo* 傳染病研究所).[39]

Hou Yuwen had been trained in Western medicine in Japan and was something of an evangelist for a national organization of public health on the grounds that 'a nation without a health administration cannot be said to have a complete political [system]; a nation without sanitary laws cannot be said to have a complete legal [system].'[40] In the same editorial he recommended the establishment of a tiered system of national health care provision in China, with health stations of decreasing size and complexity at national, provincial, county, and village levels. This would enable China to be independent in sanitary matters, an independence Hou thought was more important to the Chinese state than judicial independence. (By judicial independence, Hou was referring to the movement in China for the abolition of extraterritorial rights for foreigners and the return of judicial control of the treaty ports and leased areas to China.) Hou's tiered system, which he proposed in 1924 to extend basic health service into the rural villages, antedates the League of Nations proposals for a similar system, first mooted in December 1929, and was also many decades ahead of the much-vaunted 'Barefoot Doctor Movement' of the Maoist Cultural Revolution.[41] Hou drew his inspiration from the Japanese medical system that had been applied to the Japanese colony of Taiwan since 1895 and that, in turn, was based on a German model. This Japanese influence on Chinese primary health care reform has usually been overlooked.[42] Hou was also the president of the Chinese Republican Medical and Pharmaceutical Association, formed under his leadership in 1915, which was the preferred association of those doctors who had received their Western medical training in Japan. As such it was a rival of the National Medical Association, also founded in 1915 (on the initiative of Wu Lien-teh), which catered mainly to doctors who had trained in the West or in Western-run medical schools in China.

In spite of these criticisms, the Central Epidemic Prevention Bureau, with its staff of only 'six experts and 45 assistants, all technical members having received special training in America, Europe or Japan,'[43] was able to identify infectious diseases and provide vaccines, sera, and antitoxins for sale to local administrations in the event of disease epidemics. When, in 1927, Chiang Kai-shek's Northern Expedition succeeded in bringing a significant number of the provincial warlords under central government control, the bureau was transferred to the new national capital in Nanjing, where it continued its activities until the Japanese invasion in 1937.

To sum up the Chinese government's attempts at public health work in China on the eve of the Nanjing Decade, it is convenient here to cite propaganda from the Nanjing administration, produced in 1937:

> Public health machinery was practically non-existent prior to the establishment of the National Government at Nanking [Nanjing] in

1928. There was a nominal sanitary bureau under the Ministry of Interior of the defunct Peking Government. Earlier attempts to initiate this phase of health work were made by the North Manchurian Plague Prevention Bureau in Harbin, the National Epidemic Prevention Bureau in Peiping [Beijing], the municipal health departments in Canton and Shanghai, and the health demonstration station in Peiping. Owing to the limitation of health personnel and financial resources, the facilities provided by these health machineries proved to be inadequate in meeting the growing demand of the country, although they were quite efficient in tackling the problems within their circumscribed areas.[44]

Although this assessment was written with the deliberate intent of providing a favourable comparison with the new government's activities since 1928, its conclusion regarding the limited impact of these services is certainly accurate. What it fails to mention is that a major motivation for even these few limited services was to represent the emerging modern Chinese state as assuming the public health responsibilities that the international community expected of it – even if all this meant in practice was that there were a few shiny new laboratories for foreign delegations to visit. It was in China's interest to make an effort to meet these expectations because the machinery of trade and communication – and therefore government revenue – was in the control of these foreign powers. This machinery included railways, telegraphs, major international trading ports, and control of the Chinese Customs Service. Because of these connections, the first few steps towards public health provision were inseparable from Chinese efforts to regain national sovereignty.

The Secondary Importance of Rural Health

If public health initiatives in Republican China were primarily undertaken in order to gain credibility among the international community, it should follow that the provision of public health facilities in remote rural areas would not be a high priority in Chinese government circles. And this is indeed what the evidence suggests. This is not to say that there were no attempts to promote public health in rural areas, but all such attempts were still very much in the initial stages by the time of the Japanese invasion of 1937 and the subsequent retreat of the government to Chongqing.[45]

From the date of the First National Health Conference in April 1934, the Chinese government was starting to turn its attention towards rural health provision. The head of the administrative department of the government (*xingzhengyuan* 行政院), Wang Jingwei 汪精衛 (1883-1944), apologized in his address to the conference for the previous lack of government support for the establishment of Western medicine in China. He put the extension of modern health care into rural areas on the top of his list of priorities for the development of medicine in China. (His other priority was the 'scientification' of Chinese medicine, to be undertaken only by persons qualified in Western medicine.)[46] The same year, the Chinese Medical Association's Council on Public Health carried out a survey on modern rural public health practice. It found seventeen rural public health centres: Tangshan (which was government-funded), two that were funded by local administrations, nine that were funded jointly by local administrations and other agencies (such as missionary medical schools), and five that were wholly privately funded or entirely maintained by mission funds.[47]

Several more rural health centres were founded in the last years of the Nanjing regime, some funded by the Rockfeller Foundation's China Program for the promotion of rural reconstruction. By 1936 there were 181 *xian* health centres – that is, small establishments for Western medicine that typically had thirty to forty beds, the services of up to three physicians with varying standards of medical education, and a few nurses and midwives. Although they were small in relation to their county-wide catchment areas, it is clear that substantial rural public health investments had taken place since the 1934 survey.[48] Additionally, several Chinese cities, starting with the foreign-run treaty ports, had established their own public health administrations, and most of these were in Chinese hands by the 1930s.[49] Although closer examination of these initiatives is beyond the scope of this book, we may note that the extension of medical facilities into rural areas, where it did occur, was often primarily an exercise in state penetration and that it involved general medical activities rather than those restricted to public health. This was the case, for instance, when the Nationalist government regained control of former Communist territory in Jiangxi Province in 1934. It set up new 'rural welfare centres,' designed to match or improve on the basic health and welfare facilities that the evacuated Communists had provided. By January 1936, ten such centres were up and running. However, they were estimated to reach a maximum of only 400,000 people; in order to reach the rest of even this one province's population, an additional 292 centres would have been necessary.[50]

Additional evidence of the state's involvement in local health matters comes from the way these local centres were staffed. Since rural doctors were often imposed on a given rural district from outside, and since they relied on support from the Ministry of Health and the National Public Health Administration (which, in turn, received funds and advice from the League of Nations Health Organization), and on their foreign funding agencies, their relationships with local administrations were problematic. At the fourth general conference of the China Medical Association in Shanghai in 1937, Dr. Liu Ruiheng 劉瑞恆 (Harry Liu, or Dr. J. Heng Liu in English, 1890-1961), who by this time was director of the National Health Administration, appealed to missionary doctors in rural areas 'not to be discouraged by local situations in matters of co-operation in public health work but rather *to keep in close touch with the National Public Health Administration* as to what to do and how to do it.'[51] This comment shows how the Nationalist government deployed foreign missionary doctors to extend the level of state penetration in public health matters further into the rural areas than the native Chinese medical elite were prepared to go. In return for bringing 'state' medicine to remote areas, the government promised to give them direct support, if necessary over the heads of local government officials.

The change from a form of 'liturgical governance' to a politically self-serving adaptation of 'survival of the fittest' was nearly complete. Government public health activities in late Qing and early Republican China had the primary aim of meeting international expectations of the activities of a modern nation-state. The main difference between the Chinese government's concept of public health and the West's was that, in Republican China, public health activities were, first and foremost, *tools* of government. Towards the end of the Nanjing Decade, as the Nationalist government consolidated its rule, medical writings increasingly referred to public health and rural health care provision in terms of government *responsibility*. Large-scale public health works were also beginning to appear affordable. The concept of public health in China would change again over the next two decades, and this is discussed in Chapter 7, when we look at the rise of new institutions.

For now, the stage is set. Western missionaries increased Chinese exposure to different medical practices and concepts, allowing China the opportunity to reflect on its indigenous medicine. Japan provided China with an example of an Asian nation able to garner admiration beyond its region, with methods and practices that advocates of both traditional and Western medicine found useful. A plague outbreak and political pressure provided China with the chance to show that it could build a healthy nation fit for survival.

None of these elements forced China to modernize its medicine. None determined whether Western medicine would dominate indigenous practices. None defined the shape of a distinct Chinese medicine. Rather, these factors formed a substrate that joined with individual and institutional aims in an interplay that we now recognize as 'modern.' We now turn our attention to examples of those individual and institutional drives by examining the lives of five individuals who were active during this period, the rise of new medicine-related institutions, and changes in medical theories and practices.

Medical Lives

6

> On the opening day ... a dozen or so of the very poorest of the people made their appearance in the waiting-room ... they were desperately poor, and they had no money with which to pay the native doctors' fees or buy the medicines they might prescribe ... They would all of them preferred [sic] not to have come here to consult this foreigner, but they were afflicted with diseases that their own physicians could not cure.
>
> – J. MACGOWAN, *HOW ENGLAND SAVED CHINA*

Western medicine had only limited credibility with Chinese during the nineteenth century. The first Chinese to learn any Western medicine were the 'native assistants' employed by the early medical missionaries, starting in 1836 when Peter Parker took on his first assistant.[1] Without accredited status of any sort, after leaving the missionaries' employment, the best that former assistants could do was to set themselves up in the unregulated market as medical entrepreneurs by combining techniques they had learned from the missionaries with traditional medicine. In recognition of this problem, a Dr. Myers, working in Formosa in 1888, managed to have three of his native pupils certified as competent by a specially convened examining board in Hong Kong. However, even with their diplomas they 'could not obtain suitable posts in China and settled in the Straits Settlements.'[2]

The situation was not much better for the early graduates of the Viceroy's Hospital Medical School in Tianjin. Established at the end of 1881, with Dr. John Kenneth MacKenzie, originally of the London Missionary Society, responsible for most of the teaching, it was completely funded by Viceroy Li Hongzhang 李鴻章 (1823-1901), who was perhaps the greatest enthusiast of Western science and technology in the late Qing government. Although the first graduates were awarded high (fifth and sixth) rank in the Chinese civil service, attempts to employ these home-grown Western doctors in the Chinese armed services met with problems of drug supply, greater cost, and prejudice against Western medicine from their commanding officers. Patients of traditional practitioners paid for their own drugs and the doctor was paid only seven taels (*liang*, silver dollars) a month. In the 1880s, Western practitioners still had to dispense their own drugs and therefore cost the armed services the much greater sum of thirty taels a month.[3]

In their 1911 *Diseases of China*, Jeffreys and Maxwell describe the opportunities for Western physicians in China at that time:

> For the conscientious private practitioner, native practice is not yet available as a life work. It is the missionary physician, the port health officer, the customs surgeon, who are in 'native practice' or in a position to study the conditions thereof; men whose support is not dependent on native fees. The trained native assistant with his certificate of proficiency, and even the Chinese student with his degree taken in Europe or America, is hardly yet able to make a living in practice.[4]

Most of the viable career opportunities for Western-trained physicians before the establishment of the Republic of China in 1912 were in the gift of Westerners. Those ports with health officers were the foreign treaty ports, where the surgeons of the Imperial Maritime Customs Service, although nominally employed by the Chinese, were hired and fired by the inspector-general of customs, who was also a Westerner.[5]

In summary, at the end of the nineteenth century, a few Chinese were able to enter the Western medical profession through studying abroad or at one of the small Western-run medical schools in China. The first president of the Republic of China, Sun Yat-sen, exemplifies this kind of student. He was a member of the first class to graduate from the Hong Kong Medical School in 1892, having been taught by Dr. (later Sir) James Cantlie, and Dr. (later Sir) Patrick Manson. However, this profession was firmly in Western hands and inextricably linked with Christian missionary work. Even the professional organization of Western doctors in China was called the China Medical Missionary Association.

Just as these unpromising beginnings nonetheless developed into movements for modernization on a national level, as seen in Chapters 4 and 5, the international power relations that influenced the Chinese government to implement modern public health initiatives also influenced the actions of individual Chinese. The Qing government's decision to abolish the traditional civil service examinations in 1905, and to award civil service rank to graduates of recognized modern schools and foreign and Chinese universities, provided a further incentive for the study of Western medicine to scholars who might otherwise have continued with a classical education.

Qiu Jin

Today Qiu Jin 秋瑾 (1875-1907) is celebrated in China as a martyr to the cause of the 1911 Revolution and as an early champion of women's rights. At a time when respectable Chinese women were expected to confine themselves to the home, Qiu divorced her husband and left China to study in Japan. On her return to China, she earned her living as a teacher and journalist. She also became a leader within the network of secret organizations working for the overthrow of the Qing dynasty and was jointly responsible for planning the ultimately unsuccessful armed uprising that led to her execution in July 1907.

When Qiu Jin left China and her husband and children in 1904, she enrolled at Shimoda Utako's Girls' Practical School in Tokyo to study teaching and technology and was particularly interested in nursing as a profession.[6] However, her main interests lay in revolutionary activity and the position of women in society. She joined Sun Yat-sen's Revolutionary Alliance (*tongmeng hui* 同盟會), worked with a women's association in Japan that was active in the support of Japan's Red Cross Society, and co-founded the *Vernacular Journal* (*Baihua bao* 白話報), which openly advocated the overthrow of the Qing imperial house.[7]

On her return to Shanghai in 1906 she founded and wrote for the *Chinese Women's Journal* (*Zhongguo nübao* 中國女報); continued her anti-Qing activities; taught Japanese, physiology, and hygiene in a local girls' school; and translated Japanese texts on nursing.[8] One of these translations, *A Course in Nursing* (*Kanhuxue jiaocheng* 看護學教程), was serialized in the *Chinese Women's Journal*. In this, Qiu advocated female employment in the nursing profession on both nationalistic and economic grounds. At the time, nursing as an occupation for women was new and unusual. Moreover, it was not the kind of activity that any respectable family would want for its daughters. The idea of women as active workers outside the family home was still shocking.[9] Yet, as Mary Rankin shows, elite attitudes towards education for girls had already begun to change, especially in Qiu Jin's native region, the lower Yangzi valley area.[10] Several Chinese novelists had satirized the treatment of women in their own society, the most famous of these being Li Ruzhen in his popular novel *Flowers in the Mirror* (*Jinghua yuan* 鏡花緣), first published in 1827.[11] The famous leaders of the 1898 Reform Movement, Kang Youwei 康有為 (1858-1927) and Liang Qichao 梁啟超 (1873-1929), had called for women to be freed from their confinement and allowed to be economically active. They expressed social Darwinist concerns that the economic waste represented by keeping women at home, and the effect this was having on the health of China's children, was making China unfit for the international struggle for survival.[12] Qiu Jin's strategy for achieving change was different. She emphasized how traditional 'womanly' qualities made women uniquely qualified for the few work opportunities available at the time, including Western-style nursing.

In her introduction to *A Course in Nursing*, Qiu Jin's argument for nursing as a profession for women relies on the strong links between nursing and philanthropic work in the West and the acknowledged value of women nurses in wartime:

> Restrained by social custom, it is common to regard nursing as a 'base occupation' – this is a very grave error ... Since [nurses] are able to protect the tranquillity of society in peacetime and add to the nation's advantage in wartime, it would be no exaggeration to call [nursing] a profession of advantage to the nation and convenience to the people. How can this be a 'base occupation'?[13]

The main part of Qiu Jin's short text describes some of the skills expected of nurses and shows the extent of the influence of Western medical practice at this time. About half of the discussion on skills concerns making beds and the domestic care of the sick room, while the rest describes matters like the proper arrangement of the patient's environment, feeding regimens, and how to take temperatures.[14] Thus, although the occupation of nursing was to include a fair proportion of low-status chores, the fact that it was to be undertaken in a professional working environment would dignify even those menial tasks that women of Qiu's social status would not normally undertake. When we recall that most girls and women from comfortable families in China would have had their feet bound from about the age of eight, the change in attitude is striking.

As if this were not revolutionary enough, the text of the *Course in Nursing* introduced concepts that were very much at variance with traditional Chinese views of the workings of the body. For instance, in the section on temperature-taking, Qiu Jin's translation states: 'The vital functions of humans and many other kinds of animals are always due to the body's inner warmth; this is called body heat.'[15] To most Chinese, however, vital functions were possible because of the presence of *qi*, something akin to vital essence: 'warmth' or 'heat' can hardly have been very convincing alternatives.

In the section on 'patients' diets' (*bingren zhi yinshi* 病人之飲食), Qiu translates several Western dietary ideas without explanation or comment. For instance, she praises cow's milk as a good source of many dietary requirements but suggests that, since it will turn sour on keeping, nurses should first boil it and then add a little bicarbonate of soda. Although she adds the English words 'bicarbonate of soda' after the unfamiliar and imported chemical neologism *chongtansuan caoda* 重炭酸曹達, fresh cow's milk was unavailable in most, if not all, Chinese cities at this time. Even powdered milk from Europe – which was sold in China from the early twentieth century and advertised as a cure-all tonic, much as ginseng is advertised in the West today – was still a rarity in Qiu Jin's time.[16]

Similarly, in her discussion of water for drinking purposes she recommends giving patients cold water and iced water to drink – something that is anathema to most Chinese, who consider cold drinks as damaging to the digestion. Again, Qiu translates without comment. The section on the importance of open windows for cleansing the air and preventing aerial poisons and bacteria from invading the body must also have confused many readers since it, too, contains almost no explanations. True, the word 'bacteria' is rendered three ways – in English, in its Japanese translation *(xijun)*, and phonetically (*ba-ke-te-lüe* 巴喀特略) – but there is no attempt to explain what bacteria are and why they might be damaging to the body.

It seems that promoting a thorough understanding of the principles of Western nursing was not sufficiently high on Qiu Jin's agenda for her to devote much effort to it. Rather, the issues at stake for Qiu and her fellow activists for women's rights and revolution were the salvation of the Chinese nation-state and, with it, the economic independence and social status of women: 'Alas! My sisters, in the whole world there is not a single person who is willing to accept the title "slave," why do you accept it calmly and not consider it a disgrace?'[17] Qiu issues this more militant, forceful call for women's economic independence in her article 'A Warning to My Sisters' (*Jinggao jiemeimen* 警告姊妹們), published in the first issue of the *Chinese Women's Journal*. Dropping the diplomatically persuasive style of the introduction to her *Course in Nursing,* she clearly intends to goad her women readers:

> Nowadays, girls' schools and women's occupations are springing up, but if we can study science and technology, become teachers and start up factories, why shouldn't we support ourselves? At least we would not be idle mouths, a burden on our menfolk. Firstly, this would help family businesses to prosper, and secondly, it would earn men's

respect. By clearing our names of uselessness, we would gain the joy of freedom.[18]

Qiu was not alone in her mission. Two years after her death the *Medical News*, which aimed to promote Western medical knowledge, was also keen to establish the respectability of nursing as a profession and expressed some embarrassment at China's backwardness in its training of nurses and midwives: 'Because there are not yet many schools for girls, it is difficult to recruit many literate female nursing students. In China, midwifery is regarded as a base occupation, so any prospective students are bound to be from the lower levels of society, and are even less likely to be literate.'[19]

This clearly shows a convergence of interest between promoters of Western-style medicine and promoters of women's emancipation. Nursing, along with Western medicine, was part of the modernization that reformers and revolutionaries alike were keen to espouse. The name coined for nurses reflects this desire to upgrade women's work: the original term for the word 'nurse' in Chinese, *kanhu shi* 看護士, means 'scholars (or soldiers) who watch and guard.'[20]

Nursing, then, while it may have trampled many Chinese ideas about the proper activities of respectable women, also offered the new generation a route to emancipation. In this, as in so many other fields, Chinese people were ready and able to adapt a Western import to their own interests and needs. If the short-cropped hair and unbound feet of Qiu Jin's generation of women workers were shocking to the establishment of their day, within a generation they were to become an everyday sight in urban China.

Chen Yuan

Chen Yuan 陳垣 (styled Yuanan 援庵, 1880-1971) was another active promoter of the overthrow of the Manchu Qing dynasty in the first decade of the twentieth century. In contrast to Qiu, however, Chen Yuan limited his battles to those fought with the pen. He eventually became the director of several Beijing universities, including Beijing Normal University. He is celebrated today on both sides of the Taiwan Strait mainly for his later career as a cultural historian who pioneered the writing of religious history in China; developed new methods for dating manuscripts, such as using patterns of name avoidances; and generally oriented modern Chinese historiography towards empirical questions.

Born in Xin'an County, Guangdong Province, in 1880, Chen originally aspired to be an imperial official and nearly made it. In 1897 he travelled to Beijing to sit for the triennial second degree examination (*xiangshi* 鄉試) but failed.[21] After a spell working as a schoolteacher, in 1904 he and a friend started a journal in Guangzhou, the openly anti-Qing *Affairs of the Age Pictorial* (*Shishi huabao* 時事畫報). For instance, after the execution of Qiu Jin and her cousin Xu Xilin in Zhejiang Province, he published an article castigating the government for persecuting the people and causing rebellion through its own incompetence.[22] In order to further agitate anti-Qing sentiment, Chen also selected and published passages from the official 'veritable records' (*zhengshi wenjian* 正式文件) of the dynasty that exhibited language or edicts that discriminated against, or were deprecating towards, Han Chinese. Even though their reproduction in print was clearly inflammatory, there was little the authorities could do because the documents were part of the dynasty's official record.[23]

Chen Yuan also helped write and distribute anti-American propaganda during the 1904-5 boycott of American goods in retaliation for US government action against Chinese emigration to the United States and for American discrimination against Chinese communities on American soil.[24] This patriotic sentiment also induced him to leave the South China Medical College (*Boji yixuetang* 博濟醫學堂), which the China Medical Missionary Society ran with substantial financial help from the Chinese community. Chen, along with several of his fellow students, was incensed by the attitude that American staff members displayed towards their Chinese colleagues. In 1908, several of the Chinese students left to found their own school of Western medicine, the Guanghua Medical College, taking the Chinese members of the teaching staff (six out of ten) with them. This brought teaching at the missionary college to a halt until 1909.[25] Chen completed the four-year, Cantonese-taught course at Guanghua in 1911 and stayed on at the college as a teacher. While there, he was also an active editor of the *Journal of Medicine and Hygiene* (*Yixue weisheng bao* 醫學衛生保),

which published ten issues between 1908 and 1909, and the *Guanghua Journal of Medicine and Hygiene* (*Guanghua yixue weisheng zazhi* 光華醫學衛生雜誌), which published at least eight issues with contributions from Chen Yuan between 1910 and 1913.[26]

Western medicine may seem an odd vehicle for the expression of revolutionary zeal such as Chen Yuan's. After all, the profession was firmly in the hands of foreign imperialists, except for the school Chen had himself helped to found. How then did Chen see medicine as contributing to his goal of regaining Chinese sovereignty from both the 'alien' Manchus and the foreign imperialists?

In his focus on medicine, Chen was following a logical line of thinking that was spurred by his desire to end extraterritoriality on Chinese soil. Recall that extraterritoriality meant that foreigners and their belongings were not subject to Chinese law and that any suspected foreign criminal could be tried only in a foreign court. These privileges even extended to Chinese converts to Roman Catholicism and to all Chinese residents within foreign-leased territories, such as the foreign settlements in Shanghai, Tianjin, and the other treaty ports. The clauses in the Treaty of Nanjing that established the precedent for foreign extraterritoriality in China had been inserted in order to protect foreign traders from having to pay Chinese taxes and also because foreign governments disapproved of the Chinese use of torture for extracting confessions from suspected criminals.

The essential first step towards persuading foreign powers to agree to the abolition of extraterritoriality was to enact a legal code that was in accordance with international law.[27] Chen Yuan saw that, if a Chinese legal code were to gain international approval, then it would need the services of doctors of (Western) forensic medicine in addition to lawyers trained in international law. The New Policies (*xinzheng*) reforms of 1901-11 failed to provide for this necessary expertise. Chen, who was already fiercely anti-Qing, was caustic in his condemnation of these efforts. In 1909, he published an article about reforms to the qualifications for coroners, showing the connection between forensics and international law. In the past, the legal examination of the bodies of victims of violence had been carried out by a local specialist called a *wuzuo* 仵作, which Lu and Needham render as 'ostensor' to indicate the lowly status of the occupation. The ostensor would examine the body at the request of the local magistrate and report his or her findings orally. Midwives were sometimes called in to examine female corpses.[28] This was a hereditary post without official rank and required no qualifications beyond the memorization of the Song dynasty classic of forensic medicine, *The Washing Away of Wrongs* (*Xi yuan lu* 洗冤錄). During the *xinzheng* reforms, the governor general of Manchuria had sent a memorial to the throne to suggest that this post be abolished since most of those who held it were uneducated and unable to explain the meaning of the text they had memorized. He suggested that the position should be replaced with that of 'coroner' (*jianyan li* 檢驗吏). In order to qualify for this status, candidates would have to successfully complete an eighteen-month course in anatomy and physiology as well as demonstrate mastery of *The Washing Away of Wrongs* and its modern commentaries. The memorial was explicit with regard to how unfavourably Chinese ostensors fared in comparison with the organized and professionally qualified practitioners of forensic medicine in foreign countries. It also emphasized that recognized forensic experts would be necessary in order to abolish foreign extraterritoriality in China.

The memorial was approved and circulated to all the provincial capitals of China with instructions to establish such courses. Chen Yuan scorned the lack of understanding of international relations it revealed:

> If you want to abolish extraterritoriality, it can't be done without making your legal system the same as other nations ... Suppose there is a case involving the death of a foreign national: the foreigners will want to verify the approved findings of our coroner. Will they not need corroboration from a physician with an education in forensic medicine? ... This [reform] still retains *The Washing Away of Wrongs* as a textbook, and requires the learning of no more than the most general and superficial physiology and anatomy. It is certainly insufficient to convince others.[29]

Chen was nothing if not consistent in his criticism of reforms that did not go far enough. In 1909, Duanfang 端方, the reform-minded

Manchu governor of Liangjiang, instigated China's first general medical licensing examination in the area under his jurisdiction. Chen Yuan wrote another long piece criticizing this initiative, which, he said, was a useless piece of state interference since, without state provision of a uniform and regulated medical education system, the examination certificates proved almost nothing.[30]

Thus, for Chen Yuan, Western medicine was an essential tool of modern government that China needed to use in order to regain national sovereignty as well as the health and prosperity of its people. Not surprisingly, Chen was also critical of Chinese medicine, which he saw as an obstacle to the modernization of China. After the Chinese Revolution, Chen was elected to the first National Assembly in 1913, and, on moving to Beijing to take up his new post, he gave up the teaching and practice of medicine. For him, it had served its purpose, and he was ready to turn to more direct means of helping to build the modern Chinese state.

Ding Fubao

Unlike Qiu Jin and Chen Yuan, Ding Fubao 丁福保 (styled Zhonghu 仲祜, 1874-1952) was not a revolutionary. On the contrary, he was a monarchist who supported the same 'New Policies' that Chen Yuan was so quick to denounce. Between 1909 and 1921, Ding translated, collated, and published at least eighty-three medical titles, the majority of which were translations from Japanese works on Western medicine.[31] He also contributed to almost all of the medical journals of the time, so that his writings dominated the market for information about Western medicine. Given Ding's influence on the processes through which Western medicine became established in China, his actions and motivations deserve special attention.

Most of what we know about Ding is contained in his own writings. In addition to his many translations and publications in medical periodicals, the main sources of information concerning his personal activities are his autobiographical works. Principal among these are his *Autobiography of the Lay Buddhist of Mathematical Mysteries* (*Chouyin jushi zizhuan* 疇隱居士自傳), published in Shanghai in 1948 (hereafter *Autobiography*), and the *Annalistic Autobiography of the Lay Buddhist of*

Mathematical Mysteries (*Chouyin jushi ziding nianpu* 疇隱居士自訂年普), published around 1937 (hereafter *Annals*). The *Annals* also exists in a slightly different published version of circa 1930. Shorter versions also appear at the front of some of his major compilations, such as the *Collected Glosses on the Shuowen Dictionary* (*Shuowen jiezi gulin* 說文解字詁林) and the *Encyclopaedic Dictionary of Buddhism* (*Fojiao da cidian* 佛教大辭典).[32]

In 1896, Ding took and passed the first degree in the imperial civil service examination system – the district examinations – earning the title of 'government student' (*shengyuan* 生員). The next year, aged twenty-three and in his third year at the prestigious Nanjing Academy in Jiangyin, he began to study mathematics in addition to the traditional canons and histories. Later in 1897, both Ding and his elder brother went to the provincial capital, Nanjing, to take the provincial civil service examinations. After an absence of about two weeks, they returned to find that their father, who had been suffering from tuberculosis (Ding uses the Japanese-coined neologism *fei jiehe* 肺結核 for this disease), had died during their absence. As a mark of filial respect, Ding decided never again to sit for the imperial examinations.[33]

This decision not to retake the civil service examinations was less of a change of career direction than it might appear. Barry Keenan notes that there were over fifty-three thousand holders of the *shengyuan* status in Jiangsu Province in the years between the suppression of the Taiping Rebellion in 1864-65 and the end of the century. Of these, only eighty-seven were admitted to second degree status ('provincial graduate' *juren* 舉人) every three years. As Keenan notes: 'The remainder were left as a rural intelligentisia naturally interested in educational innovations or management opportunities that could utilize its talents.'[34] Moreover, Ding married the same year, so his decision to abandon the very expensive pursuit of a bureaucratic career may also have been influenced by the need to support a family without the assistance of his father.

In 1898, Ding returned to the Nanjing Academy to specialize in mathematics, and he also took a job as a teacher of mathematics at the nearby 'Await Results' School 俟實學堂.[35] Ding's mathematics teacher at the Nanjing Academy was Hua Shifang 華世芳 (1853-1904), younger brother of the famous late Qing mathematician and popularizer of

Western mathematics Hua Hengfang 華衡芳 (1833-1902) and a native of Ding's home region, the Wuxi area of Jiangsu Province.

The following year, suffering a long and debilitating bout of an unspecified illness in relative poverty, Ding determined to become wealthy. In 1900, he published his first books, *An Annotated Bibliography of Mathematical Books* and *Questions and Answers Concerning Hygiene* (*Weishengxue wenda* 衛生學問答). This primer of general medical knowledge was later approved as a new school text during the New Policies reforms and was reprinted several times. Towards the end of 1900, Ding visited Shanghai, where Hua Shifang introduced him to Hua's cousin Zhao Yuanyi, who was to be a significant figure in Ding's future career. Zhao Yuanyi 趙元益 (styled Jinghan 靜涵, 1840-1902) not only was a provincial graduate, and therefore a successful classical scholar, but had also studied both Chinese and Western medicine. He had even accompanied the Chinese minister Xue Fucheng 薛福成 (1838-94) on a diplomatic tour of Europe in 1888. He was therefore unusually well versed in the ways of the West and in Western medicine. Zhao is even reported to have met the famous German bacteriologist Robert Koch while on this trip. After his return to China, Zhao was employed at the Jiangnan Arsenal in Shanghai, where he collaborated with John Fryer and Alexander Wylie in translating Western medical textbooks.[36] Perhaps it is no surprise that Zhao and even Ambassador Xue also hailed from the Wuxi area in Jiangsu Province.

In 1901, at the age of twenty-seven, Ding left his job at the 'Await Results' School and enrolled to study English at Suzhou University, which was run by the American Southern Methodists, but he had to abandon his course in the summer because of tuberculosis. After that, he went to Shanghai, where Zhao Yuanyi invited him to recuperate at his house and also taught him Western medicine. As a result of his connections with Hua Hengfang and Zhao, Ding enrolled at the Jiangnan Arsenal Polytechnic Institute (*Jiangnan zhizaoju gongyi xuetang* 江南製造局工藝學堂) to study chemistry. The same year, he also took and passed the first entrance examination for the new School of Japanese (*Dongwen xuetang* 東文學堂), which was set up in Shanghai by the prominent government official and industrialist Sheng Xuanhuai (盛宣懷,

1844-1916), who was then at the height of his powers.[37] Sheng's patronage was to influence the development of Ding's career. He even contributed a postscript to the second edition of Ding's *Questions and Answers Concerning Hygiene*. As a result of his preparation for this exam, Ding was able to publish a compilation titled *Questions and Answers on Japanese Literature (Dongwendian wenda* 東文典問答), which sold very well.[38]

At this time Ding's writing, editing, and publishing ventures were still financially disappointing. Probably because of this financial embarrassment, he accepted an invitation to teach at the translation bureau of the new Metropolitan University in Beijing for a monthly salary of one hundred *yuan*. He started there in May of 1903 as a teacher of mathematics and physiology.[39] However, he did not enjoy his work in Beijing and resigned at the end of the summer vacation in 1905, returning first to Shanghai and then to Wuxi.[40]

Returning to Shanghai in 1908, Ding decided to raise capital on his own for his publishing house. He also started to work as a medical doctor in the autumn but, after several months, had saved only thirty *yuan* from his medical practice. (At this time, there were no restrictions on medical practice – anyone could prescribe remedies for whatever fee they were able to command.) He did, however, succeed in publishing ten medical titles in this first year of independent publishing. Several of the works he published between 1908 and 1910 suggest that Ding still had a strong interest in the classical medical tradition at that time: *Ancient Prescriptions for Today; The Contents of Medical Works through the Ages; A Survey of the 'Inner Canon' and the 'Canon of Difficult Issues'; A Survey of the 'Treatise on Cold-damage Disorders'; Biographies of Famous Physicians through the Ages;* and *The Medical Section of the 'Annotated Catalogue of the Four Treasuries [Encyclopaedia].'*[41]

Early in 1909, Duanfang, the Manchu governor-general of the two lower Yangzi provinces (*Liangjiang* 兩江), decided that medical licensing examinations should be held in order to credential competent doctors – this was the same initiative criticized by Chen Yuan (see above). Those who did not practise, or who treated only close relatives for no fee, or were medical graduates of foreign medical colleges, did not need to attend.[42]

Ding went to Nanjing to sit the exams in the fourth month. The questions, as shown by Ding's summary, were remarkable for the fact that they demanded the candidates be familiar with much of the classical medical literature as well as up-to-date with Western medical developments:

1 Describe the advantages and disadvantages of Chinese and Western pulse-taking.
2 Describe the similarities and differences between Chinese and Western pharmacy.
3 Discuss the use of anaesthetic drugs in ancient times.
4 Discuss the properties and uses of X-rays.
5 Discuss Chinese and Western needling techniques.
6 Discuss the cause and treatment of rat-borne plague.
7 Discuss the character '*cong* 刿' in the context of the theory that consciousness belongs to the brain.[43]

This examination is the first recorded attempt in China to enforce medical licensing on *all* practising physicians in any area outside of the imperial bureaucracy. It preceded the formation of the Chinese (Western-) Medical Association by seven years. Not surprisingly, some influential figures in the Chinese-medical world found it distressing. He Lianchen 何廉臣 (1861-1929), one of the founding editors of the *Shaoxing Journal of Medicine and Pharmacy*, a friend of Ding Fubao and co-vice-president with him of the Chinese Medicine Society, wrote in the journal's front page editorial:

> The greatest pity in all this is that those [practitioners] who have diagnosed very many [patients], and whose experience is refined and profound, or whose manual skills are precise and skillful, but who are unable to express themselves in writing, will on this account fail the exams and so the government will stop them from practising.[44]

He Lianchen used the social Darwinist terms coined by Yan Fu to compare the examination to a violent struggle for existence, in which 'the superior vanquish and the inferior perish,' and he urged his colleagues not to join the battleground. His response is interesting because it shows clearly that, at this time, there was as yet no consensus among its elite practitioners that Chinese medicine would have to be upgraded and standardized.

Ding received the top score in this examination, a result that was reported widely in the medical journals of the time – along with his model answers. (It is not unlikely that the questions were set by Ding's friend Zhao Yuanyi, although this is just speculation.) Duanfang, the governor general who had ordered the examination, decided to reward Ding by sending him to Japan to report on the medical reforms that had been carried out there since the start of the Meiji Restoration in 1868. He instructed Ding to report on the legislation employed, the training of doctors, the organization of medical schools, and the use of Chinese herbal drugs. In addition, Sheng Xuanhuai gave Ding a letter of introduction to the Chinese ambassador in Japan, instructing him to give Ding one thousand Japanese *yen* for books and Western drugs.

Ding's reports of his five-week study trip to Japan seem to have attracted little official attention on his return. However, he did publish a summary of his findings in a travel diary and in the *Medical News* of 1909. He also published twenty-five medical titles that year, some of which were translations of books he had bought in Japan.

By the time Ding returned from his trip to Japan, he had become a supporter of the Westernization of medicine in China. On the very day of his return to Shanghai, he responded to a letter from his colleague He Lianchen:

Although most doctors in the [Japanese] capital look down on Chinese medicine, all of them welcome Chinese-medical drugs. Their interpretations of their experiments on Chinese-medical drugs are in scientific terms and not in terms of *yin* and *yang* and the Five Phases. Although Chinese-medical drugs really have excellent [raw] materials [in them], yet in not a few cases, their true qualities have remained hidden beneath erroneous theories. This is truly regrettable.[45]

Not all of Ding's colleagues were prepared to accept Chinese-medical theories as erroneous. Things came to a head later in 1909 in a dispute over the editorship of the *Medical News*.[46] Ding and He Lianchen decided that the *News* should be edited by Ding's student, Gu Mingsheng 顧鳴聲, in place of the existing editor, Wang Wenqiao 王問樵, who was a student of Cai Xiaoxiang 蔡小香, the chairman of the Chinese Medical Society (*Zhongguo yixue hui* 中國醫學會), of which they were all members. One of the stated aims of the society was the reform of Chinese medicine along scientific lines, and the *Medical News* was its official organ of publication. This was not just a trial of personal political strength but also an issue of editorial principle. Ding and his colleagues insisted that the reform of Chinese medicine necessitated abandoning most Chinese medical theory and concentrating on the scientific analysis of Chinese drugs. Cai and Wang accused Ding and Gu of slavishly copying the foreigners (in this case, the Japanese). Wang also pointed out that, in view of the scarcity of physicians with adequate instruction in both systems of medicine, Ding was advocating the impossible. Unable to settle the issue amicably, the two sides eventually took their cases to the Shanghai magistrate, who decided against Ding. This was in 1910, by which time Ding had already established his Sino-Western Medical Research Society. He promptly made Gu Mingsheng editor of the society's journal, the *Journal of Sino-Western Medicine* (*Zhong-xi yixue bao* 中西醫學報), withdrawing his considerable financial support from the *Medical News,* which folded after only a few more months.[47]

By contrast, Ding's Sino-Western Medical Research Society quickly attracted several hundred members. Ding's personal prestige was high, as he had previously taught at the nation's foremost academy, the Metropolitan University, and had gained publicity due to his success in Duanfang's medical exam. Clearly, Ding's views on the scientification of medicine in China did not lack an audience. However, the supporters of an intact Chinese medicine continued to regard him with great suspicion. The Nanjing Medical Society (*Nanjing yixue hui* 南京醫學會) even went so far as to resolve to have no dealings with him.[48]

In 1911, when the Qing government fell to the revolutionary armies, Ding noted that he, too, 'cut off his queue.' In fact, the revolution was a potential disaster for Ding since he owed his success to the patronage of prominent Qing officials. Ding expressed some of his views of the change in a poem titled 'Autumn Feelings':

Things of the past cause me so much pain
I cannot bear to look at the tattered banner
Swords and spears penetrate the whole world
Where is Chang'an?[49]

From 1912 on, Ding immersed himself in his commercial publishing activities, which included a series called Mr. Ding's Medical Compendium, containing translations from Japanese works on Western medicine. Ding submitted the Compendium to the League of Nations Health Organization's competitions in Rome and Berlin, where it won first prize. Ding used his knowledge of Japanese and of Western medicine to survive in the absence of his former mentors – and to achieve success, a certain amount of fame, and the wealth he had desired.

We have devoted considerable attention to Ding Fubao's story in order to show the path he took to becoming the leading source of information about Western medicine in the first decades of the Republic of China. The best efforts of Western medical missionaries and of Western-educated Chinese physicians were not able to supersede Ding's prodigious output until the late 1920s at the earliest. A look at his views of Western medicine completes the picture of his position during this phase of modernization.

Ding described himself as being interested in any and all kinds of medicine due to his own frequent and long illnesses as well as to the deaths from illness that he saw around him. Although he recovered from tuberculosis, he lost at least twelve family members to that disease, including his father and one of his sons.[50] We may conclude that one of the main reasons Ding devoted so much attention to Western medicine had to do with the fact that he genuinely believed it to be more effective than the Chinese treatments he had tried and found wanting. Of course, many in the Chinese-medical world disagreed with him, but in this period of the high tide of Western imperialist expansion and of scientism in China, Ding's Western-medical publications were thoroughly in tune with current concerns.

Ding Fubao's only formal qualification in Western medicine was the certificate he gained as a result of sitting Duanfang's medical registration exam in 1909. As Chen Yuan so caustically noted at the time, this was insufficient to qualify Ding in the eyes of either foreigners or the Western-educated physicians of the day. Ding's position within the medical world reflected this ambiguity. He remained a member of several associations of Chinese-medical physicians while maintaining that most Chinese-medical theory was useless and should be discarded. In the preface to his translation of Wada Keijūrō's *Iron Spear of the Medical World* (*Yijie zhi tiezhui* 醫界之鐵椎), published in 1911, he writes:

> Western medical arts have not yet advanced to a state of completion; some of China's drugs and prescriptions surpass Western ones ... If we exert ourselves to the utmost to investigate Chinese drugs, there are bound to be new discoveries. These will enable Western drugs to be replaced and illnesses to be cured that Western medicine is unable to cure. It will be justified to call them discoveries of world significance.[51]

It is clear from Ding's writings that 'to investigate Chinese drugs' meant scientific investigation. In his 1939 editorial in the first issue of *The New Voice of National Drugs* (*Guoyao xinsheng* 國藥新聲), Ding writes: 'For forty years I have been advocating that the synthesis of Chinese and Western medicine must proceed from the scientization of Chinese medicine.'[52] Ding's publications on the subject of the Chinese pharmacopeia emphasize this point. For instance, in his *Simple Chinese Pharmacy* he classifies herbal drugs under Western rubrics ('febrifugals,' 'diuretics,' 'analgesics,' stimulants,' 'antihelminthics,' etc.). He also includes in each entry the alternative names of each herbal drug, their botanical descriptions, results of chemical analysis, and their applications (using SI units of measurement and Western disease nomenclature).[53] Ding's attitude, like that of the Japanese researchers, was rather similar to that of pharmacognosists of today, who regard the traditional pharmacopeiae of the world as so much raw material for analysis in their search for such 'lead compounds' as may facilitate the development of new Western-medical drugs.

Ding Fubao had his own clinic for many years, and an account of his clinical activities is preserved in the long preface to his *Encyclopaedia of Modern Internal Medicine* (*Jinshi neike quanshu* 近世內科全書), first published in 1914. The preface was written by Lu Jusheng, a former director of the prestigious Nanjing Academy in Wuxi, where Ding had studied. In the preface, Lu records several consultations that he had observed. These short case records are interesting for the rare glimpse they offer of the kinds of diagnostic tools and therapies Western-medical practitioners used at this time. It is noteworthy that Ding used the tuberculin test on only one of the two suspected cases recorded here – the test was not wasted on the poorer, less educated patient. The range of procedures Ding employed clearly varied according to the educational and social status of the patient. The cases are summarized below.

[CASE HISTORY 1]: Lu accompanied his elder brother to seek a consultation with Ding Fubao because the brother was fat, listless, and impotent. On examining the brother's urine, Ding found sugar and diagnosed diabetes. He prescribed some drugs and forbade the patient to eat cereals and sugary foods, which were to be replaced with animal food products. After several months of this drug and food regimen, the illness was cured.

[CASE HISTORY 2]: Lu's nephew, aged twelve *sui*, was suffering from swelling of his entire body, but particularly of his scrotum. Ding examined the boy's urine, which contained protein, and diagnosed acute nephritis. He ordered bedrest, and the drinking of only cow's milk, and prescribed a strong purgative. The patient was cured.

[CASE HISTORY 3]: A woman whose surname was Li came to Ding with a painful abdomen. Ding examined her chest and her stool, in which he found fly larvae and eggs. He thought he could cure the painful abdomen, but since the lung extremities sounded waterlogged, he also diagnosed pulmonary tuberculosis, which was bound to become worse. After the abdominal pain was cured, the patient refused to believe she had tuberculosis, and the next year, sure enough, she died of it.

[CASE HISTORY 4]: An old woman suffered from headaches, vomiting, and high fever. Ding examined her lymph glands and a blood sample, and diagnosed plague. He ordered her to go quickly to the Ministry of Works' Infectious Disease Hospital, but she didn't obey. The next day, she died, as did several of those who lived with her. This was the first news of plague in Shanghai.

[CASE HISTORY 5]: Mr. Zhou Xueqiao (1870-1910, founder of the *Medical News*) was suffering from a stomach complaint, bringing up blood, and producing noxious sweat over his whole body. Ding diagnosed stomach cancer and said that it should be operated on quickly or it would be incurable. Mr Zhou was unable to reach a decision and, as a result, died two years later.

[CASE HISTORY 6]: Mr. Song Gengfu had a hacking cough and brought up blood. Ding introduced tuberculosis serum (i.e., Koch's tuberculin) into his shoulder in the same way as one inoculates with cowpox (to treat smallpox). About twenty-four hours later the shoulder showed a tuberculous reaction. Ding also examined Song's phlegm under the microscope and found tuberculosis bacteria. Accordingly, he diagnosed pulmonary tuberculosis. Using a combination of injected and oral drugs, in a little over four months Song was completely cured.

Lu continues:

> These few are all cases I saw and heard myself, and I marvel that none of today's diagnosticians are up to Ding Fubao ... Now I saw that Ding Fubao's treatments and methods are not recorded in the ancient books. So I questioned him minutely on the sources of his medical practices. Ding replied: 'My treatment of ailments comes primarily from the *Encyclopedia of Modern Internal Medicine:* I have no diagnoses or prescriptions that are not drawn from this book.'
>
> On hearing this I was extremely happy – at first I'd thought that Ding's treatments were his own ingenuity ... Now [I discovered] there was already a book with which to follow established methods

... The original book is by a Japanese author, Hashimoto Sessai, in 11 chapters.[54]

Lu is wonderfully explicit in his praise of the methods transmitted by Ding Fubao: what he admires most is the relative consistency of the Japanese book and its usefulness in generating precise diagnoses. This enabled Ding to make accurate prognoses even though fully half of the cases related by Lu were fatal. It was the standardized and accessible nature of the Western medical approach – which promised, even though it could not yet deliver, the ability to control disease – that appealed to Lu and to many others of his generation. They had been brought up with a medical system in which a successful physician would normally jealously guard the identity of the most efficacious remedies in order to maintain an advantage over the competition. There is no mention of the use of any Chinese-medical procedures or drugs in any of Lu's account.

Zhang Xichun

Western and Chinese understandings of disease were combined in the service of Chinese medicine by another hugely successful author, whose magnum opus is regularly reprinted even today. Zhang Xichun 張錫純 (1860-1933) spent much of his life fighting against the uncritical replacement of Chinese learning with Western ideologies.[55] In 1900, Zhang even supported the Boxer Rebellion, which had the expulsion of foreigners from Chinese soil as one of its explicit aims. As a result, he was forced to take refuge with a relative in the treaty port sanctuary of Tianjin for about a year. Later, the first print run of his book was financed by a study society devoted to the refutation of Western knowledge.[56] In 1918, the first installment of Zhang Xichun's *The Assimilation of Western to Chinese in Medicine* was published to rave reviews; the final installment was published in 1934.

Zhang had gained access to Japanese Western medical books through Ding Fubao's translations, and his use of Benjamin Hobson's medical terms in Chinese (from Hobson's 1850s series on Western medicine and natural philosophy) indicates that he had also read some missionary translations.[57] The discussions of Western medicine in his book were scarcely uncritical, however. Zhang was consistent in viewing disease and therapy from a Chinese-medical point of view, and it was his aim to make Western ideas comprehensible from within a Chinese-medical epistemology.

Zhang came from a scholarly family and had clearly been taught the Qing dynasty rationalistic tradition of Chinese medicine, much as had Qiu Jisheng, who surveyed the range of popular medical practices described in Chapter 1. Zhang's secular Chinese medicine was well suited to his agenda of judging Western medicine by how well it coincided with, or could be explained by, Chinese medicine. For example, his discussion of the Western concept of tuberculosis came in his first chapter, 'Prescriptions for Treating *Yin*-Depleted Exhaustion (or Wasting) Fever.' Here, he refers neither to the 'wasting worms' (*laochong* 勞蟲) of popular understandings of consumption nor to theories of Five Phases correspondence.[58] Instead, he describes how consumption (*laozhai* 勞瘵) is a result of depletion of the *yin* aspect of the body's *yinyang* economy. This depletion originates either in the lungs or the kidneys, the latter also being responsible, in Chinese medical thought, for reproductive and sexual functions. He explains: 'These are the cases that Westerners ascribe to "excessive lust."' In Chinese medicine, excessive sexual intercourse endangers the kidney system, which might lead to *yin*-depletion diseases, which is a neat match with the Western association of tuberculosis with pathologically heightened sexual desire.

Zhang described the tubercles, which Westerners considered characteristic of the disease, using Hobson's transliteration of *dubikali* (都比迦力) for 'tubercle.' He then explained that the Japanese had expanded on the Western understanding: they called the disease *fei jiehe* 肺結核 (meaning 'lung tubercles') and considered it to be the result of infection by a bacterium. Since the Japanese works were the only ones Zhang knew that discussed tuberculosis in terms of bacterial etiology, he seems to have concluded that the tuberculosis bacterium was a Japanese discovery. Zhang did not dismiss germ theory, but he did argue that germs alone were not a sufficient cause of the consumption (*laozhai*) he was describing.

In the case studies that follow this discussion, Zhang invented several new treatments, some of which combine Chinese and Western therapy. In one of these, after preliminary treatment with herbs, he decided to use aspirin to induce sweating and then continued by treating his patient with pills made from two Western drugs – creosote and menthol combined in a base of bean flour. He recorded that, after five to six days, the coughing started to improve and the patient began to recover.[59]

Creosote (in a 1 percent solution) was an orthodox and common Western medical treatment for tuberculosis at the time, but Zhang evaluated it in terms common to Chinese pharmacy, giving it a 'nature' *(xing)* and a 'taste' *(wei)*, and explaining that, although it was smelly and unpleasant, when taken with menthol, which he assessed as having a 'cooling' nature and 'pungent' taste, the prescription would be well balanced. It was, he said, a fast and effective treatment for cases of pulmonary tuberculosis.

Aspirin, too, was assessed by Zhang in Chinese pharmaceutical terms as 'cooling' in nature and 'slightly sour' in taste. It was, he said, especially useful for dissipating the fever of tuberculosis but could lead to excessive sweating. Because of this, he quoted Ding Fubao to the effect that the doses listed in Western works needed to be halved when treating Chinese.[60] Ding had explained that in Europe the ground is cold, and people are accustomed to eating lots of meat from an early age, so their organs and *qi* are very robust. In China, this not being the case, it was necessary to halve the dose and to add sweat-inhibiting herbs if perspiration became prolific. This kind of view of racial/cultural difference was common in both China and Europe at the time.[61]

From this example of the treatment of tuberculosis in Zhang Xichun's work we can see how Chinese and Western disease entities were mapped so that drug treatments for Chinese lung-wasting disease could be seamlessly combined with Western treatments for pulmonary tuberculosis. Zhang Xichun was virtually the only medical author of the period to display a sound knowledge of Western medical writings and to consistently assess them from the standpoint of Chinese medicine. This strategy is the reverse of that employed by Western laboratory researchers, who take Chinese herbs and attempt to analyze them in terms of the pharmaceutical activity of their 'active principles.' Zhang Xichun's writ-ings were very influential in Republican Chinese medicine, and he became something of a medical hero. In 1918, the head of Shenyang's Tax Bureau, with the help of the governor of Liaoning Province, built and funded a school of Chinese medicine for him, inviting him to be its director.[62]

Xie Guan

Xie Guan (謝觀, styled Liheng 利恆, 1880-1950) was a native of Wujin County in Jiangsu Province. His grandfather, Xie Baochu 謝葆初, is recognized as part of the local Menghe medical current recently studied by Volker Scheid,[63] and his father, Xie Zhongying 謝仲英, was a locally renowned scholar who specialized in historical geography. As a youth, Xie Guan studied at home, as was normal practice for members of a gentry family, and, by the age of twelve, he was reputed to have not only mastered the Four Books and Five Classics but also to know the courses of China's rivers and the locations and histories of China's towns and cities. He was also able to recite the medical classics by heart. Xie's ado-lescence came during the Sino-Japanese War of 1894-95, when many debated the casues of China's weakness and the need for reform. At the age of twenty, as Ding Fubao had briefly done before him, he entered Suzhou University (run by American Southern Methodists) but aban-doned his studies in order to observe the three-year mourning period after his father's death.[64]

We are not told how long he studied at Suzhou, but it was charac-teristic of Chinese students at the missionary schools of this period to attend out of a desire to discover the available sources of information about the West rather than out of a desire to seek a foreign degree. In general, the drop-out rate at these colleges was very high, not out of any lack of ability but, rather, out of the students' impatience to move on and study material of more immediate use to their careers and surroundings.[65]

In 1905, Xie took a post teaching geography at one of the new middle schools in Guangzhou (Canton), some twelve hundred kilometres south of Shanghai. It is likely that he went at the invitation of Lu Erkui 陸爾奎 (1862-1935), who was also from Wujin and later became Xie's colleague at the Commercial Press. Lu had been invited to take charge of middle school education in Guangzhou, and it would have been normal practice for him to have employed some of his personal contacts.[66] Xie was reputedly a great success, but his mother and wife 'did not accustom themselves' to life in the far South, so he resigned and returned to Jiangsu, becoming a geography editor for the Commercial Press in Shanghai. Xie also ran a private college in Shanghai for a while, and, after the 1911 revolution, his growing reputation as an educator caused him to be appointed director of education in his home county of Wujin. During the next two years, Xie presided over a massive expansion of the local educational system, taking it from thirty schools to 158, and from about four thousand students to well over sixty thousand. When the Ministry of Education compiled a league table of educational standards across the country, Wujin was ranked second overall. In recognition of Xie's competence, President Yuan Shikai offered him the job of director of the Provincial Education Bureau in 1914, but Xie, 'anticipating Yuan's attempt to make himself emperor,' declined. Instead, he accepted the post of chief geography editor for the Commercial Press and saw more than thirty titles to publication there, including the first Chinese-medical dictionary, which we discuss in the next chapter.

In 1917, two of Xie's contemporaries from Wujin, Ding Ganren 丁甘仁 and his son Ding Zhongying 丁仲英, collaborated with the Shanghai physician Xia Shaoting 夏紹庭 to establish the Shanghai Technical College of Chinese Medicine (*Shanghai zhongyi zhuanmen xuexiao* 上海中醫專門學校), one of the first colleges of Chinese medicine in the country. Xie accepted their invitation to lecture there, becoming responsible for setting the curriculum and editing lecture courses. In 1925, the Shenzhou (All China) Medical Association established the Chinese-medical University (*Zhongyi daxue*) in the Zhabei area of Shanghai. Xie Guan was asked to be director and to create a research program designed to raise the standard of Chinese medicine. This university venture failed in less than two years when the school was burned in the factional fighting between the Nationalists and the Communists. However, after its closure, Xie continued to teach students privately. Chen Cunren reports having seen at least sixteen 'end-of-term' photographs of these private groups, indicating that he continued to teach in this way for several years.[67]

There were many medical organizations in the Shanghai region at this time – one scholar has counted forty in 1929 – representing widely differing views.[68] Traditional-style elite physicians had begun to organize themselves into associations in order to share information about Western medicine and to protect themselves from modernizers who were attempting to discredit 'old' culture, including Chinese medicine. However, as in so many fields of activity, these associations tended to unite people from one geographical area of China only.[69] While this style of organization may have been effective in promoting its members' interests locally, when the fragmented political structure of the warlord period was replaced with Chiang Kai-shek's Nationalist government in 1928, the new national administration posed a significantly greater threat to practitioners of Chinese medicine. In Shanghai, the only non-parochial association was the *Zhongyi xiehui* 中醫協會 (Chinese Medicine Union), which had been formed from the merger of three previous associations. Xie Guan was one of its more prominent members. The association quickly declared its opposition to Yu Yunxiu's 1929 resolution to abolish Chinese medicine (described in Chapter 4) and called a national congress of medical and pharmaceutical societies. The congress was held on 17 March, with 262 delegates taking part, representing 132 societies from fifteen provinces. Shanghai drugstore owners staged a half-day strike to coincide with the congress, which discussed over a hundred resolutions and resulted in the formation of the National Federation of Medical and Pharmaceutical Associations (*Quanguo yiyao tuanti lianhe hui* 全國醫藥團體聯合會). The seventeenth of March was named 'National Medicine Day,' and Xie Guan was chosen to lead a five-man delegation to petition the new national government in Nanjing to reject the resolution to abolish Chinese medicine. As a result of these activities and the large amount of public support they generated, the resolution was never implemented.[70]

Chen Cunren 陳存仁 (1908-90), the youngest member of the delegation, provides a report that is quite revealing. When the delegation reached the government offices in Nanjing, it was met in person by Minister of Heath Xue Dubi薛篤弼. Chen records that the minister appeared embarrassed, and he attributes this to the fierce opposition that the abolition resolution had already encountered, most notably from the famously progressive provincial governor Feng Yuxiang 馮玉祥. After Xie Guan delivered the delegation's address, Minister Xue replied: 'The Ministry of Health has absolutely no intention of abolishing Chinese medicine, and as for the resolution of the National Health Congress, it is awaiting a decision from the Ministry's Executive Committee. Please be reassured, and convey this to your colleagues nationally, so that there will be no misunderstanding.'[71]

That same evening, Xue Dubi invited the delegates to a meal of Chinese food set with Western table-settings, to which he had also invited a prominent foreign geographer. Worriedly, the minister hinted to Xie and his group that it wouldn't be helpful to criticize the abolition resolution over dinner, for fear of inciting the foreigner's ridicule. When the meal was over, the foreigner rose and delivered a lecture on his geographical researches in Tibet and western China, describing the origin and historical courses of Chinese rivers and illustrating his talk with slides. When he finished, Xie Guan also rose and politely filled in some of the gaps in the foreigner's knowledge, citing his Chinese maps and sources as he went, and specifically refuting his priority claim for the discovery of the source of the Jiangchuan River, showing that the source had been recorded in a particular Qing dynasty work. Surprised and impressed by this display of knowledge, the foreign guest complimented Xie, saying that he had met very few Chinese who knew much of the geography of China and none as well-informed as Xie Guan. According to Chen Cunren's (admittedly partisan) account, Minister Xue was cheered and relieved by this praise from the foreign expert, and his attitude towards the Chinese medicine delegates improved markedly.[72]

This anecdote reveals a good deal about the value of Xie Guan's involvement in the struggle to re-establish Chinese medicine as a high-status occupation. The minister was concerned to present China as a modernizing world power at a time when the most influential Chinese were those who had returned from overseas study, preferably with foreign qualifications. The continued existence of Chinese medicine was a source of potential embarrassment to these people in their dealings with Westerners. Xie Guan, by contrast, represented the best of the native tradition of scholarship and was even able to employ his home-grown expertise to correct the rather arrogant foreigner's assumption that his findings were completely new. (I can't help being reminded of a Kenyan fellow student's outrage at being taught, as a schoolgirl, the geography of Kenya from an English textbook that naïvely recorded the 'discovery' of a local Kenyan mountain by an Englishman in 1910.) Xie Guan remained committed to the value of Chinese scholarship on its own terms, which included resisting the popular trend towards the accommodation of Western medical knowledge within Chinese medicine.

Xie continued to be prominent in the ongoing struggle to develop Chinese-medical education in the face of strong opposition from the Westernizing faction in government, which persistently opposed including Chinese medicine in any government-sanctioned activity on the grounds that it was unscientific and an obstacle to national progress. Xie was consistently elected to the executive committees and sometimes to the chairs of the national organizations that spearheaded the opposition. By the time of his death in 1950, the Shanghai Municipal Sanitary Bureau had carried out licensing examinations for Chinese-medical doctors eleven times: every time, Xie had been on the Examination Committee.

When the Institute of National Medicine (*Guoyi guan* 國醫館) was founded in 1931, Xie Guan was elected to its standing committee. However, the institute had the reform of Chinese medicine according to scientific principles as part of its remit, a task that generated a good deal of bad feeling. In his 1935 book, Xie wrote this of the Nanjing Decade:

> Since the restoration of the Republic, the propagation of Japanese-Western medicine (*dong-xi yi* 東西醫) in China has gradually spread. The Chinese people have been infected by it and Chinese-medical physicians have encountered its influence. Therefore they have joined together in associations to provide for research; they have established academies to extend training and published journals to provide publicity. They have been promoting it in many ways. New forces have sprung up, holding high the banner of 'New Chinese Medicine.'

I suppose their initial intentions were to use scientific methods to put the old medical works in order ... However, their successes were hardly outstanding and in their complacency they gave the impression of going in as masters and emerging as slaves.[73]

In his own writings, Xie describes Chinese medicine without scientific or linguistic borrowings from the West or Japan. There is no better example of a scholar, teacher, administrator, and delegate who preferred to promote Chinese medicine on its own terms.

Conclusion

Four of the five individuals described here valued the new medicine from the West but *not* primarily for its medical efficacy. This may come as something of a surprise. It is normal to assume that modern medicine has spread around the world at least partly because it works, even after taking the context of imperialism into account. By looking at the lives of four Chinese who were influential in modern Chinese history and who were also active in adapting Western medicine to the Chinese context, we see that the curative efficacy of modern medicine was not its main appeal. Even Ding Fubao, perhaps Western medicine's most effective evangelist in the early twentieth century, admitted: 'Western medical arts have not yet advanced to a state of completion; some of China's drugs and prescriptions surpass Western ones.' So why did these people integrate medicine into their programs for social and political change?

The women nurses observed by Qiu Jin in 1905-6 were potent agents of Japanese government propaganda. Japan had signed the Geneva Conventions in 1887, and the International Committee of the Red Cross recognized Japan's Red Cross Society the following year. In spite of the Empress's early support for women as nurses, it was not until the aftermath of the Sino-Japanese War of 1894-95 that nursing became a respectable woman's profession. At that time Japanese war widows were recruited to be Red Cross nurses, something that transformed them from burdens on their families into respected professionals, able to contribute to both their families and society.[74] In 1900, Japanese troops were members of the 'eight nations alliance' that quelled the Boxer

Rebellion in China, and Britain signed the Anglo-Japanese Alliance in 1902. Japanese military organization was displayed to even greater effect during the Russo-Japanese War in 1904-5, in which the Japanese Red Cross was able to deploy two hospital steamships, four hospitals, 369 surgeons, 2,874 female nurses, and 1,544 male nurses.[75] The Japanese Red Cross won international acclaim for its humanitarian treatment of the seventy thousand prisoners of war, even providing prosthetic arms, legs, and eyes for 175 of the wounded Russians.

Qiu Jin's motives were not the same as those of the Japanese government. Her primary agenda was to battle the forces of female repression, and she saw paid employment as a necessary step in women's emancipation. Many Chinese considered it disgraceful for a woman to work outside the home, but the example of Red Cross nurses working for both themselves and their country's national defence presented Qiu Jin with powerful arguments in favour of female employment. So for her, Western medicine and nursing were means towards achieving full citizenship and employment for Chinese women, goals that she saw as fully consonant with throwing off the feudal social order and creating a modern Chinese republic.

Chen Yuan was also inspired by Japan's successful assimilation of Western medicine, and he, like Qiu, wanted to use modern medicine to make China stronger on the international stage. However, Chen's admiration was tempered with an awareness of the potential uses of medicine as a tool of empire. When Germany announced that it would open a medical school in its leased territory at Qingdao, Chen wrote that Germany was extending its 'rights to educate' (*jiaoyu quan* 教育權) in China, thereby competing with the United States, Britain, and France, who also claimed the right to set up educational establishments on Chinese soil. When the king of Korea dismissed most of his traditional-style court physicians in favour of a single Japanese-educated MD, Chen wrote that Japan was using medicine to 'pay back' Korea for having been a source of medical knowledge in the past and that, if China did not pay attention, Japan would soon be using medicine to 'pay back' China, with potentially dire consequences for China's national sovereignty.[76]

Chen's medical publications often stressed the importance of public health and personal hygiene in preventing disease. For him, spreading this knowledge was important not only for personal health but also for the success of modern institutions like schools, railways, and armies, and, ultimately, for China's survival as an independent nation. The Qing government's failure to see medical politics in these stark terms was, for Chen, evidence of its inadequacy and further justification for revolutionary action.

Ding Fubao learned his Western medicine in a Qing government institution and also greatly admired the new Japanese medical system. This is interesting because, as we have seen, he was a monarchist who supported the Qing efforts to reform from within. As the most influential of these five reformers in effecting medical change, Ding's case reminds us that Western medicine could be deployed in the service of diametrically opposed agendas.

Neither Qiu Jin nor Chen Yuan had any patience with Chinese medicine. Ding Fubao began as a reformer of Chinese medicine but, after seeing Japan's new medical system, restricted his support to the scientific analysis of herbal drugs. Zhang Xichun shared Ding's interest in pharmacology, but for Zhang the direction of research flowed in the opposite direction. Knowledge about Western drug treatments could be used to formulate improved Chinese herbal formulae, and, in the process, the new ingredients would lose their foreign associations. Zhang turned to Western science in such a way that he confirmed and justified his secular interpretation of the Chinese classical tradition in medicine. This interpretation was similar to that of *kanpō* supporters in Japan, who, like Zhang Xichun, emphasized Zhang Ji's Han dynasty classic texts *On Cold Damage and Miscellaneous Disorders* (*Shanghan zabing lun* 傷寒雜病論) and *Essential Prescriptions of the Golden Casket* (*Jinkui yaolüe fang* 金匱要略方). Zhang Xichun's solution to political weakness at home and imperialist encroachments from abroad was to use Western science to demonstrate the strength and adaptability of indigenous medicine. His writings are still very popular today in spite of the fact that many of the Western-medical treatments he discusses (such as giving creosote for tuberculosis) are obsolete. Indeed, perhaps that is the secret of his book's success. In contrast to the temporary fixes offered in Western medicine, Zhang adapted classic prescriptions to incorporate new ingredients without losing the inherent logic of the original formulae. As we saw in Chapter 2, medical missionaries spent much energy trying to do the same thing when they ran out of pharmaceutical supplies and were forced to make local substitutions, using Chinese drugs to formulate Western-style prescriptions.

Our fifth individual, Xie Guan, serves as a salutary reminder that not all scholars of this period embraced Western medicine, even as a means to bolster the case for Chinese medicine. Xie believed that Chinese medicine, like Chinese geographic knowledge, could be judged on its own merits, that it need not be subordinated to Western concepts. That Xie went on to write and compile the first dictionary of Chinese medicine – a work that would remain popular for decades and is still in print – suggests that his views were not so extreme as to be isolating.

In the jargon of science studies, what these medical lives demonstrate is that the meanings of Western medicine in China were 'underdetermined': different individuals used new medical knowledge to argue for revolution or against it, for women's emancipation or for the preservation of traditional culture. It is also striking that all five individuals were deeply impressed by the example of Japanese medical modernization and its relation to military success.

New Medical Institutions   **7**

The different views on Western medicine and Chinese medicine advanced by the individuals discussed in the previous chapter were also reflected in the institutions created to support medical endeavours. To make the situation more comprehensible, I examine these in two parts: those dedicated to Western medicine and those dedicated to Chinese medicine. Since many of the latter institutions came about in dialogue with Chinese use of Western medicine, I begin with Western-medical institutions.

The Institutionalization of Western Medicine in China

As we have seen, the China Medical Missionary Association, formed in China in 1837, was run by and for medical missionaries. Chinese graduates of Western medical colleges could be admitted as honorary (non-voting) members only. When, in the wake of the Sino-Japanese War of 1894-95 and the Boxer Rebellion of 1900, the Qing government announced the New Policies reforms, including a new school system and the replacement of the old civil service examinations with selection based partly on competence in sciences and languages, many aspiring bureaucrats went to study in Japan.[1]

Japan's early encounters with Western medicine had been mediated by Dutch traders, as a result of which the first Japanese medical students to study abroad were sent to colleges in Continental Europe, mainly in Germany. (In the late nineenth century, Dutch medical works were usually written in German.) The wave of Chinese students who went to Japan to study in the first years of the twentieth century were therefore taught German-style medicine. On the other hand, Chinese students sent abroad through connections with medical missionaries were usually trained in Britain or North America. There was also a Chinese regional difference: students who came from South China tended to move south to Hong Kong, learn English, and study medicine in English, whereas students from North China were more likely to study medicine in Japan or Germany. This was because the Jiaozhou Peninsula was a German concession and because, after 1895, Japan had a constant presence in Manchuria. Right from the beginning, then, there was latent factionalism between members of the first generations of returnee medical graduates. In practical terms, the major difference was that German-Japanese medicine was already much more laboratory-based than Anglo-American medicine in the years before the First World War.[2]

These differences between returnee Chinese medics were soon institutionalized with the 1907 formation of the Chinese Pharmaceutical Association (*Zhongguo yaoxue hui* 中國藥學會), which was composed entirely of students who had studied in Japan, and the 1915 formation of the Chinese Medical and Pharmaceutical Association (*Zhonghuaminguo yiyaoxue hui* 中華民國醫藥學會), which was also composed entirely of graduates of Japanese schools. The National Medical Association (*Zhonghua yixue hui* 中華醫學會), also established in 1915, was by contrast almost entirely composed of medical graduates from the English-speaking world.[3]

The establishment of these medical associations by Chinese and for Chinese marks the first decisive step towards the creation of an indigenous Western medical profession in China. However, the early members of these associations were so convinced of the medical and technical superiority of the foreign institutions that had trained them that, in their efforts to establish and maintain their own prestige as foreign medical graduates, they often failed to join forces with other, less prestigiously educated compatriots. For instance, the first constitution of the National Medical Association (NMA) of 1915 provided for three classes of membership:

1 *Regular members* being (a) graduates in medicine of recognised foreign universities or colleges; (b) graduates of medical colleges in China recognised by the Association who have a good reading and writing knowledge of at least one Western language.
2 *Associate members,* being graduates from recognised medical colleges in China who possess no knowledge of a Western language. These were to enjoy the same privileges as the regular members except eligibility as officers ...
3 *Honorary members.*[4]

Doctors who fulfilled the language conditions for admission to the NMA as regular members would inevitably have been students at one of the foreign-run medical schools in China if they had not qualified abroad. This may be seen from the fact that, among the fifteen Western medical colleges in China recorded as admitting students in 1915, nine were run by foreigners and seven of these by missionary societies. Of the six schools operating under Chinese patronage, all but two were set up with the help of foreigners and had Westerners or Japanese on the teaching staff. Because the schools run without foreign help also taught in Chinese only, their graduates could only qualify for associate membership in the NMA.[5]

These discriminatory admission regulations were calculated to repulse medical imperialism rather than to collaborate with it. Wu Lien-teh, who had risen to national prominence through his handling of the Manchurian plague epidemic of 1910-11,[6] was a driving force behind the establishment of the NMA in 1915. In an article written that same year, he described the condition of the Western medical profession in China and his proposals for improving it. First of all, he said, it was shameful that, at the recent 1913 international medical conference in London, China had sent only two delegates, compared to Japan's sixty and more than five hundred each from Germany and the United States. Then he went on to describe how the poor level of basic sanitary education in China made it the laughingstock of the Westerners. Moreover, medical qualifications obtained by graduates of the Chinese state-run (*gongli* 公立) medical schools were not standardized, with the result that foreigners did not recognize them. Since foreigners still controlled the Chinese customs, railways, and quarantine medical services, these Chinese medical graduates had trouble obtaining employment even in state enterprises in China. Wu then urged the establishment of a national governing body for the Western medical profession so that other nations would recognize Chinese medical graduates' qualifications, thereby allowing the Chinese to regain control over state medical facilities. Only then could the trust of local populations be won over for Western medicine and hygiene. The establishment of a basic standard of 'national hygiene' was essential to the survival of an independent China. 'Strengthening the nation, strengthening the [Chinese] race and purging foreigners' contempt all depend on this,' he concluded.[7]

Strengthening the Chinese nation and purging foreigners' contempt – if not foreigners altogether – were aims shared by all educated Chinese at this time. These concerns are voiced frequently in the literature of the period, mostly accompanied by a concern for strengthening the Chinese race. Race as such was a familiar concept in China, but it acquired new urgency with the popularity of Western social evolutionary ideas, which first appeared in Chinese translation between 1895 and 1903.[8] Already in 1903, Zou Rong, in his famous article 'The Revolutionary Army,' stated that revolution was 'a universal rule of evolution' and maintained that the Chinese were in danger of degenerating, of atavistically moving *down* the evolutionary ladder. The famous writer Lu Xun also used this idea of degeneration to attack the backwardness of Chinese society with characteristic sarcasm: 'My fellow countrymen, to whom servility has become second nature, will degenerate day by day through natural selection through apes, birds, shellfish, seaweed and finally to a lifeless thing.'[9]

Members of the new class of Western-trained Chinese physicians, with their ready-made orientation towards public employment and civil service rather than private practice, were well placed to take advantage of Chinese fears of racial inferiority and degeneration. Time and again their arguments for the furtherance of the Western-medical enterprise are couched in such words as: 'To cure the nation first cure the people; to cure the people first cure medical theories.'[10] They repeatedly translated the foreign image of China as 'the sick old man of Asia' into '400 million sick Chinese' and advanced the establishment of a modern medical system as the solution.

A modern medical system was also represented as the mark of a strong and civilized nation. In 1924, Dr. Hou Yuwen, editor of the medical journal for the Japanese-trained medical association, opened an editorial with the remarks:

> The strength or weakness of a nation's people is related to whether medicine is advanced or not. Therefore the establishment of medical schools is currently an urgent task. If we look at our capital city, apart from the intermittent activities of the Army Medical School, only the Medical University fully qualifies ... Whereas foreign medical schools from all over the world are constantly springing up [in China].[11]

These arguments were all addressed to those with sufficient power and authority to advance the Western-medical cause, on behalf of the medical contingent of China's aspiring new mandarinate. However, the first years of Chinese Republican government failed to provide this authority. When Yuan Shikai died in 1916 after his unsuccessful attempt to re-establish a constitutional monarchy with himself as the emperor, China entered a period of little central control and growing provincial warlordism that lasted until 'the second Chinese revolution' and the establishment of the Nationalist (Guomindang) government in Nanjing in 1928. Under these circumstances, new Western-medical institutions were necessarily local in character, the majority being funded by private individuals or missionary societies. During the period 1912-27, three medical schools were set up by the national government and funded by the Ministry of Education, two more were established by provincial authorities; additionally, there were five private medical schools and seven that were run by missionary societies. The Peking Union Medical College, originally a mission school but from 1921 operated by the Rockefeller Foundation, was five times as well funded as its nearest rival, the Shandong Christian University

Medical School in Jinan.[12] In general, the foreign-run medical schools were better-funded and taught larger numbers of students, so that, by the time a central government under Chiang Kai-shek was re-established in Nanjing in 1928, foreigners had trained the majority of the Western-medical elite. Since the foreigners were still in control of China's international medical responsibilities (railway, customs, and quarantine medical officers), the only way the Chinese medical associations could hope to achieve international recognition for their members was by imposing membership qualifications that were at least as strict as those employed in the West.

In this regard, it is also important to remember that there was no universal medical licensing system in China. It was still possible for anyone to claim to be a doctor of Western medicine, so the strict entry qualifications of medical associations like the NMA were the only available guarantees of professional competence. This is in spite of the fact that regulations had been issued by the Ministry of Internal Affairs (*neizheng bu* 內政部) in 1922 that were intended to register all practising physicians as either 'physicians' (*yishi* 醫師) or 'medical scholars' (also pronounced *yishi* 醫士). The former would be qualified for government employment and to issue death certificates, and they could obtain a licence upon producing a graduation certificate from any college of Western medicine in China or abroad, or a certificate stating that they had practised medicine in a foreign hospital for at least three years. The age qualification for such doctors of Western medicine was at least twenty years. To be issued a licence to practise Chinese medicine, applicants had to be over twenty-five years of age and to have either graduated from a school of Chinese medicine, practised in a Chinese-medical or Western-medical hospital or clinic for over three years, or practised privately for over five.[13] Although some local administrations may have attempted to persuade doctors to register for these licences, there is no evidence of enforcement. The regulations are not even included in a recent compilation of medical laws enacted during the Republican period.[14] In January 1929, the Ministry of Health also issued 'Provisional Regulations on Doctors,' which empowered local police departments to register only medical school graduates, disqualifying others from practising Western medicine. Surprisingly, all the Western-medical associations opposed these regulations. Xu Xiaoqun argues that their opposition was grounded in the competition for patients between doctors of Chinese and doctors of Western medicine. Western-trained physicians feared that Western medical practice in general would lose market share to Chinese medicine if doctors who lacked formal Western-medical qualifications (such as Ding Fubao, for example) were barred from practice.[15] The primacy of the competition between Chinese-style and Western-style practitioners over efforts to maintain professional standards in Western-style practice is also borne out by the case of Chinese-medical activist Ding Ganren, who, in 1925, succeeded in having his Technical College of Chinese Medicine (*Zhongguo yiyao zhuan-men xuexiao* 中國醫藥專門學校) approved by the government in spite of the fact that it clearly did not measure up to the criteria for the appellation 'technical college.' In response, the *Republican Medical Journal* published a furious editorial complaining bitterly about the arbitrary way in which the regulations were administered.[16] In such an unpredictable political environment, with frequent cabinet and government changes, there was little hope of effective government intervention to regulate the practice of medicine of any kind.

The re-establishment of a central government in 1928 was the opportunity the medical world had been waiting for. Both traditional Chinese physicians and Western-trained medics demanded state support, although initially only Western medicine continued to be recognized by the new Nanjing regime. However, Western physicians lacked a single representative organization. They were still organized into three different professional associations: the China Medical Association (CMA), formerly the China Medical Missionary Association, for Western medical missionaries, secular doctors, and Chinese graduates of foreign or approved Far Eastern medical schools; the Chinese-run National Medical Association (*Zhonghua yixue hui*), run predominantly for Chinese graduates of British- and American-run medical schools; and the Chinese Medical and Pharmaceutical Association (CMPA) (*Zhonghua minguo yiyaoxue hui*) for graduates of Japanese-run medical schools.

Even before this point, however, signs of trouble had appeared for the CMA and the CMPA. Although Japan had been the foreign educational environment of choice for many Chinese during the first decade of the twentieth century, after the Japanese issued their Twenty-One Demands near the beginning of the First World War, attempting to force China's acceptance of a much increased imperialist presence in China, Chinese public opinion hardened against Japan. Far fewer students went to study there, and Japanese schools in central China (i.e., outside of Manchuria) had increasing difficulty in recruiting students at all.[17] The May Fourth Incident of 1919, in which students and workers protested the Paris Peace Conference's decision to award Germany's former properties and concessions in China to Japan, led to the Chinese delegation's refusal to sign the Versailles Treaty. Following this, the protest movement expanded into a broad-based effort to advance literacy and the use of the vernacular (*baihua* 白話) in written Chinese, modernize education to include science and foreign languages, and promote resistance to imperialism, particularly Japanese imperialism.

Accordingly, membership in the CMPA for Japanese-trained graduates stagnated. Anti-Japanese sentiment grew into anti-foreign sentiment in China after 30 May 1925, when British police in Shanghai opened fire on a student-worker demonstration, killing nine Chinese. Further demonstrations against this 'May Thirtieth Incident' resulted in more deaths and widespread Chinese strikes against all foreign goods. (The diplomatic corps in Beijing had rejected a Chinese accusation against Britain, blaming the demonstrators instead. Chinese indignation was therefore extended to all foreign powers.) It was in this atmosphere of general anti-foreign feeling, on 9 July 1925, that the president of the CMPA, Hou Ximin, published a plea for the merger of his shrinking society with the National Medical Association. He suggested that the combined influence of these associations would benefit both.[18]

Hou's view of events seems to have been right, since some traditional Chinese physicians claimed that the same May Thirtieth Incident of 1925 had turned public opinion against foreign medicine in general and in their favour.[19] However, the NMA made no move to cooperate with its Japanese-trained colleagues until 1928. This is significant because it was in October of 1928 that the new Nationalist government, with Chiang Kai-shek as its president, was inaugurated in Nanjing. Suddenly there was a real advantage to be had in presenting the case for Western medicine with one voice, devoid of imperialist allegiances. The Seventh Biennial Conference of the National Medical Association, held in late January 1928, had been attended by many of the members of the CMPA and had resolved to create a joint committee to work on the proposed amalgamation of the two societies. This was achieved in 1930.[20] When the new Ministry of Health was established in late 1928, the NMA further recommended that the government appoint an intermediary body, the General Medical Council, to supervise and regulate Western medical practice in China.[21]

The government declined to follow the NMA's advice and, instead, issued legislation governing the registration of medical practitioners, which was promulgated on 15 January 1929. The Western medical community was especially offended by the infringements of its professional autonomy in Articles 12 and 17, which required physicians to keep a record book of all patients and treatments for at least five years, and to allow local authorities and patients' relatives to see these records. Article 20 obliged physicians to comply 'with whatever instructions may be given them by the Court, Department of Public Safety or other local governmental organizations.' The commissioner of health in Shanghai promptly used this article to fix a limit to the fees doctors and surgeons were allowed to charge. The doctors were furious and called a national conference in Shanghai in October 1929, at which they convened the new Medical Federation of China 'as a permanent association to protect the rights of its members.' The federation was open to all Western medical graduates, wherever trained.

At this juncture, the Ministry of Health 'expressed a desire to see a unification of the various medical forces of this country so that the Government [could] deal with one compact organisation instead of several diversified elements.'[22] Wu Lien-teh's report on the next conference of the NMA in February 1930 reveals that, although the Rockefeller Foundation had contributed a grant to be used to further the amalgamation of the CMA with the NMA, this had not yet been achieved. In fact, this last unification of the two remaining associations was finally accomplished during 1932, their combined journal appearing in Chinese and English for the first time in January and the first joint conference convening at the end of September.[23] The CMA had had a membership of seven hundred, of whom about one hundred were Chinese. The NMA had been almost exclusively for Chinese, of whom, in 1931, 449 had trained in mission schools in China or in the Rockefeller-funded Peking Union Medical College (eighty-nine members), whereas 197 had trained in mainly Chinese-run schools (some schools changed hands during the period). Seventy-nine members had qualified in the United States or Canada, 34 in the United Kingdom, 15 in Germany, 13 in Japan, 5 in France, and 1 in each of Russia and Korea.[24] The new association was called the Chinese Medical Association in English, though the Chinese name remained the same as that of its Chinese parent society, *Zhonghua yixue hui*, which had previously been referred to in English as the National Medical Association.

The Western medical profession had now achieved a single voice with which to negotiate with the government. This was necessary since the government was far from unanimous in its support for Western medicine. In 1930, for instance, supporters of traditional Chinese medicine had obtained funds for the establishment of the Institute of National (i.e., 'traditional' Chinese) Medicine, much against the wishes of the Western profession. The new CMA did, however, successfully lobby against awarding the Institute of National Medicine administrative control of Chinese-medical education and licensing.

At the second conference of the new CMA in Nanjing in April 1934, Education Minister Wang Shijie announced some explicit criticisms of the Western medicine community. He berated Western-medical doctors for having lower standards of medical ethics than their traditional counterparts. The Chinese ideal was that a physician should treat poor patients for nothing and never accept a larger fee than a family could afford. Western-medical doctors, on the other hand, preferred to live in the large cities, where they could grow wealthy by treating only the urban rich. None was prepared to work in the rural areas, so that these were almost completely without modern medical care. Western drugs were also too expensive for most Chinese. While personally accepting responsibility for raising educational standards, he urged the association to exert itself to keep prices down and ethical standards up. The CMA, however, was more interested in pressing for changes in the regulations governing the availability of corpses for autopsy.[25]

Even after uniting in defence of their common purpose, professional autonomy, the fifteen hundred members of the new CMA continued to be influenced by their nationality and medical provenance. For instance, nearly all physicians of Western medicine who were prepared to work in the rural areas during the Nanjing Decade of 1928-37 were missionary doctors. Likewise, official public health initiatives in rural areas, although mainly staffed by Chinese and supported by the Ministry of Health, were run either by foreign or missionary institutions or by the Mass Education Movement under James Y.C. Yen, who was funded by the American YMCA.[26]

By contrast, the *Chinese Recorder* reported in 1937 that, in the cities, 'the inevitable competition between government and mission hospitals' was beginning to be felt.[27] The report continued: 'Nearly all mission hospitals are handicapped by small poorly paid staffs and the necessity of being self-supporting while government institutions at present are coasting along on large subsidies.'

Thus, on the eve of the Japanese invasion of 1937 that ended China's decade of national reconstruction, it is clear that those Chinese who had chosen a Western medical education had done very well for themselves. They enjoyed high incomes in city practices and staffed nearly all of the central government's health posts. They had succeeded in creating a role in the creation and maintenance of the new modernizing China. The best of the Western-trained Chinese doctors had made themselves into legitimate members of China's new mandarinate, thereby improving the Chinese government's international reputation. To borrow Eliot Freidson's words, the Chinese profession of Western medicine had succeeded in persuading the governing elite that there was special (political and economic as well as medical) value in its work.[28] However, the profession as a whole was concentrated in the large cities of China, where the most money was to be made. The members of the Nationalist administration during the Nanjing Decade, however, were far from united in their support for only Western medicine, and little progress had been made in the licensing of medical practitioners. It remained the case that anyone could practise medicine, and even call him or herself a doctor of Western medicine, without much fear of official censure.[29] In these respects, the government clearly regarded the practice of modern medicine as less vital to national survival than modern law, which it regulated much more rigorously.[30]

As Dr. Wu Lien-teh put it for the most Westernized city in China, Shanghai, in 1934:

> Although a medical register is now kept by the Health Commissioner of the International Settlement containing a list of about 900 practitioners, who voluntarily register themselves, the authorities still have no power to discipline those who behave unprofessionally, as is done in other countries. The result is that the newspapers, both foreign and Chinese, publish regularly the names of all sorts of 'specialists,' some of whom 'guarantee' cures – for a consideration of course. This should not be allowed.[31]

At the same time, a united association of practitioners of Western medicine was useful when the government wanted to parade a modern China before the imperial powers. Building on the work done to promote public health as a tool of the state (see Chapter 5), the establishment of the Chinese Quarantine Service shows the value of Western-medical connections. We conclude this look at Western-medical institutions with the story of this service.

The Chinese Quarantine Service

Before the inauguration of the Chinese Quarantine Service on 30 June 1930, quarantine inspections at Chinese ports had been carried out on an ad hoc basis by the port medical officers of the Chinese Customs. These port medical officers, almost always British, had been assumed to have the formal status of port health officers and therefore to have both the right to inspect passengers and shipping and the responsibility to enforce quarantine restrictions in cases of infectious disease. The fact that this was a mistaken assumption is spelled out clearly in a memorandum of September 1931, written by Frederick Maze, inspector-general of Chinese Customs, in which he also instructed port commissioners and medical officers to hand over control of quarantine organization to Dr. Wu Lien-teh, the service director under the National Health Administration of the Ministry of the Interior, when requested to do so.[32]

China had no ports that met international standards for inspection and quarantine of shipping until the 1930s, with the exception of Shanghai, which boasted a rudimentary thirty-bed quarantine hospital erected in 1912 and the services of a private company that carried out fumigation and disinfection.[33] The reason for this apparent indifference was to be found in the 1842 Treaty of Nanking (Nanjing) and in later treaties, which gave exemption from Chinese jurisdiction (i.e., extraterritoriality) to all nationals of the signatory states *and their goods.* As a result, the Chinese government had no right to impose quarantine restrictions on foreign shipping. When a severe cholera outbreak occurred in Indochina in 1873, the foreign commissioners of Chinese Customs at Amoy (present-day Xiamen) and Shanghai drew up regulations for inspection and quarantine of all vessels. These regulations, ratified by the foreign consuls the following year, became the sanitary guidelines for the containment of cholera at all treaty ports up until the Chinese Revolution of 1911. The authority to decide which ports were to be considered infected and acted on was ceded to the superintendent of Chinese Customs and the foreign consuls at each port. Although all employees of the Customs Service were nominally in the service of the Chinese government, foreigners filled the positions of customs commissioners and port health officers. Quarantine and other preventive measures against disease in China thereby became the exclusive prerogative of foreigners. The Customs Service medical officers were able to make large profits from their charges both to ships and to individual emigrating Chinese for certificates of good health. They generally blocked the employment of Chinese doctors who had qualified in China on the grounds that their training was inadequate.[34]

At first, the Chinese Revolution of 1911 made little difference to these arrangements. Extraterritoriality for foreigners continued, making Chinese enforcement of epidemic control measures on foreign shipping virtually impossible. The lack of an effective authority meant that no one was prepared to build the necessary hospitals or to buy disinfecting equipment. Even when Customs proposed measures for particular ports, they were likely to be rejected by the local 'consular body,' for instance on the grounds that quarantine measures discriminated against foreign trade when the volume of local Chinese shipping (mainly junk traffic) was so much greater and impossible to control.[35]

This lack of Chinese action to control cholera excited little controversy until after the First World War. It was the impressive modernization of Japan's quarantine and public health services before and during the First World War, most visible to the international community in the form of Japan's Red Cross Society, that provided an unfavourable contrast with the Chinese case. In 1921, a Japanese delegate to the League of Nations Health Committee suggested that the Health Section of the League Secretariat survey the incidence of epidemic diseases and the provisions for quarantine in the Far East. Japan, eager for recognition as a modern world power, clearly wished to display its own modern public health facilities to the international community. Acting on this suggestion, Dr. Norman White was sent to conduct such a survey. The resulting 1923 report noted the relative lack of sanitary facilities at most Chinese ports, leading the League to establish the Far Eastern Epidemiological Bureau at Singapore for the purpose of collating and broadcasting information to international shipping on the incidence of infectious disease throughout East Asia.[36]

After Chiang Kai-shek formed the Nationalist government, the vice-minister of the new Ministry of Health, Dr. J. Heng Liu – a graduate of Harvard Medical School – invited Dr. Ludwik Rajchman, director of the Health Section of the League of Nations, to join a new 'international advisory council' established by the Chinese Ministry of Health in 1929. Liu hoped to build on Dr. White's work by conducting a 'sanitary mission' on behalf of the League of Nations into port health and maritime quarantine in China.

Liu was anxious to gain the approval of the treaty powers for a new Chinese-run national quarantine service as a prerequisite for the return of the Customs Service to Chinese control and, thence, to Chinese recovery of tariff autonomy (the right to set its own levels of taxes, including import and export levies). The Customs Service was the source of fully 50 percent of the income of the new Nanjing government,[37] but, if the Chinese were to regain control of its administration, they would have to convince the treaty powers of their competence in preventing the spread of epidemic diseases from their ports. The new Quarantine Service's efforts at preventing the spread of cholera may legitimately be regarded as an important and integral part of Nationalist China's rights recovery movement. The officers of the League were also told that the new Quarantine Service 'would serve as a nucleus for the setting-up of a modern public health service.'[38]

Rajchman visited in 1929 and, as a result of his report, the League assumed an advisory and training role in the establishment of the Chinese National Quarantine Service. It also advised China on other model public health initiatives, such as the Central Field Health Station, devoted to experimenting with ways of providing and funding rural health care, and the Central Hospital in Nanking, a model training and research centre for medical personnel. Wu Lien-teh drew up the blueprint for the new National Quarantine Service with the help of Dr. C.L. Park, a previous head of Australia's Quarantine Service then serving as the chief of the Epidemiological Section of the League of Nations, which oversaw the inauguration of the service.[39] The regulations of the service were modelled on the 1926 International Sanitary Convention of Paris.[40] In other words, the Chinese government used the League advisors as guarantors of the standard of those essential medical services that were of interest to the international community.

The nations of the League, for their parts, were primarily concerned with preventing the importation of cholera from Chinese shipping. The *North China Herald* quotes from the published correspondence from Rajchman to Chinese health minister Liu: 'The continued prevalence of cholera in Shanghai during the last 25 years (on 15 occasions in 25 years) is a serious pre-occupation of the sanitary administrations of various countries, particularly since 1919, when cholera broke out in every year except 1924 and 1928.'[41]

One of Rajchman's chief preoccupations on behalf of the League was to have *foreign-trained* Chinese officials at the head of the new quarantine administration. His correspondence specified several names of people he wished to see appointed, all of whom had been trained abroad.[42] This was no particular insult to the Chinese government of the day since many of its ministers were also graduates of foreign universities.[43]

So, on 1 July 1930, the National Quarantine Service of the Republic of China was established, at first taking over responsibility only for Shanghai (the source of half the Customs Service revenue), other ports being successfully phased in over the next two years. The Service, like most other 'modernizing' projects in Republican China, was funded with revenue from the Maritime Customs. As mentioned, foreigners ran the Maritime Customs in the name of the Chinese government, and it constituted one of the very few sources of income available to the Chinese state that were reliable enough to be used as security against development loans from foreign banks.[44] The head of the Quarantine Service, Wu Lien-teh, was ideally qualified for this high-profile post, in which effective epidemic containment was again – as in Manchuria two decades previously – very much a political tool with which to prove China's administrative competence.

Although Wu's many publications in English rarely mention the political implications of his medical work (his English-speaking audience being more interested in scientific competence than in Chinese national sovereignty), in Chinese he was more explicit. Already in 1915 he had castigated his compatriots for not adopting modern methods of epidemic prevention and educating a better class of modern physician. He stressed the importance of the roles of Customs Service medical officers and railway and port medical officers, and pointed out how foreign physicians almost always occupied these posts in China because Westerners considered graduates of medical colleges in China to be inadequately qualified. With better-educated doctors, he said, other nations would acknowledge their competence and: 'Through the positions of customs service, railway and port medical officers, we will be able to regain national sovereignty.'[45]

One of Wu's first actions on taking up his duties was to treat the managers of all the international shipping companies based in Shanghai to a ceremonial dinner, during which he paraded his own qualifications and those of his staff. He also explained to his guests the new procedures to be followed in order to clear customs and assured them of the speed with which these would be carried out.[46] This propaganda exercise was necessary because 'foreign shipowners looked upon these services as non-Chinese and were loath to see them transferred by the Government of China to the Ministry of Health.'[47]

Thus it was the concern to regain control over territory and the lucrative Customs Service that lay at the heart of Chinese efforts to convince the foreign community of Chinese competence in Western methods of disease control. However, since the main danger of epidemic spread came from cholera, which broke out among the local inhabitants of Chinese ports nearly annually, the Chinese government and its new Quarantine Service were soon persuaded of the necessity of diverting some of their attention to domestic cholera prevention. In Shanghai, under the leadership (again) of Dr. Wu Lien-teh, the different municipal authorities of the International Settlement, the French Concession, and the Chinese city all agreed to coordinate their prophylactic efforts under the single umbrella of the Shanghai Central Cholera Bureau, funded by all three municipalities and with extra funds from the Ministry of Health.[48]

Transferring responsibility for quarantine inspection and port health matters to China was a great success both for the nascent Chinese profession of Western medicine and for the Nationalist government. By 1933, the government had regained full control over the Maritime Customs Service as well as the Salt Revenue Administration and the Chinese Post Office, and it was then able to exert full tariff autonomy. Even after the headquarters of the Quarantine Service were destroyed in the Japanese bombing of Shanghai in 1932, Wu Lien-teh was quick to re-establish operations. Originally, it had been planned to assume control of quarantine inspection at all Chinese treaty ports within two years. In fact, even allowing for the Japanese bombardment of Shanghai and invasion of Manchuria, it took only three years to effect the transfer of responsibility, starting with Shanghai in 1930. During the period from 1928 to 1937, the Chinese government also succeeded in having the treaty port status of twenty of the original thirty-three foreign concessionary areas withdrawn, thereby returning them to Chinese control. However, with the escalation of Japanese aggression, the government decided that it would be wiser to leave the remaining thirteen ports under foreign sovereignty as a brake on future Japanese action. Further talks with the Western powers on the renegotiation of the 'unequal treaties' were quietly suspended in 1932.[49]

The New Institutions of Chinese Medicine

Before the Communist era, much of the Chinese literature about the new societies, journals, schools, and hospitals in China was devoted to discussion of *Western* medicine. The theories, practices, and institutions of Western medicine constituted the external standard to which all innovations in Chinese medicine were compared. The fact that Western medicine often came off the worse in these comparisons did not change its status as the standard of reference.

The driving force behind the institutionalization of Chinese medicine was not Western medicine as such, however. In several cases, Chinese who disapproved of Western medicine established Chinese-medical schools, as we saw Zhang Xichun doing in the previous chapter. As with the advance of Western-medical ideas in China, these institutional innovations were primarily propelled by an ideology of modernization that involved the establishment of professional standards in several walks of life. The widespread popularity of social Darwinism had become tied to the idea of civilizational progress and also to a fear of racial degeneration. Chinese concern for the standardization of medicine was particularly driven by a desire to improve the health of the Chinese race, which was perceived as being in a dangerous state of decline.[50] We have seen how these ideologies influenced the development of Western-medical institutions in China, but they also affected Chinese perceptions of how best to develop Chinese medicine.

There were few formal institutions for teaching Chinese medicine in Imperial China. All kinds of medical specialists, from the illiterate itinerant to the local midwife and the scholar-physician, tended to acquire practical medical knowledge through teacher-pupil relationships that sometimes had the character of formal apprenticeships (*yishi daitu* 以師帶徒). For a literate Chinese physician, medical authority rested ultimately on the correct interpretation of the ancient canonical works. These works gave rise to a large body of exegetical and supplementary literature. Most medical authors presented themselves as relying on at least one of the canonical works in significant ways. The considerable variation both within and between canonical texts allowed for a variety of approaches to etiology and therapy, and also for significant innovations. Transmission of the knowledge, both canonical and derivative, contained in these texts was a kind of 'vertical' transmission from teacher to pupil that was closely modelled on family structures and that was often superimposed on them.[51] Members of each medical lineage had an obligation to preserve and pass on the learning of their teachers to worthy successors. Because of this, even the medical authority enshrined in the canons was expressed in decidedly local variants. In this sense, it is common to speak of the currents of medicine of different regions and famous physician-teachers.[52]

Another path to scholarly medicine was through self-study of the medical classics and commentaries. A general interest in practical topics such as medicine was expected of the scholarly gentleman, and the biographies of many famous physicians state that they started their careers as aspiring bureaucrats, only later moving to medicine, often after failing the imperial civil service examinations or after tending sick parents. The Chinese scholars Liu Xiaobin and Deng Tietao found that, of 157 physicians in Qing dynasty Guangdong Province, 51 percent had studied with a teacher as a planned route to a medical occupation and another 27 percent were found to be 'Confucian physicians' (*ruyi*), that is, individuals who practised medicine only after first acquiring a scholarly education. They further argued that the many theoretical medical works produced during the Qing were often written with the express purpose of instructing pupils or apprentices. For example, the physician Chen Dingtai 陳定泰, whose only book was published in 1844, is known to have taught his four sons and at least twenty-seven other pupils from it.[53]

The Imperial Medical Academy (*Tai yi yuan* 太醫院) in the Forbidden City was of course a major exception to these generalizations. At the beginning of the Qing dynasty in 1644, eleven medical specialties were taught there: major disorders, minor disorders, cold-damage disorders, women's medicine, ulcers, acupuncture, ophthalmology, dentistry, throat medicine, bone-setting, and pox treatment.[54] This list differed from that taught under the previous dynasty, the Ming (1368-1644), in that pox treatment was new and the three disciplines of military traumatology, 'incantation therapy,' and massage had been deleted from the curriculum.[55] In 1799, pox treatment was subsumed under 'minor disorders,' and throat medicine and dentistry were combined into one subdiscipline. In 1822, acupuncture was removed from the curriculum and its practice discontinued within the Forbidden City, an event to which we will return in the next chapter.[56]

In addition to the Imperial Medical Academy, Zhu Chao notes that the *Statutes and Ordinances of the Qing Dynasty* (*Daqing hui dian* 大清會典) initially provided for medical schools throughout the empire at the prefecture, provincial, and county levels. All three levels of school were to teach from the *Annotated Commentary to the Yellow Emperor's [Inner Canon]* (*Neijing zhushi* 內經諸釋), the *Treatise on Cold Damage* (*Shanghan lun* 傷寒論), and the *Systematic Materia Medica* (*Bencao gangmu* 本草綱目).[57] However, there appear to be no records of these institutions in action, and they are not mentioned in other histories of Chinese medicine.

Starting in the late nineteenth century, new, privately run schools for teaching Chinese medicine alongside pre-clinical Western sciences such as anatomy and physiology began to emerge. By the first years of the twentieth century, medical societies with the aims of reforming and protecting Chinese medicine and teaching basic Western medicine were also starting to be established, as were the first medical journals in Chinese (which had the same aims). The rise of these new Chinese-medical institutions took place in the broader context of the period's educational politics.

The period of the 'self-strengthening movement' (1860-95) saw the establishment of the first modern school of Chinese medicine, the *Liji Yixuetang* 利濟醫學堂, founded in Ruian County, Zhejiang Province, in 1885 by Chen Qiu 陳虬 (1851-1904). The school published its own textbooks and issued its students the *Catalogue of Medical Texts*, which included descriptions of forty-eight Western medical titles along with over a hundred Chinese medical works. The college's journal also included reviews of Western medical works in Chinese translation.

This school had a strict examination system and, in the ten or so years of its operation certified over three hundred graduates. Although the teaching included the subject 'organ appearance' (*zangxiang* 臟像), there is now no way of knowing for certain whether this interest in the shape of the organs derived from the new Western anatomical translations. What is certain is that the course duration of five or six years, and the attempt to establish the status of the school's graduates with certificates, heralded the beginning of a long struggle to establish professional status for the literate, elite practitioners of Chinese medicine in the private sector.[58]

Another school established during this period was the Jiangxi Modern School of Chinese Medicine (*Jiangxi zhongyi xuetang* 江西中醫學堂), established in Nanchang in 1901 by Chen Rixin 陳日新, a secretary (*zhushi* 主事, usually ranked 6a) on the Qing Board of Punishments. This school was run until its closure in 1906 as an official technical school under the same system as that devised for the new Metropolitan University in Beijing. The constitution of the school stated the relationship between Chinese and Western medicine very clearly: 'There are two kinds of medical works: Chinese-medical and Western-medical. Where the art has been lost in Chinese medicine, use Western learning to restore it; where Chinese learning is incomplete, use Western learning to supplement it. The task is to apply Western learning in the service of Chinese medicine, and not the other way around.'[59] The curriculum taught eight classes from different Chinese medical texts, plus the 'Western' subjects of chemistry, anatomy, optics, acoustics, pharmacology, *qixue* 氣學 (likely physics), and *rexue* 熱學 (literally, 'heat studies,' or calorimetry), also a physical science.[60]

The models for the next generation of schools of Chinese medicine were to come from the modern school system established in China as part of the New Policies of 1901-11. Ever since China's defeat in the Sino-French War of 1885, which was fought over control of Indo-China, some high officials had started to argue that the scope of the self-strengthening movement was not broad enough to effect the military and organizational modernization necessary to withstand foreign imperialism. These criticisms became widespread after China's defeat in the Sino-Japanese War in 1895 and led directly to the abortive 'Hundred Days Reform' of 1898. As Jerome Ch'en puts it:

> Summing up the state of Western studies in China, Liang Ch'i-ch'ao [Liang Qichao] compiled and published his *Catalogue of Books on the West (Hsi-hsüeh shu-mu piao)* in 1896, a year after China's defeat by Japan and a year after the first publication in a limited edition of Yen Fu's translation of Thomas Huxley's *Essays on Evolution and Ethics.* The defeat made the Chinese mind more receptive to new ideas and theories and Yen's exquisite style made social Darwinism more appealing. The impact of both the defeat and of the theory of evolution was shattering. China suddenly found that she was only one of many states in the world, and to make things even worse, she was not even 'fit to survive' in the Darwinian sense.[61]

However rude the awakening to China's literati, it was the fact that a foreign allied expeditionary force relieved Beijing from the Boxer Rebellion in 1900, forcing the court to retreat to Xi'an and leading to capitulation to foreign demands and the payment of a crippling indemnity, that finally persuaded the Chinese government of the modernizing imperative. Widespread reforms were announced on 29 January 1901, and in November of that year instructions were issued calling for all traditional academies (*shuyuan* 書院) to be converted into modern schools (*xuetang* 學堂) and to teach a broader range of subjects, including geography, foreign languages, and modern science. The modern schools were no longer to train students in the composition of the 'eight-legged essay,' the required compositional form for the imperial civil service exams.[62] Beijing's new Metropolitan University, founded in 1898, was reorganized in 1902 as the highest institution in the new education system, with seven faculties, one of which was medicine.[63] In fact, the medical curriculum at the university was almost entirely Western, with only one of twenty-nine medical courses and one of seventeen pharmacy courses devoted to Chinese medicine.[64]

While the traditional civil service examination system persisted, students in the new schools who had ambitions of government employment were in a difficult position. As Reynolds notes, 'for three or four months at a time during civil service examination periods, ambitious students would absent themselves from their *xuetang* ... in order to return to their provinces to sit for the provincial examinations of that year.'[65] However, in September of 1905, at the urging of Zhang Zhidong, Yuan Shikai, and others, an imperial edict abolished the examinations system. From 1906 on, official employment would be on the basis of the candidate's qualifications, as attested by diplomas and graduation certificates. In that year, each province was also obliged to appoint a commissioner of education, all of whom were promptly sent to Japan for a study tour. In fact, the whole new educational system was closely modelled on Japan's, which had drawn heavily from the German example.[66]

This new educational system, created to promote practical studies (*shixue*) such as mathematics and science, was the critical stimulus to the Chinese-medical world. When it became clear that qualifications gained in the new 'modern schools' were to be the only measures of competence that the government would recognize (apart from degrees gained at foreign institutions), state recognition of these schools became crucial both to the viability of the schools and to the employment prospects of graduates. Thus, for reasons of status, it suddenly became imperative that Chinese medicine be taught in schools in which a significant section of the curriculum was devoted to such modern subjects as anatomy, pathology, foreign languages, and physical education.

Further institutionalization of Chinese medicine proceeded fairly slowly and along differing paths. For example, in Hong Kong a consortium of Chinese guilds had been running the Tung Wah Hospital of Chinese medicine since 1870. This consortium had even briefly experimented with a scheme to train students in Chinese and Western medicine on the premises.[67] Just north of Hong Kong, in Guangdong Province, Western medicine had its highest presence, with nine hospitals of Western medicine (all established before 1911), twenty-five Western medical translations published locally and in circulation, and more Western physicians than in any other province.[68] Here, one of the first new educational institutions for Chinese medicine was founded in 1906. The Guangdong Medical Benevolent Society (*Guangdong yixue qiuyishe* 廣東醫學求益社) was organized by a group of Confucian physicians and

philanthropic associations from Nanhai County with the aim of promoting Chinese medicine. While the establishment of the society clearly
reflected the native-place association of ten out of the eleven founding
members, its principles declared more far-reaching ambitions: 'Although
initiated by locals of Nanhai County, in fact [this society] is established
with the intention of promoting world medicine, and protecting and
preserving Chinese medicine and the national essence.'[69]

Although this society was not a formal medical college but, rather,
a cooperative teaching institution, it is noteworthy for its aims and for
the Western medical content of its activities. On the first of every month
all members were sent three essay questions, two based on the classical
Chinese medical texts and the third relying on familiarity with Western
medicine. Society members could choose to answer one or more of
the questions, with the member who wrote the best essay for a given
month becoming the examiner of the next month's essays. Every year,
the society published the five best essays from each month for internal
circulation to all its members.[70] The society had a flourishing membership in Guangzhou and was the parent organization of several later
medical colleges throughout the Republican period. These colleges
relied for their establishment on financial support from the same
philanthropic organizations as did the Guangdong Medical Benevolent Society.[71]

Xu Xiaoqun's study of the rise of professional associations in Shanghai shows the establishment, in 1904, of an early but short-lived society
whose purpose was to improve native medicine. In 1908, its founder,
Li Pingshu, went on to organize a private hospital in Shanghai, which
employed doctors of both Western medicine and Chinese medicine and
was funded by local merchants and gentry.[72]

The idea of establishing medical societies to improve the exchange
of knowledge between Chinese and Western-style physicians was apparently promoted by the Qing government. In January 1906, an edict stated
that the promotion of medical education was important for the state,
but it admitted that the government lacked the funds to establish medical
schools. Therefore, regional governors were to promote the establishment of medical societies for the exchange of views between Chinese

and Western medicine. This measure would both promote hygiene and strengthen the people.[73]

The question of how to improve the status of Chinese medicine became more acute after the establishment of the Republic of China on 1 January 1912. Symbolizing its attitude towards modernization, the new Republican government adopted the Western calendar and founded the Republic of China on the first day of the Western year. This new government was much more uncritically scientistic than its Manchu predecessor and drew up a new set of regulations for the national educational system. Chinese medicine was not one of the subjects to receive official support, even in the form of a nominal class offered in government medical schools, as had been the case in the late Qing. So, in late 1913, representatives of many of the new Chinese-medical associations from nineteen provinces across China, organized by the All-China Medical and Pharmaceutical Association (*Shenzhou yiyaoxue zonghui* 神州醫藥學總會), a confederation of several regional medical associations, sent a delegation to Beijing to plead for the inclusion of Chinese medicine in the national educational system and for Chinese-medical schools to qualify for government licences. Education Minister Wang Daxie 汪大燮 (1860-1929), retorted that he had 'decided in future to abolish Chinese medicine and also not to use Chinese drugs,'[74] a remark that has often been taken as the beginning of an official campaign to abolish Chinese medicine.[75] Zhao Hongjun, in his path-breaking study of medical polemics in China, cites other documents describing this encounter, and these suggest that, whatever Minister Wang's personal position may have been, the government's refusal to include Chinese medicine in the national educational system did not imply any intention to abolish Chinese medicine as such. In fact, the Ministry of State issued a statement explicitly rejecting this idea.[76] Chinese medicine was to be left pretty much to itself.

What is clear is that the status of Chinese medicine certainly suffered from the comparison with Western medicine. Even back in 1908, when both the Guangxu emperor and the Empress Dowager Cixi died on 14 and 15 November, respectively, several palace physicians were sacked and a new department of Western medicine, complete with a

Table 1   Establishment of modern schools of Chinese medicine

Date of establishment	No. of schools according to:		
	Zhen and Fu (1991)	*Zhao (1989)*	*Deng and Cheng (2000)*
Before 1912	3	9	7
1912-19	5	8	8
1919-27	10	16	8
1928-37	58	54	33

Western pharmacy, was installed in the Imperial Medical Academy alongside its traditional counterpart.[77] This had deprived Chinese medicine of its official monopoly postion at court, but now the new Republic simply deprived Chinese medicine of any official role at all.

Against this backdrop, advocates of Chinese medicine had to present their case for it as a modern discipline, with students receiving preclinical and clinical teaching and, if possible, practical experience in a clinic or hospital. The aim was not to make Chinese medicine resemble Western medicine but, rather, to establish standards of education that would entitle the holders of the new Chinese-medical school diplomas to professional status and respect. At the same time, new schools of Chinese medicine had to be seen as part of the modernization of China. Since it was virtually impossible for schools of Chinese medicine to obtain a government licence for much of this period, data on the numbers of Chinese-medical schools are bound to be incomplete. However, statistics from three sources reveal clear trends. (Table 1)

These data show that the number of schools of Chinese medicine grew steadily even during the culturally iconoclastic May Fourth Movement, which started in 1919, suggesting that the vocal antagonism towards Chinese medicine in this period had less effect than one might have supposed. After the establishment of the Nanjing government in 1928, however, many more schools were founded, suggesting that Chinese-medical educators were looking to the state to endorse their teaching activities and their graduates' qualifications.

It will come as no surprise that many of these schools taught several Western scientific subjects as part of the Chinese-medical curriculum. The Shanghai School of Chinese Medicine taught physiology (*shenglixue* 生理學); the Zhejiang School of Chinese Medicine, founded in Hangzhou in 1916, taught both anatomy (*jiepouxue* 解剖學) and physiology; the Guangdong School of Chinese Medicine and Pharmacy, which started teaching in Guangdong in 1924, taught both Western and Chinese physiology, Western and Chinese diagnostics, anatomy, pathology, chemistry, 'essential Western pharmacy' (*Xiyao gaiyao* 西藥概要), and nursing, along with Japanese language and physical education.[78]

At one extreme was the medical school associated with the Research Society for the Advancement of Chinese Medicine (*Zhongyi gaijin yanjiu hui* 中醫改進研究會). The school, founded in Taiyuan in 1921, had a four-year curriculum that included the essential courses of Western medicine, a full range of Chinese-medical courses, and classes in English, German, and Japanese. Some criticized such a broad approach to Chinese-medical education as being impossibly ambitious.[79] Shanxi governor Yan Xishan 閻錫山 (1883-1960), who was famous throughout China for his efforts to promote primary education and literacy campaigns among adults, funded the school and its hospital to protect the important source of revenue generated by domestic and international trade in Chinese drugs and to improve the people's health by promoting the modern education of Chinese-medical physicians. His interest had been aroused by a three-month stay in a Western hospital, where he saw X-rays, which he said allowed the Westerners to see inside their own bodies like the legendary Daoist adepts of old, and microscopes, which facilitated the detection of otherwise invisible micro-organisms. Western medicine, he said, was like a train, able to cover a thousand *li* in a single day. Even though Chinese medicine could never dream of achieving such rapid progress, by learning particular skills from Western medicine, it could be made 'responsive to world trends and into a systematic science.'[80] The particular skills that Yan thought Chinese physicians ought to learn were as follows: a standardized system of diagnosis, which was to replace the highly personal interpretations of (mainly) pulse diagnosis that prevailed in Chinese medicine; sanitary science, which was to include bacteriology, so that Chinese physicians would be as competent in taking preventive measures against the spread of epidemics as their Western counterparts; surgical skills, including obstetric surgery; the use of diagnostic instruments; and thorough scientific research into each of the traditional specialties of Chinese medicine.[81]

With the teaching of Chinese medicine came the requirement for teaching materials. Obviously, the new scientific subjects – such as anatomy, physiology, and pathology – could be taught straight from specialist textbooks, often translations of Japanese works, which, in some cases, were themselves translations of German texts. The teaching of a scientific Chinese medicine was more complicated, however, and was a recurring subject in the medical press. Although medical students today may be surprised to hear it, Western medical textbooks seemed *simple* to understand when compared with the classical texts of Chinese medicine. However, Zhou Xiaonong 周小農 (1876-1942), one of the younger generation of reformers of Chinese medicine at this time, complained in 1915 that the frequent double translation of Western anatomical books from European languages into Japanese, and then from Japanese into Chinese, could render the medical content incomprehensible.[82] So when, in 1916, He Lianchen announced his intention to publish new textbooks of Chinese medicine with expositions of the medical classics, he received several letters urging him to apply scientific principles to his expositions, to write in the vernacular, and to organize his teaching material in a clear and progressive manner.[83] This may be the beginning of the format of Chinese-medical textbooks so familiar to the student of Chinese medicine today, in which quotations from the classics are usually short and pithy, employed to reinforce an internally consistent formulation of 'Chinese medical theory' that is actually a modern construct.

A further problem for Chinese-medical educators was how to interpret the extensive body of existing medical literature. One solution adopted by the prime movers in the Shaoxing Medical Association, He Lianchen and Qiu Jisheng (whom we met in Chapter 2), was to compile, edit, and republish medical works that had previously been rare or circulated only in manuscript form or that were, in their opinion, of such primary importance that they merited wider circulation. Qiu published a collection of ninety-nine such titles in 1924 under the title *Double Three Medical Books* (*San, san yi shu* 三三醫書). In 1936, he published a second collection of ninety titles, *Compilation of Valuable Medical Works* (*Zhen ben yi shu jicheng* 珍本醫書集成). In the prefatory general principles (*fanli* 凡例) section, he stated that the main criterion for inclusion was 'whether [a book] was entirely suitable for practical use or for reference.' He listed several titles of medical works associated with esoteric medicine and Daoist practices, which, even though they were rare and valuable editions, he had omitted on the grounds of their unsuitability for modern practice.[84] This, too, anticipated the approach of modern Chinese medicine, which eschews association with 'superstitious' healing practices.

Similarly, 1936 saw the publication of *Great Achievements of Chinese Medicine* (*Zhongguo yixue da cheng* 中國醫學大成), compiled by Cao Bingzhang 曹炳章 (1877-1956), whose preface openly discusses the reasons for such large republication projects: 'My intention is that this will succeed in destroying the esoteric arts of national medicine that are secretly transmitted through families. It will launch a new beginning for the great achievements of more than four thousand years of national medicine.'[85]

Cao also devotes space to discussing the many rival theories of disease causation in Chinese medicine. He concludes that the theories prevalent in different dynasties reflect the fact that the 'national *qi*' is different in each age, giving rise to different diseases and therefore different ways of coping with them. 'In recent years,' he writes:

Communications have been increasingly convenient, and the ailments of each locality have travelled rapidly back and forth. The habits and customs of daily life are also very different from of old. As a result, many of the people's ailments were unknown to earlier ages. In this environment, how can it be permissible for physicians to adhere to the ways of 'one lineage, one school of thought'?[86]

Cao, like many of his generation, was concerned to establish recognizable standards in Chinese medicine. This meant turning away from local interpretations of disease in favour of newly constructed universal disease categories (much as had occurred in Western medicine as a result of germ theory: many local 'fevers' were discovered to be caused by the same bacterium and were reclassified accordingly).[87] His compilations of relatively secular medical works from the past attempted to identify a new corpus of semi-canonical literature that would be easily accessible to all students of Chinese medicine and would therefore form part of their shared professional education.

But professional learning is shared not just by common textbooks and professorial teaching but also by keeping current on the state of knowledge and practice, which is one of the roles of the professional journal. Western missionaries introduced periodical publications to China in the mid-nineteenth century along with metallic movable type. Before then, the cost of engraving wooden blocks in order to print would have been too high to support periodical literature.[88] Since the

Table 2   Medical journals founded in China to 1935

Year	Western-medical	Chinese-medical
To 1905	5	2
1906-11 (6 years)	13	7
1912-15 (4 years)	9	7
1916-20 (5 years)	14	7
1921-26 (6 years)	22	15
1927 (1 year)	7	3
1928 (1 year)	10	3
1929 (1 year)	16	11
1930 (1 year)	12	10
1927-30 (4 years)	45	27
1931-35 (5 years)	45	41
Total to 1935 (including journals of unknown launch date)	171 (56.25 %)	133 (43.75 %)

Note: I follow the system used by the authors and categorize the journals into those that espouse Chinese medicine and those that espouse Western medicine. However, it is important to remember that journals of Western medicine were likely to carry articles that discussed the value of Chinese medicine and to publish the most recent results of pharmacological analyses of Chinese drugs, just as journals of Chinese medicine frequently discussed Western-medical subjects.

first wholly Chinese-run medical journal was launched in Guangdong in 1886, we can surmise that, by that time, the cost of producing such literature was within the reach of wealthy Chinese. Thereafter, and especially after the establishment of the Nationalist government in 1928, the number of medical journals mushroomed. Table 2 shows the number of medical journals founded in China to 1935, from data collected by Song and Shen.[89]

The number of new journals of Western medicine increased more quickly than those of Chinese medicine during the May Fourth period (1919-27), which is what one might expect given the scientism of the time. But note the sizeable increase in medical journal publication for both approaches to medicine between 1927 and 1935, roughly corresponding to the Nanjing Decade (1928-37). Although this period witnessed rapid growth in the publishing industry generally, this suggests an increasing market for these publications during a time of relatively consolidated central rule. Once the number of journals of unknown launch date has been added to the total, we see that, although more journals of Western medicine were launched during the Chinese Republic, support for Chinese medicine, as judged by the number of new titles of Chinese-medical journals, remained robust throughout the period. Unfortunately, we have no data for circulation, so it is impossible to estimate the relative size of the audiences for these publications.

Of course, these journals of 'Chinese' medicine differed from their Western-medical counterparts only insofar as their publishers wished to apply the new scientific medicine to the modernization of Chinese medicine. Both groups agreed that the learning of Western medicine was necessary and desirable, but they differed in the extent to which they thought Western medicine should replace Chinese medicine.

The *Shaoxing Journal of Medicine and Pharmacy* provides a fine example of this distinction. This was the first of the journals founded with the explicit aim of promoting Chinese medicine as opposed to explaining the new Western medicine to those with a medical interest. It was published from 1908 in Shaoxing, Zhejiang Province, a place with rich local medical traditions since late imperial times. The first issue defines the desired relationship between Chinese and Western medicine: 'AIMS: This society is devoted to research into Chinese, Western and Japanese medical and pharmaceutical science, taking as its aim the exchange of knowledge and the import of new theories for the purpose of the elaboration and development of China's own medicine and pharmacy.'

The editor, He Lianchen, explained that, with the exception of the *Medical News (Yixue bao)*,[90] there were no journals devoted to explaining Western medicine to the uninitiated. Recently, a Japanese medical journal had become available for sale in China, but its technical language and theoretical complexity made it virtually unintelligible. The aim of the *Shaoxing Journal*, he reiterated, was to 'commend those aspects of national medical learning that were worth preserving, advance those aspects of Western medicine that were worth assimilating, and to carefully edit and collate the relative merits and drawbacks of both Chinese and Western medicine.'[91]

He also discussed other reasons for the formation of the society and for the publication of the journal. These included reforming the contemporary 'corrupt' state of Chinese medicine, with its reliance on such 'absurd doctrines' as the five colours, five tastes, and the movements of the five phases; general ignorance of physiology, pathology, bacteriology, physics, and chemistry; over-reliance on pulse-feeling in diagnosis; belief in demon possession as a cause of epidemics; rote-learning of medical texts; and the adulteration of Chinese drugs.[92] He Lianchen may have been a stalwart and energetic proponent of Chinese medicine, but he and many others were acutely aware of its shortcomings when viewed through the new lenses of modern science.

In fact, journals of Chinese medicine dedicated significant space to discussions of how to rid Chinese medicine of superstition and 'corrupt' practices. During Yuan Shikai's governor-generalship of Zhili (the area around Beijing) and Shandong provinces at the turn of the twentieth century, in a drive to create a secular, modern administration, government agents destroyed or appropriated many temples (with the cooperation of local gentry) in order to house the new schools. This anti-religion, anti-superstition drive was repeated in the lower Yangzi region in the early years of the Nanjing administration (1928 to around 1930).[93] As with public health initiatives, the intended audience for these moves towards secularization was the international community. Prasenjit Duara quotes the 'Standards for Preserving and Abandoning Gods and

Shrines' in the *Collection of Laws of the Chinese Republic* as speaking of 'religious authority as being obsolete in the age of popular sovereignty,' of 'superstition as an obstacle to progress,' and of the superstitious nation becoming 'the laughing stock of the scientific world.'[94]

He Lianchen shared these concerns. His friend and colleague Qiu Jisheng wrote in the *Shaoxing Journal of Medicine and Pharmacy* that, every time He met reputable physicians

> discussing the rise and fall of *yin* and *yang*, the mutual production and control of the Five Phases, the cyclical flow of *qi* and other empty and extravagant talk, he contented himself with real therapeutic measures, and clear and uncomplicated theories ... He often sighed 'How is it that the enlightened physicians of our fatherland are few and solitary like the morning star?'[95]

Specifically, the would-be reformers of Chinese medicine were most concerned to distance themselves from the kind of medical practice that occurred in temples. In many temples, statues of the 'Medicine King' (*yaowang* 藥王), often identified with the Tang dynasty physician Sun Simiao, stood waiting for sufferers' appeals. Other temples and shrines were devoted exclusively to medical deities, and these and many more eclectic temples were host to the divinatory procedures described in Chapter 2. The *Shaoxing Journal of Medicine and Pharmacy* reported in 1917 that the Shaoxing Police Department had prohibited the sale of booklets containing instructions for and interpretations of such divination. The local news urged residents to consult physicians rather than to pray in temples if they were sick, reminding them that, if they did not, they could be fined.[96]

This concern about easily identifiable, temple-based superstition was matched by a much more controversial discussion of whether Five Phase theory was admissible in the new scientific Chinese medicine. The *Shaoxing Journal* contained several articles both for and against during the period between 1908 and 1917. The editorial foreword of the *National Medicine Critic* of 1933 advocated excising such 'unhealthy medicine' as Five Phase theory by 'placing Chinese medicine on the operating table' and 'cutting out these malign tumours.'[97] Perhaps most telling is an article in the *Double Three Medical Journal* of 1925, which cites the great political reformer Liang Qichao as saying: 'Abolition of the unstable and confused Five Phases ... would be a good sign of the progress of medicine.'[98] Indeed, many prominent Chinese-medical authors of the Republican period seem to have come to the same conclusion. The writings of such authors as He Lianchen, Zhu Weiju, Zhang Xichun, and many others are all devoid of any mention of the Five Phases in relation to disease. Chen Bangxian 陳邦賢 (1889-1976), famous for his histories of Chinese medicine, castigated Five Phase theory as 'legend' (*shenhua* 神話) in the first (1919) edition of his history.[99]

By contrast, Yun Tieqiao 惲鐵樵 (1878-1935), a respected Chinese-medical author and teacher, mounted a defence of Five Phase theory. He argued that the Five Phases were cosmologically equivalent to the seasons in ancient Chinese philosophy, so that the organization of the internal organs, senses, and functions of the body into corresponding sets of five had little to do with the actual structures of these objects. The Five Phases were to be best understood as a conceptual framework for medical theory, not as a description of reality. This is an argument frequently rehearsed today, and it is one that finds its apologists in the Western literature on Chinese medicine. Yun Tieqiao appears to have been the first Chinese physician to formulate it.[100]

The First Dictionary of Chinese Medicine

We conclude with an often overlooked institution – the dictionary. Dictionaries codify knowledge. They represent the terms in which knowledge of a field may be discussed at a particular time. What they exclude, what they include, and how they describe their contents provide clues to the accepted knowledge of their compilers and users. We return to Xie Guan, whom we met in Chapter 6, for the first dictionary of Chinese medicine.

The first edition of the *Encyclopaedic Dictionary of Chinese Medicine* (*Zhongguo yixue da cidian* 中國醫學大辭典) appeared in 1921.[101] Although many dictionaries of modern Western medicine as well as bilingual medical dictionaries were in print at this time, it appears that Xie's *Dictionary* was not only the first but also the only such reference work of this kind for Chinese medicine until at least the 1950s.

Published in four volumes, Xie's *Dictionary* contains over seventy thousand entries. He claimed to have referred to over two thousand different works in its compilation, including scattered titles extant only in Korea and Japan. By March 1927, it was already in its fifth printing, and by 1954 it had been reprinted thirty-one times, having sold over a million copies.[102] Reprints of the second edition of 1926 are still readily available. We can safely conclude from this that the work was – and is – a financial success for its publishers, the Commercial Press of Shanghai. Since there were Chinese-medical texts in print before 1921, it seems strange that the first appearance of a dictionary of Chinese medicine should have taken so long. Understanding the activities of its publisher will help explain this anomaly.

The Commercial Press of Shanghai was the largest Chinese publishing company throughout the Republican era, but in 1912 the editor of two of its most successful textbook series left the firm to set up his own press, taking both series with him.[103] The Commercial Press worked hard to recover the lost ground and, in the same year, published the *New Character Dictionary* (*Xin zidian* 新字典) under the editorship of Xie Guan's friend and mentor from Wujin, Lu Erkui 陸爾奎 (1862-1935). This dictionary included many of the new characters coined by missionaries and Japanese to translate scientific terms as well as some characters used to indicate dialect words, which the purely literary dictionaries of the past had ignored. It specifically aimed to replace the 1716 *Kangxi Dictionary* (*Kangxi zidian* 康熙字典), the standard dictionary for the Qing dynasty, in which the character definitions were intended to facilitate comprehension of ancient Chinese texts rather than to reflect current oral usage.[104]

Chief editor Lu Erkui continued with another dictionary project for the Commercial Press that was much more ambitious. The new dictionary was to be the first to give two-character and multi-character words ('colocations,' or 'polymorphemes') as separate entries. This dictionary, the *Word Source* (*Ciyuan* 詞源), published in 1915, represented a major break with the past in this respect since multi-character words were a feature of both spoken Chinese and of the new technical terms but were rare in classical Chinese. However, their frequency in written Chinese had been increasing rapidly as more and more students went to Japan for a modern education and imported the Japanese two- and four-character neologisms back into China. The geography editor for this dictionary project was Lu's old friend Xie Guan.[105]

The Commercial Press was also busy publishing other kinds of dictionary in this period and commissioned Xie to work on one for Chinese medicine. The first edition of Xie Guan's *Dictionary* was compiled by a team of twelve people. Of these, two died of consumption during the project and another four suffered serious illnesses along the way.[106] Xie's project was clearly less well funded than was his friend Lu Erkui's *Ciyuan* project, which took seven years but had a team consisting of over fifty compilers.[107]

The 1921 first edition of the *Encyclopaedic Dictionary of Chinese Medicine* must have run into criticism quite early because Xie quickly decided to carry out a revision, using his students at the Chinese Medical University as collaborators. Their names are listed at the front of the second edition of 1926, whereas those of the members of the Commercial Press staff are not. The second edition also sported a new supplementary character index at the back that used Wang Yunwu's new four-corner method for indexing characters.[108] Even with these revisions, the dictionary's major shortcomings were quickly apparent. One review in the *National Medical Critic* of July 1933 complained that none of the ten or so dictionaries recently produced by the Commercial Press were entirely satisfactory but that the *Encyclopaedic Dictionary of Chinese Medicine* was the worst of the lot.[109]

The reviewer went on to ascribe the problems to the fact that Xie had employed his own students and that students of Chinese medicine were not the best calibre. In fact, he suggested that not a few of them were completely illiterate. Some of the concrete failings of the dictionary included phrases that were seldom referenced to their source. Furthermore, even when a source such as the *Yellow Emperor's Inner Canon* was cited, to give the title of such large works without also referring to the chapter and section from which the dictionary entry was drawn was, in the reviewer's opinion, as good as giving no source at all. As if this were not enough, several of the entries had alternative explanations and meanings that were not recorded in the dictionary; other character entries had been mistaken for similar characters and misinterpreted accordingly; the identities of Chinese herbal drugs were often confused; several of the most important Japanese works of Chinese medicine had been left out altogether; and the old-fashioned phraseology used to explain terms that referred to bodily processes showed a complete ignorance of modern physiology. This aggressively critical attitude can be related to the diametrically opposing strategies of the journal editors and Xie Guan. For the editors of the *National Medical Critic*, only modern science could validate medical knowledge, so the omission of important Japanese treatments of Chinese medicine written by physicians already qualified in Western science was a grave error. Since the editors held Western anatomy and physiology to be self-evidently true, Xie's lack of any concession to these sciences in his explications of classical theoretical terms rendered him, in their eyes, reactionary and backward.

However, this review was not an isolated diatribe from the pens of extremists. Even the writer of the otherwise highly laudatory biographical entry in Zhang Zanchen's *Sketch History of Chinese Medicine through the Ages,* Chen Cunren, wrote that the dictionary failed to match up to the scholarly expectations of the age but that Xie Guan would have had to have spent a lifetime on it in order to silence all his critics. On the issue of modern (Western scientific) knowledge and nomenclature, Xie evidently would not have wanted to try. The first paragraph in the 'User's guide' section of the dictionary states explicitly that dictionary entries would be restricted to those occurring in 'China's original medical works.' It is clear that Xie was consistent in sticking to his traditional guns.

Despite its shortcomings, Xie Guan's *Encyclopaedic Dictionary of Chinese Medicine* sold well and must have represented quite a financial success. This can partly be accounted for by the extensive distribution system of the Commercial Press, but the work also clearly filled a niche in the market. It was the first, and for a long time the only, dictionary of Chinese medicine. As such it was an innovation in the Chinese-medical world. Yet by looking at Xie's career and opinions, we can conclude that his dictionary was a tool for the entrenchment of a particular kind of traditional scholarship. Intended to codify Chinese medical knowledge as a kind of national heritage, it expressly offered resistance to the frequent calls to unify Chinese medicine with modern knowledge.

Conclusion

The new institutions of Western medicine and Chinese medicine had different aims and were initially directed at different audiences. The first professional associations of modern medicine were oriented entirely towards the foreign professional communities that had trained them: the China Medical Missionary Association was initially open only to foreign medical missionaries, and the NMPA and the NMA looked towards either Japan and Germany or Europe and America for professional validation. It was a combination of rising anti-foreign sentiment in the 1920s and pressure from the new Nationalist government after 1928 that finally effected a unification of Western-medical professionals in 1930. Thereafter, the Chinese Medical Association would represent the interests of its members to the Chinese government while also assisting that government to defend its legitimacy in the international arena.

The Chinese National Quarantine Service was part of that effort. With ship bills of health and health certificates for individual emigrants now issued by Chinese doctors holding internationally recognized qualifications, Chinese shipowners and coolies alike could be spared the indignity of having foreigners inspect their levels of hygiene. At the same time, the Quarantine Service was an essential element in the government's campaign to show that the 'unequal treaties' were not only unjust but also unnecessary.

For the Chinese-medical community, the early medical journals, book publication projects (including Xie Guan's dictionary), study societies, and schools of Chinese medicine were intended to make it less of an esoteric art and more of a science and a profession. Creating an accessible literature of respectable texts was crucial to this endeavour, as sociologist Bruno Latour argues for sciences in general: 'No matter if people talk about quasars, Gross National Products, statistics on anthrax epizootic microbes, DNA or subparticle physics; the only way they can talk and not be undermined by counter-arguments is if, and only if, they can make the things they say they are talking about easily readable.'[110]

Thus the new texts eschewed discussion of medical deities, spirits, or temple medicine, and the early journals ran impassioned debates over whether the ideas of *yin* and *yang* and the Five Phases could be retained in a modernized Chinese medicine. The rejection of superstition was thoroughly in tune with the Nationalist government's agenda: after 1928 both city and national governments repeatedly issued bans on 'superstitious persons,' including geomancers, blind fortune-tellers, diviners, Daoist priests, and spirit-mediums.[111] So the acceptable face of 'Chinese' medicine was to be the secular medicine of the elite classes, not the popular practices of ordinary people.

The fact that this separation of elite Chinese medicine from popular medical practices was a successful strategy for medical elites is confirmed by the establishment of the state-sponsored Institute of National Medicine in 1931, a result of the successful defence against Yu Yunxiu's attempts to have Chinese medicine banned in 1929. However, this state support was conditional on an agenda of reform through science: the first article of the new institute's constitution reads: 'This institute has the objective of choosing scientific methods to put in order Chinese medicine and pharmacy, improve treatment of disease, and improve methods of manufacturing drugs.'[112]

If 'scientific medicine' had been awarded epistemic priority at the new Institute of National Medicine, comparison with other institutions reinforces the idea that this status was a function of government rather than of patient preference. Elisabeth Sinn describes how the Tung Wah Hospital in Hong Kong, established by Chinese philanthropists and a key institution mediating between the British colonial government and Chinese elites, began to employ one or two doctors of Western medicine in the 1890s to satisfy government requirements for mortality statistics in biomedical terms and also to give patients therapeutic choice. Overwhelmingly, they preferred to see Chinese-medical doctors.[113] The Chinese Red Cross Society's various branches regularly employed a single Western-medical doctor to work alongside Chinese-medical doctors, and, as we saw in Chapter 2, as late as 1915, local governments such as Shaoxing's were employing Chinese-style doctors in local posts (such as orphanage and prison doctors) and Western-style doctors in more public roles (such as school medical officers).

The CMA continued to view Chinese medicine as dangerous competition. This is borne out by the social medicine movement headed by Drs. Yan Fuqing, Chen Zhiqian (C.C. Chen), and others during the Nanjing Decade. One of the reasons these leaders of modern medicine in China advocated a national socialized, single-payer health system was that such an arrangement could exclude doctors of Chinese medicine from reimbursement, giving MDs a virtual monopoly.[114]

Drugstore owners had their own institutions, often rooted in native-place associations that privileged business relations between speakers of the same dialect. For example, the inventor of 'Tiger Balm,' Aw Boon-haw, used his network of Hakka minority Fujianese from Yongding County to build a business empire that spread from Burma, Singapore, and Thailand to stores throughout urban China. Just as his most famous product combined drug ingredients from both Western and Chinese traditions, drugstores were often neutral when it came to what kind of medicine they sold: the main thing was that it sold.[115]

In the end, reformers of Chinese medicine started a far-reaching series of institutional changes and also won the right, in 1936, to have practitioners of Chinese medicine licensed as physicians. During the Republican period, however, they failed to have Chinese medicine included in the national educational system and were still a long way from achieving their aim of having Western medicine and Chinese medicine accorded equal status. More positively, they did succeed in moulding an image of learned Chinese medicine that was intellectual and secular, if not yet entirely consistent. The Communist government's adoption of Chinese medicine in the 1950s, and its reinterpretation of *yin* and *yang* as a form of primitive dialectical materialism, could not have been achieved without these efforts to fit Chinese medicine into modern institutional forms, thereby creating some distance between 'modern, rational' Chinese medicine and 'ignorant superstition.'

From New Theories to New Practices

We have seen how the desire to remove superstition and perceived corruption from Chinese medicine led to the founding of institutions designed to change the transmission of Chinese-medical knowledge. A complementary movement took place in the way Chinese-medical physicians recorded their encounters with patients. We will see how this change helped make individual virtuosity in Chinese medicine more transparent, reproducible, and teachable. To conclude the chapter, we move beyond the bureaucratic function of record-keeping to examine how Chinese-medical physicians used Western anatomy to relocate the acupuncture points in relation to the visible structures of nerves, muscles, and blood vessels. This also marked a shift of emphasis in acupuncture away from bloodletting and minor surgery and towards the manipulation of *qi* through the use of filiform needles that were understood to stimulate the nervous system. This redefinition of the aims and methods of needling in acupuncture, which has become the accepted norm in acupuncture schools and colleges in Mainland China, also marks nothing less than the creation of a new Chinese-medical body.

From Case Records to Case Histories[1]

Throughout most of Chinese history, physicians recorded their consultations. In late Imperial China, it was normal practice for a visiting physician to write down his diagnosis and analysis of a patient's case along with the recommended prescription. This record, or *an* 案, was left with the patient, who chose whether or not to act on its recommendations. (In Chinese, the phrase for this action is *tou an* 投案, literally, 'submit a record,' which even more clearly conveys the deciding role of the patient as consumer.) There are many recorded instances of families inviting (and presumably paying) several physicians in turn to submit their analyses and then choosing which to follow. The doctors themselves frequently described this process in their own collections of case records, clearly with the aim of explaining why their own analysis was superior.

The historian's access to case records is rarely mediated by patients or their families, however; our sources are overwhelmingly drawn from published collections of physicians' own records. Since most of these are compiled either by the physicians themselves or by their close relatives or personal students, there is a strong bias in the available literature towards cases that offer a display of the practitioner's virtuosity. Cases of failure are relatively rare, and death is most often recorded in order to demonstrate the veracity of the physician's prognoses. In recent years, professional historians in China have supplemented these highly selective collections by publishing all the available case documents of famous doctors for whom the material is still available. These supplementary records make it possible to gain an insight into both the kinds of ailment and therapy considered particularly interesting by the individual physician and those so mundane as to not merit a full description.

Since such case collections are necessarily the products of the educated elite, they also create an image of Chinese medicine that is distorted in favour of secular, 'Confucian' medicine. Folk and popular medical practices only appear on the rare occasions when a doctor finds cause to criticize the family for having used this kind of treatment. Regrettably, case records are also silent on the crucial matter of the physician's fee. On the other hand, these records provide unique insights into patient-physician interactions. The many records that cover repeated visits to a particular case are also a valuable guide to the therapeutic process in Chinese medicine.

The structure of these records varies tremendously, the simplest being a brief note to remind the doctor of the treatment dispensed. Here is an example from a collection of the unpublished case records of the famous Qing dynasty physician Ye Gui 葉桂 (courtesy name Tianshi 天土, 1667-1746). It consists of only two lines of text in Chinese:

Left *cun* [pulse] accelerated.
Radix Rehmanniae Praeparata; Radix Asparagi; Radix Glehniae; Sclerotium Poriae Cocos Pararadicis; Herba Dendrobium off.; Radix Ophiogonis.[2]

Although this is little more than the physician's notes to himself, there is a great deal of information embedded in it.[3] For instance, the accelerated pulse indicates excess of *yang*, with associated heat. The *cun*, or index finger position on the left wrist, correlates to the heart and small intestine pulses. The principal drug, *Radix Rehmanniae Praeparata*, *Shu di[huang]*, is attributive to the heart, liver, and kidney tracts, the pulses of all of which are felt on the left wrist, and this drug has the effect of nourishing *yin*, moisturizing dryness, and strengthening the heart. Already we may deduce that Ye Tianshi considered the excess of *yang* influence manifested in the accelerated pulse to be due to a deficiency of *yin*, and his mention of the specific pulse site indicates that the organ most affected by the resultant overheating was the heart. This deduction is borne out by examining the properties of the other drugs. *Radix Asparagi, Radix Glehniae, Herba Dendrobium,* and *Radix Ophiogonis* are all found in handbooks of Chinese *materia medica* under the heading 'drugs that tonify *yin*.' Three of the four are also used to moisturize dryness. Two of the drugs also clear away heat or 'heart-fire.' The last drug, *Sclerotium Poriae Cocos Pararadicis,* is a specific for heart depletion (*xin xu* 心虛) and has the effect of calming the spirit (*an shen* 安神). So, working from the very terse case record, it is possible to deduce that Ye Tianshi was treating a case of *yin* depletion that had damaged the body fluids and heart. This had caused symptoms of heat and *yang* excess, such as the accelerated pulse, and most probably also low fever and lung-dryness symptoms such as a hacking cough, with possibly other symptoms related to heart tract disease such as insomnia or over-anxiety. Although two or more of the *yin*-tonifying drugs often appear together in standard prescriptions, this particular combination of drugs seems to have been Ye's own invention.

Today, several modern reference works on Chinese drugs and common prescriptions published in English and Chinese facilitate this sort of deduction. Such aids were not available in the early Qing dynasty, however, so any case descriptions as terse as this would only have been of use to other physicians with substantial experience and knowledge of the medical canon. The prescription also omits the relative proportions of the drugs, again underlining the importance of tacit knowledge when interpreting this kind of case record.

At the other end of the spectrum we find long and detailed accounts of the merits of various therapies used on a single patient over time or on several patients with similar symptoms. The discursive type is often called the 'notebook' (*biji* 筆記) form of case record, usually written down after the consultation, perhaps from notes taken there, but relying mainly on the physician's (or the physician's student's) memory. This was the kind of case record most often used to advance particular theoretical standpoints. Such records often served to explain how particularly complicated cases were worked out and treated and, as such, are valuable guides to the processes of inference and deduction in Chinese therapy as well as a testaments to the physician's great skill and erudition.[4]

Somewhere between these two extremes lies the 'didactic' case record.[5] To be of value to a physician's students, a record needed to include basic information about the patient, information derived from diagnostic procedures, an account of the treatment applied, and notes on the effect of that treatment. Of even more value were the descriptions of how the diagnosis was reached and explanations of why particular therapies were chosen. It is the standardization of these kinds of didactic records that interests us as an example of the modernization of medical practice.

Here is an example of a traditional didactic case record, kept by the famous Shanghai physician Ding Zesheng 丁澤生, usually known by his style of Ganren 甘仁 (1865-1926). Ding Ganren's writings show no evidence of Western diagnostic methods or of Western therapeutics, though Volker Scheid argues that his participation in the Chinese-medical community of reformers in Shanghai was important in the elaboration of his eclectic Menghe style of treatment.[6] This case concerns an epidemic disease known in Chinese as *housha* 喉痧, literally, 'throat-pox,' the symptoms of which overlap with the Western disease entity known as scarlet fever.

> Throat-Pox with Fever, Aversion to Cold and Difficulty Swallowing: [Mr] Fu, aged 20-odd, had been suffering from throat-pox for eight days. He was feverish without sweating and had a slight aversion to cold. It was unclear whether there were spots or numbness; [these symptoms] were dispersed and indistinct. His face was dark purple and the throat was swollen and putrid. He had trouble swallowing even trickles of water and experienced restlessness and nausea, with no respite day or night. The Fu family had several households, but only [this] one son, so his old mother and young wife were weeping bitterly as they begged me to save him. I said: 'Although the condition is critical, his normal *qi* is not yet defeated, so he could still recover.' On diagnosis his pulse was obstructed, accelerated and not clearly distinguishable; when I read the prescriptions he had taken earlier, sure enough, they were [mistakenly] of the 'nurturing *yin* and clearing the lungs decoction' type. Thereupon I prescribed 'decoction for penetrating pox and dispelling poison,' with added *Fructus Aurantii Immaturus* (immature orange fruits) and *Caulis Bambusae in Taeniam* (bamboo shavings), two doses to be taken every 24 hours. I also let blood from the *shao shang* 少商 point [specific for fever, fainting, and sore and swollen throats] in order to open up the obstruction and let out the fire. After taking the medicine, he succeeded in sweating profusely, and the spots and numbness began to appear. His facial colour changed to red, and the throat swelling and pus began to recede. After taking several doses, he was cured in three to four days. 'Cases of throat-pox will survive if they sweat' – experience it and you'll believe it.[7]

This is a fairly transparent didactic case record. The physician states the nature of the ailment together with the external symptoms. Diagnosis at the pulse allows the physician to assess the condition of the patient's 'normal *qi*' and to correct previous false diagnoses. From this information the physician is able to offer a hopeful prognosis. This is then realized using a named drug decoction and bloodletting at a named site. The effects of the treatment are noted, as is the duration of the treatment, resulting in a full recovery. There is even a little rhyming couplet at the end to aid retention of the didactic message, which is that cases of *housha* must be made to sweat.[8] A student studying this record would need to know only where to look up the composition of the named decoction (if he or she had not memorized it already) and the position and effects of the named acupoint.

Compare this example with the following rendering of the same case, this time deliberately rendered in a *case history* format similar to that used to record Western-medical case histories:

A case of wind-poison throat-pox

Patient: Mr. Fu, aged in his twenties, resident of Tangshan Road, Shanghai.

Disease: Wind-poison throat-pox.

Causes of disease: Caught by infection (*chuanran* 傳染) eight days ago. Prescriptions left by doctors consulted previously were all of the 'nourish *yin* and clear the lungs' type.

Symptoms: Fever, no sweat, slight aversion to cold, [symptoms of] spots or numbness were dispersed and indistinct. Facial appearance was purple and dark, the throat swollen and putrid, and there was difficulty in swallowing even trickles of water. [The patient] experienced restlessness and nausea, with no respite day or night.

Diagnosis: The pulse was obstructed, accelerated and not clearly distinguishable, the tongue coating was greasy and yellow. I said:

'This is [a case of] throat-pox that has been misdiagnosed as *baihou* 白喉 [literally: "white throat"; symptoms similar to the Western disease entity of diphtheria].' The Fu family had several households, but only [this] one son, so his old mother and young wife were weeping bitterly as they begged me to save him. I said: 'Although the condition is critical, his normal *qi* is not yet defeated, so he could still recover.'

Treatment method: Accordingly I prescribed 'decoction for penetrating pox and dispelling poison,' with added *Fructus Aurantii Immaturus* (immature orange fruits) and *Caulis Bambusae in Taeniam* (bamboo shavings) to facilitate penetration [of the drugs] and to open up [obstructions]. I also let blood from the *shao shang* point in order to open up the obstruction and let out the fire.

Prescription: Herba Schizonepetae, 1.5 *qian; Periostracum cicadae,* 8 *fen;* powdered *Radix puerariae,* 2 *qian;* green *Fructus Forsythiae,* 2 *qian; Herba Spirodelae,* 3 *qian; Fructus Arctii,* 2 *qian;* roasted *Bombyx Batryticatus,* 3 *qian;* young *Rhizoma Belamcandae,* 1 *qian; Lasiosphaeraseu Calratia,* 8 *fen* (including liquid); *Fructus Aurantii immaturus,* 1.5 *qian; Caulis Bambusae in Taeniam,* 2 *qian;* fresh *Radix Glycyrrhizae,* 5 *fen; Radix Peucedani,* 1.5 *qian.*[9]

Results: After taking two doses of the medicine in the first 24 hours, he succeeded in sweating profusely, and the spots and numbness began to appear. His facial colour changed to red, and the throat swelling and pus began to recede. After taking several doses, he was cured in three to four days. 'Cases of throat-pox will survive if they sweat' – experience it and you'll believe it.[10]

Although the details of the case are largely unchanged in these two versions, there are some significant differences. Most striking is the organization under specific rubrics in the second version. The heading 'causes of disease' (*bingyin* 病因) brings the additional information that the affliction was 'caught by infection.' While there is plenty of evidence from pre-modern China for the concept of contagion, it is significant that the rubrics of Western-style case histories prompt the use of explanations compatible with Western medicine. Similarly, the heading of 'disease' (*bingming* 病名) forces precise classification, in this case as 'wind-poison' throat-pox, an identification omitted in the first version.

Under the rubric 'prescription,' the terse reference to a prescription in the first case record has been replaced with a very detailed description of all the drugs in the decoction, including some information on the quality of drug required, for example, 'young *Rhizoma Belamcandae.*'

The first version of this case comes from Ding Ganren's original book on 'throat-pox' published by his students in 1927, after his death in 1924; the second is the same case as it appears in a compilation of model medical case histories in Chinese medicine compiled in 1927 by He Lianchen, whom we met in Chapter 7.[11]

He Lianchen had many complaints about Chinese case records: there was no agreement on the amount of detail necessary to constitute a good record; they had no standard structure, making them difficult to interpret; the information they gave was often incomplete; they seldom reported the success or failure of the treatment; and they were often long on rhetoric and short on facts.[12]

He decided that, by following the example of Western medical case histories, Chinese physicians would be able to strengthen their case for Chinese government support and that, far from giving ground to Western medicine, this would help Chinese medicine to retain its unique character. In other words, He Lianchen wanted to standardize this aspect of Chinese medicine in order to define it; once clearly defined, it could then be effectively defended and propagated. (Recall Bruno Latour's insistence on the importance of inscription in the creation and dissemination of science, noted in the previous chapter.) It is easy to see how this could be an effective tactic given China's atmosphere of widespread scientism and the antipathy towards 'old and corrupt' elements of Chinese culture (such as traditional medicine and its association with unhygienic practices and superstition).[13] It is also now easy for us to see that this kind of medical innovation led to a mostly new Chinese medicine.

He's approach to the modernization of Chinese case records, which he promoted in the pages of the *Shaoxing Journal,* won the approval of many of his colleagues. As we have seen, Ding Ganren gave permission for him to rewrite Ding's cases to accord with the new standard format. He also took case records from the medical classics and reorganized them under his new rubrics, with the following consequences.

First of all, the prescription was transformed. In the first example above, we are given just the name of the prescription, without being given its origins or its constituents. Presumably, well-educated literati would have memorized enough medical texts to at least recognize the provenance of the prescription, so that, even if they did not know its contents by heart, they would at least know where to look them up. By contrast, the systematically reorganized case history contains detailed information about the contents of the prescription, not only naming every drug but also giving the relative proportions used. Very often, even the prescriptions given in the classic texts did not give drug proportions. This is one way in which He Lianchen's innovative use of Western-style systematization resulted in the creation of a new corpus of standardized prescriptions.

Second, by insisting on the rubric *liaofa* 療法 (method of curing), He Lianchen tried to connect theory to practice. As we have seen, one of the most frequently cited opinions about Chinese medicine in this period was that Chinese medical theory was unscientific and full of superstition. Several of the most prominent Chinese physicians of the time, including He Lianchen himself, Ding Ganren, Zhang Xichun, and Zhu Weiju, avoided referring to the Five Phases *(wuxing)* in their writings. This was not just because they were afraid of being criticized by others. They genuinely believed that a modern Chinese medicine would be better off without this particular theory, which they regarded as an obsolete relic. Another leading advocate of medical syncretism, the famous Beijing doctor Shi Jinmo 施今墨 (1884-1968), discusses this issue in his own collection of Chinese-medical case histories:

> This book is organised according to the categories of Western medicine, for convenience of reference. The systematic organisation of this book is exceptionally clear and there is also no mention of the mysterious theories of the Five Phases, so it is very suitable for patients to consult for themselves.[14]

By insisting that Chinese-medical physicians explain their reasons for employing a particular therapy, He Lianchen was defending the relevance of Chinese-medical views of the etiology of disease. At the same time, he defined the terms on which comparisons between Chinese and Western medicine should be made. The same point can also be made about his use of the rubric 'cause of disease' *(bingyin)*. Finally, these new case histories were organized under their respective *bing* (disease) names rather than by their syndromes (*zheng*), indicating a change in Chinese-medical nosology, driven by a perceived need to classify Chinese disease entities in such a way that they could be meaningfully compared with Western disease terms. In this context, the use of the word *bing* for 'disease' rather than *zheng* is significant because it avoids any commitment to a particular theoretical orientation as part of the disease-naming process.

To understand the significance of this semantic change, consider the following. In the late Qing, there were two major, competing currents of medical thought that, to some extent, determined how an individual physician would classify infectious and epidemic diseases. Labelling a disease 'warm' (*wen*) had long signalled contagion, something that most people associated with demonic influences and harm from foul *qi*.[15] During the Ming-Qing transition medical scholars from southern China had reformulated 'warm diseases' (*wenbing* 瘟病), giving them a new and secular explanation of the mass morbidity experienced during epidemic episodes: they argued that the epidemics were caused by an unseen local contaminant rather than by unseasonable *qi*.[16] Proponents of the new understanding of warm diseases considered the Han dynasty medical classic on fevers, the *Treatise on Cold Damage*, inadequate with regard to explaining the epidemics of the late imperial period. This disagreement on the causes of epidemics – unseasonable climatic *qi* versus local pestilential *qi* – led the two schools to classify epidemic diseases differently. The cold damage school classified diseases by their location in the body's tracts, or *jing*. Thus there was a class of disease called 'greater yang' (tract) disease, another called 'yang brightness' (tract) disease, and so on. Within each class, there could be subdivisions into symptom-clusters (or, for our purposes, *bing*, diseases), but the primary nosology was related to the tract structure of the body. The new warm diseases were classified differently as upper burner, middle burner, or lower burner diseases, and according to whether they had affected only the *wei* 衛, 'defensive' *qi* fraction, or penetrated through to the *ying* 營, 'constructive' fraction, represented by the blood.[17]

If we recall that both these currents of learning were producing accounts of what we would label febrile epidemic diseases, it is clear that similar clusters of symptoms might be described, discussed, and treated in very different ways, according to which school a physician followed. There is some evidence that this did actually happen. For instance, in the 1903 book *A Compass for Warm Diseases,* the section titled 'Four Principles for Differentiating Cold-Damage and Warm Diseases' says: 'When "winter-warm" first arises, there are headaches, aversion to cold and draughts, feverish body and spontaneous sweating; this is indistinguishable from the cold-factor syndrome *(zheng)* of "greater yang internal wind." This is where it is easiest to confuse the two.'[18]

The author continues to show how these two similar disease types could indeed be differentiated according to their different pulse patterns, but his comment reveals that there was a definite problem with deciding whether febrile diseases were of the cold-damage or the warm disease category unless the physician was committed to one of these approaches in advance.

However, if a case history restricts physicians to describing the symptom-cluster or the disease, *bing,* rather than the underlying syndrome, *zheng,* the matter of whether they follow the warm disease or the cold-damage orientation becomes less important. What matters most are the diagnosis of the *bing* and the details of its treatment. (And, of course, whether or not the treatment was effective.)

By the Republican period, it had become popular to assert that these two schools were the two sides of the same coin: that they both dealt in febrile epidemic diseases and that what they had in common was more important than their differences. Several prominent physicians called for *Han-wen tongyi* 寒溫統, the unification of cold-damage and warm disease theories.[19]

This shift away from particular currents of medical theory and therapy and towards a much more eclectic use of the competing medical traditions became part of the professionalization of Chinese medicine. In fact, one of the conditions of membership in He Lianchen's Shaoxing Medical and Pharmaceutical Association was that any particularly effective therapy, no matter what its source, had to be reported to the society journal so that other society members could corroborate it.[20] The priority was to identify a core of properly attested therapies by using the standardized reporting format of the new case history. In Popperian terms, He Lianchen was using the case history format to attempt to introduce the reproducibility and falsifiability of modern scientific experiments to Chinese medical treatments.

He's new format, first published as a compilation of model case histories in book form in 1927, was followed in works by Zhang Xichun 張錫純 (1860-1933). The case records in the first five installments of Zhang's *The Assimilation of Western to Chinese in Medicine,* published serially from 1918, are detailed examples of the didactic case record, usually also specifying the exact proportions of the drugs used in each prescription. This level of detail was necessary because about half of the prescriptions listed by Zhang were his own inventions. Starting with the sixth installment, published in 1931, Zhang further modernized his case records, changing the format to Western-style case histories with clearly demarcated headings almost identical to those proposed by He Lianchen. As the title of Zhang Xichun's work suggests, his aim was to use Western medicine to justify and confirm Chinese medicine. For Zhang as for He, to do this it was necessary to redefine just what should count as Chinese medicine.[21]

Thus, this attempt to identify and standardize the essential features of Chinese medicine resulted in significant changes to its theory and practice. At a time when attempts were being made to standardize many aspects of Chinese society – the standardization of pronunciation in order to create a national language, the creation of a single national currency, and the adoption of international weights and measures all spring to mind – standards had to be found by which Chinese physicians and Chinese medical practice could be assessed. A Chinese medicine based on secret remedies and individual reputations was neither consistent nor measurable enough to count as either modern or scientific. By moving from Chinese case records *(yian)* to Western-style case histories *(bing'an)*, He Lianchen and his colleagues in the late 1920s and early 1930s not only provided a useful standard around which to organize medical practice and teaching but also created a framework that encouraged, and to some extent presupposed, theoretical coherence. For Chinese medicine to have any chance of counting as scientific in the new China, it first had to be made internally consistent. A change in medical paperwork helped create this consistency.

The Advent of Scientific Acupuncture

'Acupuncture needling and moxa cautery are absolutely inappropriate to all gentlemen.' Although we can imagine this statement coming from a British physician newly arrived in China in the nineteenth century, it is in fact a Chinese slogan from the 1820s.[22] Acupuncture, the icon of Chinese medicine to the twenty-first-century Western mind, is a relatively recent development, at least in the manner it is practised today. While the history of acupuncture deserves a more complete treatment than space here allows, I now look at how this symbol of Chinese medicine came back in a new form thanks, in part, to individuals who were seeking a scientific, hence respectable, basis for it.

The teaching and practice of acupuncture and moxibustion were banned from the Imperial Medical Academy (*Taiyiyuan*), which had responsibility for the medical care of the imperial household, in 1822, during the second year of the Daoguang Emperor's reign. The edict announcing the ban cited the explanation that 'even the slightest exposure was an injury to propriety and refinement.' The reasons for this prejudice against acupuncture have long puzzled historians, and medical historian Ma Kanwen 马堪文 argues that the ban occurred in the context of popular uprisings and assassination attempts against the previous Jiaqing Emperor in 1803 and 1813. In one of these, rebels had succeeded in entering the Forbidden City before being arrested. The Daoguang Emperor experienced these attacks while a boy, and, after he ascended the throne in 1821, he ordered heightened surveillance of the area around the palace and, in 1822, commanded males of the royal clan to practise military drills, horsemanship, and archery. He also banned the private manufacture and carrying of guns. Ma Kanwen suggests that it was concern that acupuncture needles (which were much larger than today's needles) could be used as weapons of assassination that prompted the emperor to ban the practice of acupuncture in the royal household.[23]

There is evidence that acupuncture was not regularly practised by elite physicians even before the imperial ban, however. When Xu Dachun 徐大椿 (1693-1771) wrote his historical survey of Chinese medicine in 1757, 'he had to speak of acupuncture as rather a lost art, for there were then left very few experts in it, and young physicians were at a loss to find teachers to instruct them in it.' Furthermore, 'when scholars like Hsü [Xu] surveyed the ancient and medieval literature they were astonished to see how great a part acupuncture had played in it.'[24] In a similar vein, in the Ming novel *Jinpingmei* 金瓶梅 *(Plum in the Golden Vase)*, Old Woman Wang, a woman healer favoured by the female characters in the novel, is abused by the main male character as 'an old whore who will stick in needles and cauterise you at random.'[25]

For much of its early history, acupuncture involved interventions resembling minor surgery. When Sir Henry Wellcome, co-founder of the Burroughs-Wellcome Pharmaceutical Company, visited China in the 1930s, he was able to collect several sets of 'acupuncture needles,' which included straight and hooked scalpels, retractor hooks, drains, and other instruments for minor surgery. Many of the sets in the London Science Museum's collection do not contain any of the filiform needles we associate with modern acupuncture.[26] Even a cursory glance at the illustrations of the 'nine needles' of acupuncture as described in the *Canon of the Spiritual Pivot (Lingshu jing)* demonstrates the minor-surgical function of 'acupuncture' for much of its long history. And in Eugène Vincent's 1915 study of medicine in China, the 'needles of acupuncture' are depicted as part of a larger surgical kit (Figure 11).

Modern filiform needles trace their origin to Japan. As we have seen in Chapter 4, Japan provided an impetus for change in both Chinese medicine and Chinese adaptations of Western medicine. This was especially the case for mid-twentieth-century transformations in Chinese acupuncture.

Cheng Dan'an and the Relocation of the Acupuncture Points

Recent Japanese works in the Chinese-medical tradition were published in 1936 in the *Sino-Japanese Medical Collection*, edited by Chen Cunren, who was working under the auspices of the Institute of National Medicine.[27] Chen indicated that the distinguishing features of this medicine included the preservation of skills now lost on the mainland, such as bone-setting and abdominal diagnosis, certain obstetrical operations, and the relocation of acupuncture points and tracts *(jing)*, the points in Japan being limited to only seventy.

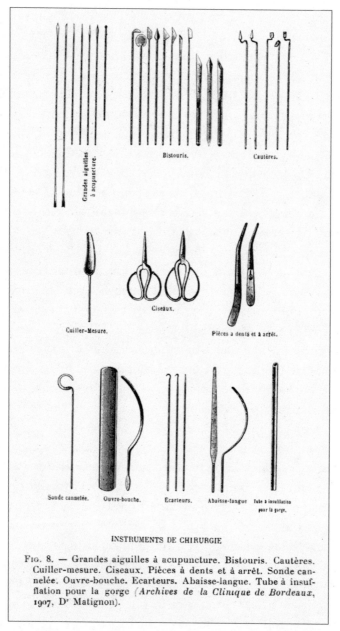

INSTRUMENTS DE CHIRURGIE

FIG. 8. — Grandes aiguilles à acupuncture. Bistouris. Cautères. Cuiller-mesure. Ciseaux. Pièces à dents et à arrêt. Sonde cannelée. Ouvre-bouche. Ecarteurs. Abaisse-langue. Tube à insufflation pour la gorge (*Archives de la Clinique de Bordeaux*, 1907, Dr Matignon).

Figure 11　A Chinese surgical kit from the turn of the twentieth century, illustrated in Eugène Vincent, *La médecine en Chine au XXe siècle* (Paris: G. Steinheil, 1915), 74. Note the group of instruments at the top left, labelled 'large needles for acupuncture.'

Source: Author's collection.

The appealing idea of reducing the number of acupoints had been raised five years earlier by Cheng Dan'an (1899-1957). Cheng had studied Chinese medicine for three years from a local Chinese physician in Jiangyin County, Jiangsu Province, before studying Western medicine in Shanghai in the early 1920s. He first studied Western medicine through the Correspondence College of Sino-Western Medicine (*Zhong-xi yi hanshou xuexiao* 中西醫函授學校) before moving to Shanghai to learn Western medicine first-hand from a private tutor in 1921. On his return home in 1923, he helped his father treat patients, having brought home a hoard of basic Western drugs and injection needles.[28] The same year, however, he developed a severe back problem that resisted Western treatment but that was apparently finally cured by his father's acupuncture. This convinced him to turn his attention to acupuncture. By 1925, his reputation was sufficiently established for him to set up his own practice, and from this time he regularly published articles on his revised acupuncture in the Chinese-medical press. In 1930, he moved to the town of Wuxi and established the Society for Research into Chinese Acupuncture, the first such Chinese institution. The society was also a correspondence college, and Cheng's later published books were written as course books. The most influential of these was his *Chinese Acupuncture and Moxibustion Therapeutics* (*Zhongguo zhenjiu zhiliao xue* 中國針灸治療學), first published in 1931.[29]

In this highly influential work, Cheng noted that acupuncture and moxibustion had virtually disappeared from China. His formula for their revival had much in common with earlier Japanese reforms of acupuncture, including using Western anatomy to redefine acupuncture points. Three years after the first publication of his book, in 1934, Cheng Dan'an also visited Japan, spending a year learning Japanese and attending the Tokyo College of Acupuncture. Drawing on Western anatomy and physiology to create a new understanding of how acupuncture worked, Cheng concluded that the tracts (or 'meridians') constituted a functional system that encompassed the nerves, blood vessels, and lymph glands of Western medicine:

The pathways of acupuncture points recorded by our forebears are mostly lacking in detail. There is even less recorded about the contents of the acupuncture pathways. This book employs scientific methods to correct this. Each acupoint must be elucidated anatomically ... In manipulating acupoints, although our forebears needled into arteries, this was still needling the nerves of that area, and certainly not [primarily] rupturing the artery ... However, when they did needle them [i.e., the arteries] the objective was [to reach] the nerves at that spot.[30]

Cheng did not reinvent the acupuncture points at will, however. He started with the points described in Wang Weiyi's *Illustrations of Acupuncture and Moxibustion Points Using the Bronze Figure* (*Tongren shuxue zhenjiu tujing* 銅人腧穴針灸圖經), a work first published in 1026 or 1027 CE during the Northern Song dynasty.[31] This manual, newly rediscovered in Japan, was republished in a high-quality edition in 1909 and appears to have been widely available. Wang Weiyi 王惟 (ca. 987-1067), a court medical official, seems to have written his book with much the same agenda as Cheng Dan'an: to compile a definitive guide to the correct position of the acupoints as a result of the prevailing profusion of alternatives.[32] The bronze figures he produced had small holes at the acupoints, which were filled with wax, and the whole model was also covered with a wax layer. The hollow bronze figure would be filled with water prior to examining the medical students of the Hanlin Medical Bureau, so that correct needling would cause drops of water to appear on the surface of the model.[33] In passing we should note that such a test required that the needles used be large and sturdy enough to poke through a wax plug, so they were obviously much larger than the filiform needles of today.

Figures 12 and 13 show the results of Cheng's redefinitions. The use of photographic representations of the acupuncture tracts mirrors the trend towards photographic illustrations in contemporary textbooks of Western medicine and was much praised by the book's reviewers. Cheng says that he used Western anatomy, for instance, to ensure that no points were placed near major blood vessels. This marks a major shift in acupuncture theory and practice. Before Cheng Dan'an, acupuncture was frequently used to let small amounts of blood in order to encourage smooth flow in the blood vessels. After Cheng had made the case for acupuncture acting through the nerves, the drawing of blood at an

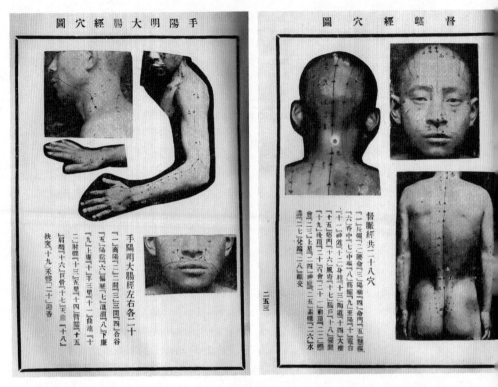

Figures 12 and 13 Cheng Dan'an redefined the paths of acupuncture channels (i.e., meridians) and moved several acupuncture points to emphasize anatomical accuracy and to argue for a mechanism of acupuncture that acted via nervous stimulation. *Source:* Courtesy of the East Asian History of Science Library, Needham Research Institute, Cambridge.

acupuncture point started to become an indication of the clumsiness and lack of experience of the acupuncturist (a view that still pertains today).

The demand for Cheng's new, scientific acupuncture was so great that the revised edition of his *Chinese Acupuncture and Moxibustion Therapeutics* appeared only a year after the appearance of the first. The new edition of 1932 was honoured by congratulatory inscriptions from twenty-two prominent Chinese physicians and included laudatory prefaces from another eleven. By May 1937, the book was in its eighth edition. Prominent Chinese medical historians have described it as 'the most influential work on acupuncture of the last hundred years.'[34]

In addition to his use of Western anatomy to create a scientific acupuncture, Cheng also rejected the idea that acupuncture treatments should be timed according to astrological and divinatory formulae. He also rejected dividing days and parts of days into *yin* and *yang*. The old idea that men should be treated on their left sides and women on their right was, according to Cheng, also a superstitious remnant.[35]

In practical terms, Cheng recommended that moxibustion not be allowed to cauterize the skin as doing so leads to ugly and traumatic cautery scars. The prevalent idea that acupuncture and moxa should not be applied at the same spot seemed to Cheng to be a product of the use of thick, coarse acupuncture needles. These needles caused such damage that combining them with moxa cautery left a considerable wound. However, if moxa were not allowed to burn the skin, and if only filiform needles were used, the two treatments could be combined to great effect.[36] Again, Cheng Dan'an was heralding a major change in the practice of acupuncture – a change that has survived to the present day. Virtually all acupuncture is now carried out with filiform metal needles of varying length, and there is none of the minor surgery or boil-lancing with small scalpels and crude bodkins that was once part of the acupuncturist's stock-in-trade.

There is no doubt that Cheng was successful in his attempts to make acupuncture scientific. In the Chinese historical literature on acupuncture, his activities are by far the most widely reported of any acupuncture specialist of the Republican period. He seems to have been the moving force behind rehabilitating acupuncture and transforming it into elite, learned Chinese medicine. In addition to founding the Wuxi Society and setting up a network of affiliated acupuncture research societies, he also started the first acupuncture journal, *Journal of Acupuncture* (*Zhenjiu zazhi* 針灸雜誌), in 1933. Research society faculty included Jiao Yitang 焦易堂, first director of the Institute of National Medicine; Xie Guan, editor of the *Encyclopaedic Dictionary of Chinese Medicine;* Zhang Zanchen, Xie's student and one of the leaders of the anti-abolition campaign; and Wang Shenxuan. By 1935, the society had at least fourteen branches in ten different provinces as well as in Hong Kong and Singapore.[37] By 1937, Cheng's school in Wuxi was running two different courses, a 'research course,' consisting of 150 hours a month of study and teaching for a year, and a 'specialist course,' consisting of 175 hours a month for two years. The same year the school built a library and re-named itself the China Acupuncture Technical College (*Zhongguo zhenjiu zhuanmen xuexiao* 中國針灸專門學校), indicating that it had won the right to award government-approved degrees.[38]

In 1938, following the Japanese invasion of China, Cheng fled Wuxi for Chongqing. On his return in 1947 he found that his school had been destroyed. After the Communist revolution in 1949, he re-established the China Acupuncture Research Society and recommenced his publish-ing activities. In 1954, he chaired the Jiangsu Provincial Congress of Chinese Medicine and was also elected to the Provincial People's Congress. In November 1954, he was also made director of the school that was soon to become the Jiangsu College of Chinese Medicine in Nanjing. In 1955, he was made a member of the Chinese Academy of Sciences and also elected vice-chairman of the Chinese Medical Association. Although he died in 1957, the society he founded is still active today.[39]

Cheng Dan'an rescued Chinese acupuncture from superstition and oblivion, paving the way for scientific acupuncture to raise the status of Chinese medicine as a whole, as it did during the Communist era. After the publication of this first book, acupuncture courses were increasingly included in the curricula of the new colleges of Chinese medicine. Of greater importance, however, is his re-envisioning of the Chinese-medical body. Cheng Dan'an used Western anatomy to describe the tracts of acupuncture (*jingluo* 經絡) as composed exclusively of the observable physical structures of the blood vessels, lymph glands, and nerves, and he explained the action of acupuncture needling exclusively in terms of nervous stimulation. Cheng recruited Western medicine in the service of the new Chinese body-image just as the newly politicized physicians, such as Wu Lien-teh, had been able to recruit Western public health measures to the service of the new Chinese state. In a nicely ironic twist, it is precisely this reformed acupuncture, previously considered the most disreputable part of the Chinese medical tradition, that Westerners now most eagerly seek out in their quest for alternative and more holistic methods of healing. The new scientific acupuncture is big business.

Cheng Dan'an's work was not without its critics, and other revisions and explanations were proposed.[40] However, with Cheng Dan'an we see, for the first time, a Chinese-medical physiology superimposed on an unambiguously Western anatomy. This composite body is represented most clearly in the modern-day equivalents of Wang Weiyi's bronze figures. Nowadays, leading schools of acupuncture in China, and particularly those that run courses for foreigners, have life-size models of the human body made of transparent plastic so that the internal organs are visible on the inside. The acupuncture points and the paths of the tracts are then also clearly visible, even where they are conceived as lying beneath the surface of the skin. Paradoxically, Cheng's success in achieving this composite view of the body is so thorough that most observers cannot see the breakthrough it represents for Chinese medicine and the struggles that it entailed.

We have considered two ways in which 'traditional Chinese medicine' was reformulated in Republican China using resources from Western medicine. Although neither He Lianchen's formula for writing case histories nor Cheng Dan'an's explanation of how acupuncture works continued unchallenged in Communist writings on Chinese medicine, both were important landmarks in the remaking of Chinese medicine.

By now it should be obvious that assimilating aspects of Western medicine into Chinese medicine did not result in a Chinese medicine that was less Chinese. Quite the opposite. The modern Chinese medicine that these innovators helped to create was public and reproducible, in contrast to the private, or even secret and experiential, practices they were designed to replace. Although a single, unified vision of traditional Chinese medicine would not be created until the publications of the national textbook series in the early 1960s, by the 1930s it was already possible to identify the characteristics of that medicine and the agenda for change had already been charted. For our purposes, all that remains is to gather these observations together to see what they reveal about the making of a modern Chinese medicine and what they suggest about the notion of modernity overall.

Conclusions: Medicine and Modernity

9

WITH DAVID L. SCHWARZKOPF

Reviewing the history of medicine in modern China, we are left with what seems to be an unusual situation: Western medicine and Chinese medicine existing side-by-side, having experienced fluctuating influence and state approval. Before offering an interpretation of this condition, let us briefly review Chinese medicine from the end of the Republican era to the present.

After the Japanese invasion of China in 1937, the Nationalist government and many of the urban elites fled to Chongqing, a major inland city on the Yangzi River in Sichuan Province. With the outcomes uncertain during both the war of resistance against Japan (1937-45) and then the Nationalist-Communist civil war (1945-49), much of the institution-building described in Chapter 7 ceased. Many of the staff of the National Health Administration were disbanded, but those who were able to reach the wartime capital established the new Chongqing Bureau of Public Health. There, an unprecedented concentration of modern medical personnel who were fired up by anti-Japanese sentiment were able to improvise a new medical infrastructure. They organized trauma hospitals and vaccination drives to combat the annual cholera outbreaks and other infectious diseases, and they built and staffed highway health centres to treat the thousands of war refugees. In Southwest China, Emergency Medical Service Training Schools, aided by US supply lines, trained Chinese paramedics and set up a system of county health stations, along models devised in the 1930s by C.C. Chen and League of Nations advisors. After the war, the Nationalist government combined the Army Medical College and the Field Service Training Schools into the National Defence Medical Centre, which is located in Shanghai. However, most of the key Nationalist medical personnel retreated to Taiwan in 1949.[1]

For its part, the Communist Red Army began to organize health care services in 1927 in the Jiangxi Soviet areas. Dr. He Cheng 贺诚 (1901-92) organized primary health care and basic public health services that set the style for future public health campaigns. After the Long March of 1934-35, the Red Army organized a health service in its base area of Yan'an, where mobile medical teams combined all available medical expertise, including practitioners of Chinese medicine and acupuncture. Doctors of Western medicine were few. On 30 October 1944, Mao Zedong gave an address titled 'The United Front in Cultural Work,' in which he acknowledged the problem that doctors of 'new medicine' were generally uninterested in practising in the rural areas. His solution was to 'unite with all the old style intellectuals, artists and doctors ... and to help, educate and remould them.'[2] In the wake of this speech, Yan'an Communist officials called medical officials together to encourage them to develop the policy of 'scientizing Chinese medicine and popularizing Western medicine.' One Western-style doctor who signed up was Zhu Lian 朱琏 (1909-78), who served in several leadership posts within the wartime medical services. She noticed that when acupuncturists accompanied mobile medical teams they used far fewer drugs. Reasoning that a scientific acupuncture would discourage uneducated villagers from resorting to the superstitious or shamanic healing methods that the Chinese Communist Party was trying to eradicate, she formulated a new approach that was eventually published as *The New Acupuncture* (*Xin zhenjiu xue* 新针灸学) in 1951. Zhu's 'new acupuncture' discarded the acupuncture channels and the concepts of *qi* (vital force), *yin* and *yang*, and the Five Phases as contrived and unscientific, instead organizing acupuncture points in military formations such as 'sections' *bu* 部 (head section, upper limbs section, etc.), 'divisions' *qu* 区 (eye division, shoulder division), and 'lines' *xian* 线 (as in battle lines, or front lines).³ Although this particular reorganization of acupuncture was relatively short-lived, falling out of favour in the 1950s, it illustrates several interesting points: first, that the CCP regarded acupuncture as a useful empirical therapy that was more 'scientific' than the popular medical practices it was trying to suppress; second, that Mao would endorse Chinese medicine when it could serve political or national ends; and finally, that the content of Chinese medicine was by no means fixed.

As Ruth Rogaski argues, the other standard of medical modernity for Chinese governments was hygiene (*weisheng* 衛生/卫生). The Chinese word *weisheng* had originally meant 'protecting life' and implied a healthy regimen and activities such as *qigong*, but under Japanese influence (as *eisei*, the Japanese pronounciation of the Chinese characters) it had been inflected with the modern meanings of hygiene in personal affairs and of sanitation in public affairs.⁴ Japanese governments had self-consciously used *weisheng* as a means of penetrating and controlling their colonies in Taiwan, Korea, and Manchuria in sanitary policing campaigns and disease eradication drives.⁵ As we saw in Chapter 5, Wu Lien-teh orchestrated similar policies both during the Manchurian plague epidemic of 1910 and as director of the Chinese Quarantine Service in the 1930s. In all of these activities, paramedical sanitary police were essential to the success of public health activities, and the CCP's incorporation of Chinese medicine by offering basic public health training to doctors of Chinese medicine was a logical extension of this.

During the early 1950s, the Ministry of Health set up a department of Chinese medicine within its Policy Bureau and also established Chinese medical institutes in major Chinese cities. He Cheng, minister of health from 1950 to 1955, began the required unification of Chinese and Western medicine by licensing Chinese-medical doctors and requiring all clinics and hospitals to adhere to standard Western-style practices in patient records and drug-labelling.⁶ In 1952, the licensing exam that had to be taken by all health personnel, including doctors, dentists, and pharmacists, contained so much modern-medical content that very few Chinese-medical practitioners were able to pass and were therefore disqualified from practice. The new health insurance system would not cover treatment from unlicensed healers and did not cover the cost of

Chinese drugs. At the same time, in twenty-six-week courses, schools for the further education of Chinese medical practitioners were teaching the essentials of Western medicine, public health, and political education according to a Soviet model. In addition to educating Chinese-medical personnel in the basics of modern primary health care, the schools were also intended, in Mao's words, to 'smash sectarianism' within Chinese medicine. The lecturers were doctors of Western medicine, who compiled teaching materials, including textbooks of acupuncture.[7]

In 1953, the policy of creating a new medicine by educating Chinese-style practitioners was reversed, and, instead, the emphasis was placed on making doctors of Western medicine study Chinese medicine. As Scheid notes, the full reasons for this change are not entirely clear, but they certainly included a desire to rectify 'the undesirable ideological tendencies of Western-trained doctors,' a need to deploy medical personnel more efficiently and to avoid social unrest from Chinese-medical doctors, and an increasing national pride. This was also the period of the Korean War and the 1952 Patriotic Hygiene Campaign, which mobilized millions of urban Chinese to clean up the streets, exterminate insects, and catch vermin in order to minimize the risk of germ warfare attacks from the United States. The intense Cold War politics of this period only increased CCP doubts about the political reliability of urban professionals. The first classes began in 1955, and the Ministry of Health initiated the production of the first national textbook of Chinese medicine, the *Zhongyixue gailun* 中医学概论 (*Outline of Chinese Medicine*), published in 1958, ironically as teaching material for these doctors of Western medicine.[8]

During the 1960s, after the disaster of the Great Leap Forward and the consequent decline in Mao's political influence, there was less emphasis on educating Western-style doctors in Chinese medicine, and scientific research into Chinese medicine was re-emphasized. At the same time the Ministry of Health agreed to allow more Chinese-medical content in the education of Chinese-style doctors, though teaching from the classical literature of medicine was almost completely replaced by teaching from the new systematic and standardized textbooks.[9]

Elisabeth Hsu observes that, since 1958, the Ministry of Health's national textbooks for Chinese medicine have consistently translated political orthodoxy into Chinese medicine. The most obvious example is the interpretation of the opposing cosmological forces of *yin* and *yang* as native Chinese materialist dialectics, which is explained in terminology borrowed from political education, such as 'the unity of opposites' and 'mutual transformation.'[10] Thus, in a repeat of the debates of the early twentieth century, the theory of *yinyang* has been retained, while the cosmology of the Five Phases has periodically been omitted from Chinese-medical texts on the grounds of being 'unscientific.'[11]

While doctors of Western-style medicine were being required to study Chinese medicine, in the rural areas Chinese healers were being mobilized to form union clinics in their townships. These clinics were self-funded and initially self-managed. With the outbreak of the Cultural Revolution in 1966, these health workers were renamed 'barefoot doctors' and put in charge of village/brigade-level 'cooperative medical services.' Union clinics became organs of the communes receiving government subsidies, and folk healers were either prohibited or incorporated into the cooperative medical services. Fang Xiaoping's recent book describes how barefoot doctors emerged as a new and dominant form of healer in the countryside. However, rather than primarily using the 'one needle and a handful of herbs' of the contemporary slogan, Fang shows how they rarely had time for traditional medicine, preferring overwhelmingly to use Western drugs and to dispense vaccinations. Barefoot doctors became the prime means of extending modern medicine into the countryside and, in the process, contributed to a steep decline in the use of Chinese medicine. Moreover, Fang's research also demonstrates that decollectivization has not been the medical disaster that it is often assumed to be. In 1968, barefoot doctors were generally characterized by their youth and their clean political backgrounds. Since rural reforms began in 1978, rural doctors have been held to higher educational standards and medical proficiency, and an increase in professional standards has resulted.[12]

Since Mao's death in 1976, ending the political chaos of the Cultural Revolution and bringing Deng Xiaoping to power, the marketplace for medical therapies has been liberalized, along with the rest of the Chinese economy. In 1988-89, ethnographer Elisabeth Hsu was able to study *qigong* 气功 therapy with a hereditary healer, apprentice herself to a Chinese medical doctor in his private practice, and study state-sanctioned Chinese medicine in the Kunming College of Traditional Chinese Medicine. In the first two of these settings the teachers had concerns about whether to transmit the secret knowledge on which their livelihoods depended, much as had been the case in the medical marketplace of the early Republic.[13]

Even though – or perhaps because – Chinese medicine has been redesigned as a modern discipline taught in colleges for the last sixty years, patients still seek out doctors with a family background in medical practice. Mei Zhan notes that over 70 percent of the Chinese-style physicians featured in a 1989 volume on famous senior doctors in Shanghai came from hereditary medical families, even while they were also celebrated for being the generation that founded the Shanghai College of Traditional Chinese Medicine in 1956 and set up its teaching hospitals. She also reports that students at the Shanghai College who also have a family background in Chinese medicine are envied by other students.[14] Volker Scheid observes that graduates find it hard to establish themselves in Chinese medicine today with only a college degree.[15] Thus, ironically, the *jingyan* 经验, or embodied experience of practice, which was contrasted favourably with the baseless superstition of Chinese-medical theory by abolitionists such as Yu Yunxiu in 1929, is once more a precious resource that the modern colleges of Chinese medicine are unable to replicate.[16]

At the same time, the Chinese state has been promoting its streamlined and standardized acupuncture as an ideal cultural export. During the 1970s, China sent medical teams to developing countries, particularly in Africa, that typically included an acupuncturist along with nine or ten biomedical professionals. Acupuncture was part of China's internationalization effort aimed at assisting the 'global proletariat.'[17] Foreigners also flock to China to study Chinese medicine, acupuncture in particular, and there are now schools of acupuncture all over the Western world. Many countries have established professional organizations for acupuncturists with government-mandated licensing.

Just as 'Western' medicine was adapted to meet the needs and concerns of Chinese patients and governments in China, 'Chinese' medicine has also been modified in its applications abroad. Mei Zhan notes how Chinese medicine in the United States is constituted as a form of 'other' knowledge to be contrasted with science, so that its efficacy becomes miraculous precisely because of this othering.[18] Linda Barnes observes how the perception of Chinese medicine as a holistic practice in contrast to reductionist biomedicine has led to the use of acupuncture for cases of 'energy blockage' that are often described in psychological terms. At the same time, some American practitioners have reinserted some religious aspects of traditional practices that were purged from "modern" Chinese medicine after reframing them as 'spiritual' rather than as 'religious' interventions.[19] These observations suggest that the contrast with an idealized modern scientific medicine is constitutive of our understanding of Chinese medicine, whether practised in China or elsewhere. Ironically, given the long history of trying to make Chinese medicine more compatible with biomedicine, this East-West contrast has sometimes been encouraged in China. Kim Taylor argues that, in 1958, the appearance of the term 'traditional' in English-language Chinese publications about Chinese medicine was, in part, a deliberate strategy to reinforce 'a front of historical continuity' in order to satisfy Western thirst for an authentically ancient healing wisdom from the Orient.[20]

In *Cultural Hybridity*, Peter Burke cautions students of cultures to describe cultural change by using different metaphors, lest we forget any single metaphor's limitations.[21] Of the many examples he presents, two should suffice to show the complexity of the history of medicine in China: cultural translation and syncretism.

One way of describing the rise of Chinese medicine is to say that, in pursuit of a goal, individuals can appropriate or translate elements of a culture differently, leaving subsequent observers to wonder how the resulting multiple forms ever came about. When one of those forms shows more signs of a folk nature or seems somehow more idiosyncratic when compared to the observer's experience, it may be a natural tendency to label that form as 'traditional' or 'native.' Thus, an outsider may be forgiven for thinking that Chinese medicine follows a line of practice that is centuries old, when we have seen that this is not the case.

In fact, we have seen that both Western medicine and Chinese medicine, as practised during the period examined in this study, included appropriations of elements of medicine available to the Chinese via missionary medical, European medical, and Japanese medical models. That Chinese and Western medicine co-exist today says more about the diversity of approaches towards China's desire to leap into the group of 'modern' nations than it does about the strength of a continuing folk tradition.

No doubt few people spend much time questioning why Western medicine should spread to non-Western lands, but, if people were to consider it, their response would likely be that Western medicine works. (We are not talking about the administrative side of the practice.) Yet, the story of Western medicine in China shows that clinical practice was not the prime motivation for the Chinese to adapt it to their practice.

Instead, the forces we have considered include missionary fervour, important in bringing nineteenth-century medicine and surgery to China, and also important in providing medical services in rural areas where other providers of Western medicine were unwilling to work. We have seen that imperialism also played an important role: Western demands for 'free' trade necessitated medical examinations of ships and their passengers; once Japan gained colonial control over Taiwan in 1895, the Japanese colonial administration self-consciously used the provision of health care and sanitary policing methods to extend its political reach and to demonstrate the superiority of Japanese rule. This policy was continued, if less intensively, in Korea and Manchuria, where Japanese army, railway, and port medical services served as evidence of Japan's high level of civilization and technological progress. Japanese politicians were even prepared to appeal to the League of Nations Health Organization to compare the port health facilities in China and Japan in order to underscore China's need of tutelage and Japan's legitimacy as an imperial power, as we saw in Chapter 7. During the Republic many foreign powers had territorial holdings and trading privileges that extended far beyond the treaty ports in a patchwork of claims to sovereignty that has aptly been called 'hypercolonial.'[22] The development of a bureaucratic and technological cadre of officials who could meet the highest international standards of professionalism – in medicine as in other fields such as law and accounting – was essential to the Chinese campaign to assert its domestic sovereignty, as we demonstrated in Chapter 5.

However, neither the missionaries nor the Western powers sharing extraterritoriality rights were able to force the Chinese to accept Western medicine. Rather, it was when the Chinese sought to show the imperial nations that they, too, were modern that they began to see Western medicine as a useful tool in this endeavour. When this occurred, there was a double translation: Chinese interpreted Western medicine in ways that distinguished China from Japan and Western nations while, at the same time, using it as a foil to Chinese medicine.

Buzan, in discussing how imperial powers can impose a 'standard of civilization' on non-Western states under the vanguardist account of the spread of international society, suggests a model under which 'China seeks to adopt selected elements of Westernization in order to increase its strength to defend its own culture against the West.'[23] This defensive modernization seems to be in line with what we observe in the rise of Chinese medicine and perhaps in the Chinese willingness to adopt Western medical practices. But it does not fully explain the co-existence of the two medicines.

What of syncretism, the other metaphor for cultural change? Buzan's summary of the syncretic account of the spread of international society bears some similarities to the story of Chinese medicine in this period.[24] Syncretism implies a two-way exchange, in this case, affecting Western and Chinese medical practices. We have seen this in the way the West grew interested in Chinese *materia medica* as the Chinese were growing interested in Western medical practices and in Western institutions useful for both Western medicine and Chinese medicine. Yet, syncretism implies a kind of mixture. Surely there is a mixing of Western and non-Western elements in China's translation of Western medicine and in its establishment of Chinese medicine, but the two medicines themselves have retained separate existences.

The shortcomings of the metaphors of translation and syncretism are obvious. For one, what exactly was translated by whom? As we have seen in Chapter 6, individuals seized on different aspects of Western medicine or Chinese medicine to further their personal goals at the same time as they were attempting to advance the state's aim to modernize. Although such individual efforts fall out of focus once we aggregate their effect under the term 'cultural translation,' it is the best we can do, particularly in a case where there is no signal event, no single leader, bringing about the change.

The role of individuals in this process underscores another important point that complicates the story of Chinese medicine. Although China's drive to show that it belonged in the league of modern nations was significant, the story is not all about the state. Individuals who supported either Chinese medicine or Western medicine helped transfer and develop knowledge, advance practice, and establish institutions for both kinds of medicine. This is why the development of Chinese medicine is 'underdetermined.' Its origin and path were not set by Western science, by the state, or by any single viewpoint or political group. It is not a 'medical system' in the structural-functionalist sense of that term. There never was and is not now a single Chinese medicine.

At this point, it is tempting to follow Marwa Elshakry's suggestion that the very notion of a 'Western' science is the relatively recent result of developments in the field of the history of science.[25] In Elshakry's view, the idea that science could be 'Western' required not just the mutual encounter of Western and non-Western approaches but also an organizing principle or ideology of the history and potential of science itself. Elshakry sees this arise in the period just before the First World War. Before this, she considers a syncretic approach dominant in China (and Egypt, her other focal point). Her observation tallies with ours, where we see the idealized opposing constructs of *xiyi*, Western medicine, and *zhongyi*, Chinese medicine, coalescing out of syncretic assimilations at the same time that Western military power and economic extortion began to pose a real threat to the survival of the Chinese state. The survival of these *two* forms of syncretic medicine, both adapted to the Chinese environment in specific ways, are reminiscent of the arguments in the famous 'Science and Philosophy of Life' debates of the 1920s.[26] Responding to the devastation wreaked by modern technology during the First World War, Zhang Junmai 張君勱 (1887-1969) argued that blind faith in science as the ultimate source of truth was what had led to catastrophe. Instead, he proposed that science should be secondary to a philosophy of life that would embody moral and societal values such as the ideals of Chinese culture. Ding Wenjiang 丁文江 (1887-1936), also a scientist, countered that it had been bad politics rather than science that had caused the conflagration of Europe. Science was the only acceptable modern epistemology.[27] Of course, science cannot exist in a moral vacuum, and Zhang Junmai was not advocating abandoning science altogether. Science and philosophy of life were presented as opposing absolutes when in fact they are mutually constitutive. We suggest that the same may be said of "Western" and "Chinese" medicines.

Thus we are left with two kinds of medicine in China, each with variants and each arising relatively recently. Each is the result of translation and assimilation, and each involved syncretism at some point in its development. Clinical efficacy seems not to have been a determining factor in the adoption or translation of Western medicine: political efficacy was more important. Clinical efficacy *was* a factor, along with nationalism and cultural chauvinism, in the robust defence of Chinese medicine in the years before 1949. Further, the state's ambitions helped in these developments, but they were not the only or last word.

This leaves us with an interesting balance, calling for a new metaphor. Chinese medicine and Western medicine can now be seen as two mirrors facing each other at a short distance. Each mirror holds the image not only of the other but also of the other's view of itself. Remove one of the mirrors from the scene and the other loses its view of itself. Just as the idea of Western science depended on the encounter with the non-West, the concept of a Chinese medicine required that the late-nineteenth-century encounter with 'Western medicine' – itself a new construct – be intelligible. If we accept this point, by extrapolation we observe that 'Western' medicine is always defined by its others. Homeopathy held up a mirror to it in the late-nineteenth- and early twentieth-century West, just as 'complementary and alternative medicines' do today. Without its unacceptable doubles, modern medicine is as incoherent an assemblage of healing technologies as any other. And, as we have seen, the same dialectic has also come into play in the history of acupuncture, which began as an unacceptable lower-class practice when compared with the herbal medicine of the gentry class; then it assimilated anatomy to become a respectably scientific practice that could be used in Communist base areas to deflect heterodox healing illusions such as shamanism.

Naturally, this metaphor also has its limitations. Cultures do not reflect; people do. Mirrors cannot see; people can. But what a person sees reflected in a mirror depends on the angle of view that person takes. In other words, there is much yet to be written about Chinese medicine from perspectives different from the one taken here. There is also much more to be reflected on, and much more to be communicated, with regard to modern science in non-Western places.

Notes

Chapter 1: Modernities and Medicines

1 Private communication from Professor Ho Peng Yoke, family friend of the Wus.
2 Ralph C. Croizier, *Traditional Medicine in Modern China: Science, Nationalism and the Tensions of Cultural Change* (Cambridge, MA: Harvard University Press, 1968), 2.
3 Bruno Latour, *We Have Never Been Modern* (Cambridge, MA: Harvard University Press, 1993).
4 Harri Englund and James Leach, 'Ethnography and the Meta-Narratives of Modernity,' *Current Anthropology* 41, 2 (2000): 225-48.
5 Kim Taylor, *Chinese Medicine in Early Communist China, 1945-63: A Medicine of Revolution* (London: RoutledgeCurzon, 2005), 111-12.
6 See Paul U. Unschuld, *Medicine in China: A History of Ideas* (Berkeley: University of California Press, 1985), 250-62 for a description, and 360-66 for a translation of a 1980 Chinese newspaper article criticizing acupuncture anaesthesia.
7 Volker Scheid, 'Kexue and Guanxixue: Plurality, Tradition and Modernity in Contemporary Chinese Medicine,' in *Plural Medicine, Tradition and Modernity, 1800-2000*, ed. Waltraud Ernst (London: Routledge, 2002), 82-83.
8 People's Daily Online, 'Constitution of the People's Republic of China,' 22 March 2004, http://english.people.com.cn/constitution/constitution.html.
9 Zhao Hongjun, *Jindai Zhong-, Xi yixue lunzheng shi* 近代中西医学论争史 [History of the controversies between Chinese and Western medicine in modern times] (Hefei: Anhui Science and Technology Press, 1989), 20-22.
10 Arthur Kleinman, *Writing at the Margin* (Berekely: University of California Press, 1997), 37-39; Eliot Freidson, *Professional Powers: A Study of the Institutionalization*

of Formal Knowledge (Chicago: University of Chicago Press, 1986); Ming-Cheng M. Lo, *Doctors within Borders: Profession, Ethnicity, and Identity in Colonial Taiwan* (Berkeley: University of California Press, 2002).

11 Dominik Wujastyk, 'Medical Error and Medical Truth: The Placebo Effect and Room for Choice in Ayurveda,' *Health, Culture and Society* 1, 1 (2011): 221-31.

12 Harry M. Marks, *The Progress of Experiment* (Cambridge: Cambridge University Press, 1997), 230.

13 Mary B. Bullock, *An American Transplant: The Rockefeller Foundation and Peking Union Medical College* (Berkeley: University of California Press, 1980), chap. 2.

14 Charlotte Furth, *A Flourishing Yin: Gender in China's Medical History, 960-1665* (Berkeley: University of California Press, 1997), 115, chap. 8; Yi-Li Wu, *Reproducing Women: Medicine, Metaphor, and Childbirth in Late Imperial China* (Berkeley: University of California Press, 2010), 18-19.

15 *Huangdi nei jing su wen* [Yellow Emperor's inner canon], chap. 2, last paragraph.

16 Robert Hymes, 'Not Quite Gentlemen? Doctors in Sung and Yuan,' *Chinese Science* 8 (1987): 44.

17 Lydia H. Liu, *The Clash of Empires: The Invention of China in Modern World Making* (Cambridge, MA: Harvard University Press, 2006), 13-14.

18 Federico Masini, *The Formation of the Modern Chinese Lexicon and Its Evolution toward a National Language: The Period from 1840 to 1898, Journal of Chinese Linguistics* monograph series 6 (Berkeley, CA: Project on Linguistic Analysis, 1993), 76, 81, 153.

19 Hugh Shapiro, 'How Different Are Western and Chinese Medicine? The Case of Nerves,' in *Medicine across Cultures: History and Practice of Medicine in Non-Western Cultures*, ed. Helaine Selin (Dordrecht: Kluwer Academic, 2003), 351-72.

20 Ralph C. Croizier, 'The Ideology of Medical Revivalism in Modern China,' in *Asian Medical Systems: A Comparative Study in Non-Western Cultures*, ed. Charles Leslie (Berkeley: University of California Press, 1977), 341-54.

21 Marianne Bastid, *Educational Reform in Early Twentieth-Century China* (Ann Arbor: Center for Chinese Studies, University of Michigan, 1988).

22 Ping Chen, *Modern Chinese: History and Sociolinguistics* (Cambridge: Cambridge University Press, 1999), 85-87.

23 See Bonnie S. McDougall and Kam Louie, *The Literature of China in the Twentieth Century* (New York: Columbia University Press, 1999).

24 For Confucianism, see Hsi-Yuan Chen, *Confucian Encounters with Religion: Rejections, Appropriations, and Transformations* (New York: Routledge, 2006); and Mayfair Mei-hui Yang, ed., *Chinese Religiosities: Afflictions of Modernity and State Formation* (Berkeley: University of California Press, 2008). For Daoism, see Xun Liu, *Daoist Modern: Innovation, Lay Practice, and the Community of Inner Alchemy in Republican Shanghai* (Cambridge, MA: Harvard University Asia Center, 2009). For Buddhism, see Don Alvin Pittman, *Toward a Modern Chinese Buddhism* (Honolulu: University of Hawai'i Press, 2001).

25 Susan L. Glosser, *Chinese Visions of Family and State, 1915-1953* (Berkeley: University of California Press, 2003); Alison W. Conner, 'Lawyers and the Legal Profession during the Republican Period,' in *Civil Law in Qing and Republican China,* ed. Kathryn Bernhardt and Philip C. Huang (Stanford: Stanford University Press, 1994) 215-48; Philip C. Huang, *Code, Custom, and Legal Practice in China* (Stanford: Stanford University Press, 2001).

26 Peter Burke, *Cultural Hybridity* (Cambridge: Polity, 2009), chap. 1.

27 Douglas R. Reynolds, *China, 1989-1912: The Xinzheng Revolution and Japan* (Cambridge, MA: Council on East Asian Studies, Harvard University, 1993).

28 Benjamin A. Elman, *On Their Own Terms: Science in China, 1550-1900* (Cambridge, MA: Harvard University Press, 2005), chap. 10. For an account of some of the scientific activities carried out at the Anqing and Jiangnan Arsenals, see David Wright, 'Careers in Western Science in Nineteenth-Century China: Xu Shou and Xu Jianyin,' *Journal of the Royal Asiatic Society of Great Britain and Ireland* 5, 1 (1995): 49-90.

29 Jack Gray, *Rebellions and Revolutions: China from the 1800s to the 1980s* (Oxford: Oxford University Press, 1990), 166.

30 James Reeve Pusey, *China and Charles Darwin* (Cambridge, MA: Harvard University Press, 1983).

31 Andrew D. Morris, *Marrow of the Nation: A History of Sport and Physical Culture in Republican China* (Berkeley: University of California Press, 2004).

32 Exceptions to this generalization in medicine include John Watt and Nicole Barnes, both of whom are working on histories of medicine in wartime China. See also Ka-che Yip, 'Disease and the Fighting Men: Nationalist Anti-Epidemic Efforts in Wartime China, 1937-1945,' in *China in the Anti-Japanese War, 1937-1945: Politics, Culture, and Society,* ed. David P. Barrett and Larry N. Shyu (New York: Peter Lang, 2001), 171-201; and Yuehtsen Juliette Chung, *Struggle for National Survival: Eugenics in Sino-Japanese Contexts, 1896-1945* (New York: Routledge, 2002). The absurdity of the lack of attention to this key period was signalled in 1995 by Prasenjit Duara, *Rescuing History from the Nation: Questioning Narratives of Modern China* (Chicago: University of Chicago Press, 1995). Since then, Hans J. van de Ven, *War and Nationalism in China, 1925-1945* (Abingdon: RoutledgeCurzon, 2003) has reasserted the nation as the subject of wartime history.

33 See Mao's speech 'The United Front in Cultural work,' discussed in Taylor, *Chinese Medicine,* 14-19.

34 Ruth Rogaski, *Hygienic Modernity: Meanings of Health and Disease in Treaty-Port China* (Berkeley: University of California Press, 2004).

Chapter 2: The Spectrum of Chinese Healing Practices

1 Bullock, *American Transplant.*

2 For the Bamboo Grove gynecologists, see Wu, *Reproducing Women,* 59-66. For martial arts and medicine, see John D. Wong, 'The Adaptable Chinese Bone: Grafting

Biomedical Technologies on Traditional Chinese Bone-setting,' unpublished paper, 2002; and Meir Shahar, *The Shaolin Monastery: History, Religion, and the Chinese Martial Arts* (Honolulu: University of Hawai'i Press, 2008).

3 Charlotte Furth, *A Flourishing Yin: Gender in China's Medical History, 960-1665* (Berkeley: University of California Press, 1997); Ping-chen Hsiung, *A Tender Voyage: Children and Childhood in Late Imperial China* (Stanford: Stanford University Press, 2007); Chia-feng Chang, 'Aspects of Smallpox and Its Significance in Chinese History' (PhD diss., School of Oriental and African Studies, University of London, History, 1996); Angela Ki-che Leung, 'Women Practicing Medicine in Pre-modern China,' in *Chinese Women in the Imperial Past: New Perspectives*, ed. Harriet T. Zurndorfer (Leiden: Brill, 1999), 101-34.

4 Dudgeon's life as a medical missionary has recently been studied by Gao Xi 高晞, *Dezhen zhuan: Yige yingguo chuanjiaoshi yu wan Qing yixue jindaihua* 德贞传：一个英国传教士与晚清医学近代化 [Biography of John Dudgeon: A British missionary and the modernization of late Qing medicine] (Shanghai: Fudan University Press, 2009). Dudgeon's views on diet and hygiene are described by Shang-jen Li, 'Eating Well in China: British Medical Practitioners on Diet and Personal Hygiene at Nineteenth-Century Chinese Treaty Ports,' in *Health and Hygiene in Chinese East Asia*, ed. Angela Ki Che Leung and Charlotte Furth (Durham, NC: Duke University Press, 2010), 109-31.

5 Qiu Jisheng, 'Shaoxing zhi yi su' 紹興之醫俗 [Medical customs of Shaoxing], in *Qiu Jisheng yi wenji* 裘吉生醫文集 [Medical writings of Qiu Jisheng], ed. Qiu Shiting 裘詩庭 (Beijing: Renmin weisheng chubanshe, 2006), 8-18.

6 Rogaski, *Hygienic Modernity*.

7 John Dudgeon, 'The Chinese Arts of Healing,' *CR* 2 (1869-70): 163-64.

8 Ibid., 167.

9 Philip A. Kuhn, *Soulstealers: The Chinese Sorcery Scare of 1768* (Cambridge, MA: Harvard University Press, 1990), 108-9; B.J. ter Haar, *The White Lotus Teachings in Chinese Religious History* (Honolulu: University of Hawai'i Press, 1992), chap. 7.

10 Arthur Kleinman gives a detailed description of shamanic healing as observed in 1970s Taiwan in *Patients and Healers in the Context of Culture: An Exploration of the Borderland between Anthropology, Medicine and Psychiatry* (Berkeley: University of California Press, 1980), 210-43.

11 Many of these practices are described in detail in Richard J. Smith, *Fortune-tellers and Philosophers: Divination in Traditional Chinese Society* (Boulder, CO: Westview Press, 1991). For a discussion of the application of divination to medicine in modern China, see Judith Farquhar, '"Medicine and the Changes Are One": An Essay on Divination Healing with Commentary,' *Chinese Science* 13 (1996): 107-34.

12 Dudgeon, 'Chinese Arts of Healing,' 186.

13 Ibid., 268-69.

14 *Zhuyou* 祝由 originally meant 'praying to understand the cause' but came to include interdictions and exorcism of demonic forces in relation to disease. Its practice at

the Imperial Medical Academy was in fact suspended after 1571, during the Ming dynasty, and not by the Manchus as Dudgeon believed. See Philip S. Cho, 'Ritual and the Occult in Chinese Medicine and Religious Healing: The Development of Zhuyou Exorcism' (PhD diss., University of Pennsylvania, 2005).

15   Dudgeon, 'Chinese Arts of Healing,' 296.

16   Ibid., 297-98.

17   Gao, *Dezhen zhuan*, 148-49; John Dudgeon, *Chinese Healing Arts: Internal Kung-Fu*, ed. William R. Berk (Burbank, CA: Unique Publications, 1986), 1-8.

18   On the partial convergence of Chinese and Western ideas of health in the 1870s, see Marta Hanson, *Speaking of Epidemics in Chinese Medicine: Disease and the Geographic Imagination in Late Imperial China* (London: Routledge, 2011), chap. 7, esp. 148-50; Rogaski, *Hygienic Modernity*, chap. 1.

19   The following is a summary of Qiu, 'Shaoxing zhi yi su,' 9-18.

20   Jean Ewen, *China Nurse, 1932-39* (Toronto: McClelland and Stewart, 1981), 25. For a description of 'child fright' as a culture-bound syndrome, see Kleinman, *Patients and Healers*, 195-98.

21   For the importance of diet as a form of healing, see Linda Chih-ling Koo, *Nourishment of Life: Health in Chinese Society* (Hong Kong: The Commercial Press, 1982); K.C. Chang, ed., *Food in Chinese Culture: Anthropological and Historical Perspectives* (New Haven: Yale University Press, 1977), in addition to the many volumes in Chinese on dietary therapy.

22   See Smith, *Fortune-tellers and Philosophers*, 235-45.

23   Adam Yuet Chau, *Miraculous Response: Doing Popular Religion in Contemporary China* (Stanford: Stanford University Press, 2006), 101-2.

24   Kleinman, *Patients and Healers*, 203-58.

25   This kind of doctor is depicted in a watercolour illustration by late Qing dynasty artist Zhou Peichun on the Wellcome Trust image website, http://medphoto.well-come.ac.uk/, image number 2044. It is this kind of doctor, a *lingyi* (bell-doctor), whose practice was described in the book *Chuanya* 串雅 by Zhao Xuemin (趙學敏, 1730-1805). See Paul U. Unschuld, *Medicine in China: A History of Ideas* (Berkeley: University of California Press, 1985), 210-12.

26   Guoyi xueshe 國醫學社 [Society for National Medicine], *Jianghu yishu mizhuan* 江湖醫術秘傳 [Transmitted secrets of 'rivers-and-lakes' medicine] (Hong Kong: Li Li Publishing 勵力出版社, 1954).

27   Yongyan Yu 永燕余, 'Jindai Zhongyi fangzhi baihoubing shilue' 近代中医防治白喉病史略 [A brief history of prevention and treatment of diphtheria in modern TCM], *CJMH* 34, 2 (2004): 79-82; Xie Guan 謝觀, *Zhongguo yixue yuan liu lun* 中國醫學源流論 [The origin and development of Chinese medicine] (Fuzhou: Fujian kexue jishu chubanshe, 1935), 88-90.

28   For the gynecology of the Bamboo Grove Monastery, see Wu, *Reproducing Women*, 59-64 and *passim*.

29   See Kleinman, *Patients and Healers*, 195-98.

30 Christopher Cullen, 'Patients and Healers in Late Imperial China: Evidence from the Jinpingmei,' *History of Science* 31, 2 (1993): 99-150.

31 Wu, *Reproducing Women*, 225-28.

32 Henrietta Harrison, 'The Experience of Illness in Early Twentieth-century Rural Shanxi,' *East Asian Science, Technology and Medicine* 33 (2013): forthcoming; Dore J. Levy, *Ideal and Actual in the Story of the Stone* (New York: Columbia University Press, 1999), chap. 3.

33 Yuan-ling Chao, *Medicine and Society in Late Imperial China: A Study of Physicians in Suzhou, 1600-1850* (New York: Peter Lang, 2009), 70-74.

34 Paul Katz, *Demon Hordes and Burning Boats: The Cult of Marshal Wen in Late Imperial Chekiang* (New York: State University of New York Press, 1995), 70-75; Carol Benedict, *Bubonic Plague in Nineteenth-Century China* (Stanford: Stanford University Press, 1996), 100-30; Rebecca Nedostup, *Superstitious Regimes: Religion and the Politics of Chinese Modernity* (Cambridge, MA: Harvard University Asia Center, 2010), 215-24; Dr. J.P. Kleiweg de Zwaan, *Völkerkundliches und Geschichtliches über die Heilkunde der Chinesen und Japaner* [Ethnographic and historical study of Chinese and Japanese healing] (Haarlem: De Erven Loosjes, 1917).

35 Unschuld, *Medicine in China*, 163-91; Unschuld reproduces images of many of these containers and advertising devices in his *Medicine in China: Historical Artifacts and Images* (Berkeley: University of California Press, 2000).

36 Sherman Cochran, *Chinese Medicine Men: Consumer Culture in China and Southeast Asia* (Cambridge, MA: Harvard University Press, 2006); Roberta Bivins, *Alternative Medicine? A History*, 1st ed. (Oxford: Oxford University Press, 2007), 171-83.

37 Caroline Reeves, 'The Changing Nature of Philanthropy in Late Imperial and Republican China,' *Papers on Chinese History, Harvard University* 5 (1996): 85; Elizabeth Sinn, *Power and Charity: The Early History of the Tung Wah Hospital, Hong Kong* (Hong Kong: Oxford University Press, 1989).

38 Paul U. Unschuld, *Forgotten Traditions of Ancient Chinese Medicine: The I Hsüeh Yüan Liu Lun of 1757 by Hsü Ta-Ch'un* (Brookline, MA: Paradigm Publications, 1990), 213; Xinzhong Yu 余新忠, 'Qingdai Jiangnan de minsu yiliao xingwei shenxi' 清代江南的民俗医疗行为探析 [Analysis of folk healing behaviour in Qing dynasty Jiangnan], in *Qing yilai de jibing, yiliao he weisheng* 清以来的疾病, 医疗和卫生 [Disease, medicine and hygiene since the Qing], ed. Xinzhong Yu (Beijing: Sanlian, 2009), 91-108.

39 Farquhar, 'Medicine and the Changes Are One,' 127-28.

Chapter 3: Missionary Medicine from the West

1 Zhang Zhongjing, Craig Mitchell, Feng Ye, and Nigel Wiseman, *Shāng Hán Lùn: On Cold Damage, Translation and Commentaries* (Boston: Paradigm Publications, 1999), 60-64.

2 Dan Bensky and Randall Barolet, *Chinese Herbal Medicine: Formulas and Strategies*, 1st ed. (Seattle: Eastland Press, 1990), 35-36.

3   W. Hale White, *Materia Medica, Pharmacy, Pharmacology and Therapeutics* (London: J. and A. Churchill, 1892), 33.

4   William G. Rothstein, *American Physicians in the 19th Century: From Sects to Science* (Baltimore: Johns Hopkins University Press, 1972), 90-91; Lawrence I. Conrad, Michael Neve, Vivian Nutton, Roy Porter, Andrew Wear, *The Western Medical Tradition, 800 BC to AD 1800* (Cambridge: Cambridge University Press, 1995), 422-23.

5   Harold Balme, *China and Modern Medicine: A Study in Medical Missionary Development* (London: United Council for Missionary Education, 1921), 1.

6   J.G.K. [Kerr], 'Chinese Materia Medica,' *CMMJ* 1, 2 (1887): 79-80.

7   B.E. Read and C.O. Lee, 'Chinese Inorganic Materia Medica,' *CMJ* 39, 1 (1925): 23-32.

8   B.C. Patterson, M.D., 'Correspondence: Substitute for Cataplasma Kaolini (USP),' *CMJ* 37, 2 (1923): 201; B.E. Read, 'Correspondence: Substitute for Cataplasma Kaolini (U.S.P.),' *CMJ* 37, 3-4 (1923): 340.

9   Anon., 'Conference Report of the Medical Missionary Conference Held at Shanghai, April 19-23, 1907, Discussion on Dr. McCartney's Paper, "The Fevers of West China,"' *CMJ* 21, 3 (1907): 163-64.

10   Henry George Greenish, *Materia Medica: Being an Account of the More Important Crude Drugs of Vegetable and Animal Origin: Designed for Students of Pharmacy and Medicine* (London: J. and A. Churchill, 1924), 10, 14.

11   M.R. Lee, 'The History of Ephedra (ma-huang),' *Journal of the Royal College of Physicians of Edinburgh* 41, 1 (2011): 78-84.

12   Peter Kiang, M.D., 'Chinese Drugs of Therapeutic Value to Western Physicians,' *CMJ* 37, 9 (1923): 742-46.

13   Sean Hsiang-Lin Lei, 'From "Changshan" to a New Anti-malarial Drug: Re-networking Chinese Drugs and Excluding Chinese Doctors,' *Social Studies of Science* 29, 3 (1999): 323-58; Margaret M. Lock, *East Asian Medicine in Urban Japan* (Berkeley: University of California Press, 1980), 65.

14   Anon., 'Progress in China: The Wheels Move Slowly in the Dragon's Empire,' *New York Times*, 11 March 1892 (emphasis in original).

15   J.K. Crellin, *A Social History of Medicines in the Twentieth Century: To Be Taken Three Times a Day* (Binghamton: Pharmaceutical Products Press, 2004), 67.

16   Anon., 'Editorial,' *CMMJ* 7, 2 (1893): 110.

17   W. Hamilton Jeffreys and James L. Maxwell, *The Diseases of China, including Formosa and Korea* (London: John Bale and Danielson, 1911), 8. The authors were not of this opinion, instead suggesting that Western surgeons who operated without anaesthetic should themselves be transformed into pincushions.

18   John Dudgeon, *The Diseases of China; Their Causes, Conditions, and Prevalence, Contrasted with Those in Europe* (Glasgow: Dunn and Wright, 1877), 53; Rogaski, *Hygienic Modernity*, 102.

19   Edward H. Hume, *Doctors East, Doctors West: An American Physician's Life in China* (New York: W.W. Norton, 1946), 54-57.

20 S.H. Chuan, 'Chinese Patients and Their Prejudices,' *CMJ* 31, 6 (1917): 504-10.

21 James Henderson, *Shanghai Hygiene: Or, Hints for the Preservation of Health in China* (Shanghai: Presbyterian Mission Press, 1863); C.A. Gordon, *An Epitome of the Reports of the Medical Officers of the China Imperial Maritime Customs Service, from 1871-1882.* (London: Baillière, Tindall and Cox, 1884); Kerrie L. Macpherson, *A Wilderness of Marshes: The Origins of Public Health in Shanghai, 1843-1893*, East Asian Historical Monographs (Oxford: Oxford University Press, 1987), 28-41.

22 Numerous examples of this are given by Michelle Renshaw, *Accommodating the Chinese: The American Hospital in China, 1880-1920* (New York: Routledge, 2005). Hugh L. Shapiro's 'The View from a Chinese Asylum: Defining Madness in 1930s Peking' (PhD diss., Harvard University, History and East Asian Languages, 1995), reproduces diagrams of the Peking Union Medical College psychiatric buildings, which were clearly built according to Chinese norms as late as the 1920s.

23 Renshaw, *Accommodating the Chinese*, 183, citing W. Hamilton Jeffreys.

24 Wong Fun to Tidman, Correspondence, 26 November 1867, School of Oriental and Asian Studies, London Missionary Society Archives.

25 See Norman Howard-Jones, *The Scientific Background of the International Sanitary Conferences, 1851-1938*, WHO History of International Public Health (Geneva: World Health Organization, 1975), 61-70. British delegates to these conferences almost always opposed any view of the etiology of cholera that might have endangered trade by imposing expensive quarantine delays. Howard-Jones cites the *Deutsche Medizinische Wochenschrift* 11 (1885): 347, on the ironic German observation of the 'surprising concordance between England's commercial interests and its scientific convictions' (58).

26 See Edwin Chadwick, 'On the Prevention of Epidemics,' in *Transactions of the Brighton Health Congress*, 24-47 (London: E. Marlborough, 1881).

27 William Ewart, *Res Medica, Res Publica: The Profession of Medicine: Its Future Work and Wage* (London: St. George's Hospital, London, 1907).

28 Lien-teh Wu, *Plague Fighter: The Autobiography of a Modern Chinese Physician* (Cambridge: Heffers, 1959), chap. 1.

29 Jeffreys and Maxwell, *Diseases of China*, 4 (emphasis in original).

30 W.G. Lennox, 'A Self-survey by Mission Hospitals in China,' *CMJ* 46, 5 (1932): 484-534.

31 James Henderson, 'The Medicine and Medical Practice of the Chinese,' *JNCBRAS* 1 (1864): 64.

32 Dudgeon, *Diseases of China*, 59-60.

33 Gordon, *Epitome*, 6.

34 'Diseases of China,' *Lancet* 110, 2821 (1877): 439-40. For more of Dudgeon's views on the relationships between Chinese culture and the relative absence of disease, see Gao, *Dezhen zhuan;* Rogaski, *Hygienic Modernity*, 101-3; Shang-jen Li, 'Jiankang De daode jingji: Dezhen lun Zhongguoren shenghuo xiguan he weisheng' [Moral economy and health: John Dudgeon on hygiene in China], *Zhongyang yanjiuyuan*

lishi yuyan yanjiusuo jikan [Bulletin of the Institute of History and Philology, Academia Sinica] 76, 3 (2005): 467-509.

35 Dr. H.D. Porter, 'From China,' in *The Medical Arm of the Missionary Service: Testimonies from the Field,* ed. E.K. Alden (Boston: American Board of Commissioners for Foreign Missions, 1894), 37-41.

36 Macpherson, *Wilderness of Marshes;* Rogaski, *Hygienic Modernity,* 195.

37 W.W. Peter, 'Appeal by Joint Council on Public Health Education in China,' *CMJ* 31, 1 (1917): 57-59.

38 Dr. S.M. Woo, 'Health Work in Amoy,' *CMJ* 32 (1918): 289-91; Carol Benedict, 'Bubonic Plague in Nineteenth-Century China' (PhD diss., Stanford University, 1992), 1.

39 Shirley S. Garrett, *Social Reformers in Urban China: The Chinese YMCA, 1895-1926,* Harvard East Asian Series (Cambridge, MA: Harvard University Press, 1970), 213-38.

40 Personal communication.

41 Editorial, 'An Obstacle to Sanitary Progress,' *CMJ* 34, 5 (1920): 523-24.

42 Sergei Tretiakov, *A Chinese Testament: The Autobiography of Tan Shih-hua* (New York: Simon and Schuster, 1934), 36.

43 Judy Slinn, 'The Development of the Pharmaceutical Industry,' in *Making Medicines: A Brief History of Pharmacy and Pharmaceuticals,* ed. Stuart Anderson (London: Pharmaceutical Press, 2005), 155-74.

Chapter 4: The Significance of Medical Reforms in Japan

1 Lu Xun, *Selected Works of Lu Hsun* (Beijing: Foreign Languages Press, 1956), 1:6.

2 Y. Fujikawa, *Japanese Medicine,* English ed., trans. from 1911 German, Clio Medica (New York: Paul B. Hoeber, 1934), 34-36; Shi Shiqin 史世勤, ed., *Zhongyi chuan Ri shilüe* 中医传日史略 [A brief history of the transmission of Chinese medicine to Japan] (Wuchang: Huazhong shifan daxue chubanshe, 1991), 81-84.

3 Otori Ranzaburō, 'The Acceptance of Western Medicine in Japan,' *Monumenta Nipponica* 19, 3-4 (1964): 20-40.

4 Noga Arikha, *Passions and Tempers: A History of the Humours* (New York: HarperCollins, 2007), 10-11.

5 Fujikawa, *Japanese Medicine,* 39.

6 John Z. Bowers, *Western Medical Pioneers in Feudal Japan* (Baltimore: Johns Hopkins University Press, 1970), 18-19.

7 Zhao, *Jindai Zhong-, Xiyixue lunzheng shi,* 283; Shi, *Zhongyi chuan Ri shilüe,* 83.

8 Ann Jannetta, *The Vaccinators: Smallpox, Medical Knowledge, and the 'Opening' of Japan* (Stanford: Stanford University Press, 2007). Shi, *Zhongyi chuan Ri shilüe,* 124-25 for the spread of variolation, and 267-70 for records of visits to Japan by Chinese physicians in the Tokugawa period.

9 Jannetta, *Vaccinators,* 31.

10 Bowers, *Western Medical Pioneers,* 67-72; Fujikawa, *Japanese Medicine,* 41-47.

11 For the increasing importance of graphic realism in Japanese scientific and popular culture in the eighteenth century, see Maki Fukuoka, *The Premise of Fidelity: Science, Visuality, and Representing the Real in Nineteenth-Century Japan* (Stanford: Stanford University Press, 2012); Timon Screech, *The Lens within the Heart: The Western Scientific Gaze and Popular Imagery in Later Edo Japan* (Honolulu: University of Hawai'i Press, 2002).

12 Togo Tsukahara, *Affinity and Shinwa Ryoku: The Introduction of Western Chemical Concepts in Early Nineteenth-Century Japan* (Amsterdam: J.C. Gieben, 1993), 79-80.

13 Ellen Gardner Nakamura, *Practical Pursuits: Takano Choei, Takahashi Keisaku, and Western Medicine in Nineteenth-Century Japan* (Cambridge, MA: Harvard University Asia Center, 2005), 4-13.

14 Screech, *Lens within the Heart*, 20-30; Susan Burns, 'Nanayama Jundō at Work: A Village Doctor and Medical Knowledge in Nineteenth Century Japan,' *East Asian Science, Technology and Medicine*, 29 (2008): 62-82.

15 William Johnston, 'Of Doctors, Women, and the Knife of Hope: The Surgical Treatment of Breast Cancer in Early Modern Japan,' in *History of Ideas in Surgery*, Proceedings of the 17th International Symposium on the Comparative History of Medicine – East and West, ed. Yosio Kawakita, Shizu Sakai, Yasuo Otsuka (Tokyo: Ishiyaku EuroAmerica, 1997), 153-80.

16 Tsukahara, *Affinity and Shinwa Ryoku*, 80-82.

17 J.L.C. Pompe van Meerdervoort, 'Dissection of a Japanese Criminal,' *JNCBRAS* 2, 1 (1860): 85-91.

18 Bowers, *Western Medical Pioneers*, 188-92.

19 Ibid., 140, quoting Sir George Sansom.

20 For a list of these schools, their founders, and their dates of establishment, see Guijuan Pan 桂娟潘 and Zhenglun Fan 正伦樊, *Riben Hanfang yixue* 日本汉方医学 [Japanese Kanpō medicine] (Beijing: Zhongguo zhongyiyao chubanshe, 1994), 178-79. These academies for medical studies (Sino-Japanese or Western) were a Japanese innovation dating from the mid-eighteenth century. See also James R. Bartholomew, *The Formation of Science in Japan: Building a Research Tradition* (New Haven: Yale University Press, 1989), 27.

21 Jin Shiying 靳士英, 'Riben fan feizhi Hanfang yu Zhongguo fan feizhi Zhongyi zhi douzheng ji qi bijiao' 日本反废止汉方与中国反废止中医之斗争及其比较 [Comparison of the Japanese and Chinese opposition to the abolition of traditional medicine], *CJMH* 1 (1993): 45-51.

22 Jannetta, *Vaccinators*, 181-87.

23 Pan and Fan, *Riben Hanfang yixue*, 253-56.

24 Zhao, *Jindai Zhong-, Xiyixue lunzheng shi*, 275.

25 Christian Oberländer, 'The Modernization of Japan's Kanpo Medicine (1850-1950),' in *East Asian Science: Tradition and Beyond*, ed. Hashimoto Keizo, Cathérine Jami, and Lowell Skar (Papers from the Seventh International Conference for the History

of Science in East Asia, Kyoto, 2-7 August 1993) (Osaka: Kansai University Press, 1993), 141-46.

26 Zhao, *Jindai Zhong-, Xiyixue lunzheng shi*, 276.

27 Christian Oberländer, *Zwischen Tradition und Moderne: Die Bewegung für den Fortbestand der Kanpō-Medizin in Japan*, 149-86; Pan and Fan, *Riben Hanfang yixue*, 263-74.

28 Ishiguro's arguments are reproduced in full in Pan and Fan, *Riben Hanfang yixue*, 274-79. On the attitudes of the International Red Cross towards Japan and China, see Olive Checkland, *Humanitarianism and the Emperor's Japan, 1877-1977* (Basingstoke: Macmillan, 1994), 45. Ishiguro's own account of the history of the Red Cross in Japan is translated in Count Shigenobu Okuma, *Fifty Years of New Japan* (London: Smith, Elder, 1909), 307-22.

29 Jin, 'Riben fan feizhi Hanfang,' 47; Zhao, *Jindai Zhong-, Xiyixue lunzheng shi*, 276-77.

30 Pan and Fan, *Riben Hanfang yixue*, 283-85.

31 Ding Fubao published Chinese translations of this book in 1911 and 1920. The 'iron spear' is an allusion to a classical story in which a lord of Han, Zhang Liang, raised an army to fight the first emperor of China, Qin Shihuang, in order to reclaim his confiscated lands. He succeeded in getting close enough to throw his spear but missed Qin Shihuang's chariot, hitting a neighbouring one instead. The message is that attacks on *kanpō* medicine were aimed at the wrong target.

32 Pan and Fan, *Riben Hanfang yixue*, 299.

33 Quoted in Jin, 'Riben fan feizhi Hanfang,' citing issue 1018 of the journal *Medical Affairs Weekly* (*Yishi zhoubao* 醫事周報), 1914.

34 Oberländer, *Zwischen Tradition und Moderne*.

35 Zhao, *Jindai Zhong-, Xiyixue lunzheng shi*, 276; Yunxiu Yu 云岫余, 'Yixue geming de guoqu gongzuo, xianzai xingshi he weilai de celue' 醫學革命的過去, 現在形勢和未來的策略 [The past work of the medical revolution, its present state and future strategy], *CMMJ* 20, 1 (1934): 17.

36 Jin, 'Riben fan feizhi Hanfang yixue,' 48.

37 Andrew Gordon, *A Modern History of Japan: From Tokugawa Times to the Present* (Oxford: Oxford University Press, 2009), 174-76.

38 Oberländer, *Zwischen Tradition und Moderne*, 205-13.

39 Zhao, *Jindai Zhong-, Xiyixue lunzheng shi*, 276-77; Jin, 'Riben fan feizhi Hanfang yixue,' 48-49.

40 For Sun's relationship with Japan and his supporters there, see Marius B. Jansen, 'Japan and the Chinese Revolution of 1911,' in *The Cambridge History of China* (Cambridge: Cambridge University Press, 1980), vol. 11, pt. 2, 339-74.

41 For the list of members, see Zhao, *Jindai Zhong-, Xiyixue lunzheng shi*, 112. Educational backgrounds checked using information given by K. Chimin Wong and Lien-teh Wu, *History of Chinese Medicine* (Shanghai: Reprinted by Southern Materials Center, Taipei, 1985 [1936]).

42 This account is based on the article by the Medical History Committee of the Shanghai Branch of the Chinese Medical Association, 'Yu Yunxiu xiansheng zhuan-lüe he nianpu' 余云岫先生传略和年谱 [Biographical sketch and chronology of the life of Mr. Yu Yunxiu], *ZHYSZZ*, 2 (1954): 81-84, an account written shortly after his death by Yu's colleagues and clearly designed to rescue his reputation from censure in a political climate that was increasingly promoting Chinese medicine. See also Yu's own accounts, as found in Yu, 'Yixue geming de guoqu gongzuo,' and Yunxiu Yu, *Yixue geming lun: chuji* 醫學革命論: 初集 [On the medical revolution: Part one] (Shanghai: Yushi yanjiushi, 1928).

43 See 'Ling, su shangdui' [Straight talk about the spiritual (pivot) and the plain (questions)], in Yu, *Yixue geming lun*, 1-5 and 46-47.

44 See, for example, Qin Danwei 秦但末, 'Chi Yu Yunxiu yixiao xitong boyi' 斥余云岫 醫校系統駁義 [A denunciation of Yu Yunxiu's disagreements with the medical school system (i.e., with the proposal to include Chinese-medical schools)], *SSYB* 3, 12 (1925): 1-2.

45 The full text of the proposal is reproduced in Zhen Zhiya 甄志亞 and Fu Weikang 傅維康, eds., *Zhongguo yixue shi* 中国医学史 [History of Chinese medicine], (Beijing: Renmin weisheng chubanshe, 1991), 497-98. English-language summaries may be found in Croizier, *Traditional Medicine in Modern China*, 91; Wu, *Plague Fighter*, 506; and Sean Hsiang-Lin Lei, 'When Chinese Medicine Encountered the State: 1910-1949' (University of Chicago, Committee on the Conceptual Foundations of Science, 1999).

46 Yu, as quoted in Zhen and Fu, *Zhongguo yixue shi*, 498.

47 Lien-teh Wu, 'The Future of Medical Research in the Orient,' *NMJC* (English section) 8, 4 (1922): 286-90.

48 Anon., 'Zhonghua yixue hui gaikuo baogao' 中華醫學會概括報告 [Summary report on the National Medical Association], *NMJC* (Chinese section) 18, 1 (1932): 175-83.

49 Yu, 'Yixue geming de guoqu gongzuo,' 16-17.

50 Zhang Zaitong, chief compiler, 张在通, *Minguo yiyao weisheng fagui xuanbian* 民国医药卫生法规选编 [Compilation of medical and sanitary laws and regulations during the Republic, 1912-1948] (Taian: Shandong University Press, 1990), 50-51 and 53-56.

51 Yu, *Yixue geming lun*, 16-17.

52 Zhang Qimin 張啟民, 'Xiandai yixue zhi guanjian' 現代醫學之關鍵 [The key to modern medicine], *Xiandai Guoyi* 現代國醫 [Modern national medicine] 2, 6 (1932): 5-10.

53 Jin Shiying 靳士英, 'Jindai Zhong, Ri liang guo de zhongyi jiaoliu' 近代中日两国的 中医交流 [Modern Sino-Japanese exchanges in Chinese medicine], *CJMH* 22, 2 (1992): 107. A similar account of Yang Shoujing's book-collecting activities is given in Fangjun Xiao's preface to Chen Cunren 陳存仁, comp., *Huanghan yixue congshu* 皇漢醫學叢書 [Sino-Japanese medical collection] (Shanghai: Shijie, shuju, 1936).

54 For Lu's use of Japanese scholarship, see Lu Yuanlei 陸淵雷, *Shanghan lun jin shi* 傷寒論今釋 [Modern exposition of the treatise on cold-damage] (Beijing: Renmin weisheng chubanshe, 1931). For the statistics, see Jin, 'Jindai Zhong,' 108-9.

55 Chen, *Huanghan yixue congshu,* editor's preface.

56 Wang Shenxuan 王慎軒, *Zhongyi xin lun huibian* 中醫新論會變 [Compilation of new essays in Chinese medicine] (Shanghai: Shanghai shudian, 1932).

57 Zhu Weiju 朱味菊, *Bingli fahui* 病理發揮 [Pathology elucidated], Mr. Zhu's Medical Collection (Shanghai: n.p., 1931).

Chapter 5: Public Health and State-Building

1 The classic reference work on the history of public health in Western countries is George Rosen, *A History of Public Health: Expanded Edition, with an Introduction by Elizabeth Fee* (Baltimore: Johns Hopkins University Press, 1993). For the relationship between industrialization and public health as a concern of the modern state, see pages 168-269. The bibliographical notes to Fee's introduction summarize the more recent literature on the history of Western public health. The state as the provider of the public's health is also the subject of Dorothy Porter, *The History of Public Health and the Modern State,* the Wellcome Institute Series in the History of Medicine (Amsterdam: Rodopi, 1994), 168-269. Porter's 'Introduction' on pages 1-44 summarizes studies of the history of public health since Rosen's day, and the chapter by Christopher Hamlin, 'State Medicine in Great Britain,' is an excellent study of the social and political forces that drove the British state's new concern for public health.

2 'Treatise on the Regulation of the Spirit by the Four "Vapours,"' Chapter 2 in the *Basic Questions* edition of the *Inner Canon.* An extensive survey of this kind of preventive medical thought in early Chinese texts is provided by Gwei-djen Lu and Joseph Needham, 'Hygiene and Preventive Medicine in Ancient China,' in *Clerks and Craftsmen in China and the West: Lectures and Addresses on the History of Science and Technology,* ed. Joseph Needham (Cambridge: Cambridge University Press, 1970), 340-78.

3 These writings are surveyed in Fan Xingzhun 范行準, *Zhongguo yufang yixue sixiang shi* 中國預防醫學思想史 [History of preventative medical thought in China] (Beijing: Renmin weisheng chubanshe, 1955), 40-80.

4 An account of Beijing's drainage system as reported by the customs medical officer for Beijing, John Dudgeon, is reproduced in Gordon, *Epitome.* On the history of Chinese urban waterworks and their uses, see Anon., *Zhongguo shuili shigao* 中国水利史搞 [A draft history of Chinese waterworks] (Beijing: Shuili dianli chubanshe, 1989), 223-25.

5 Angela Ki Che Leung, 'Organized Medicine in Ming-Qing China: State and Private Medical Institutions in the Lower Yangzi Region,' *Late Imperial China* 8, 1 (1987): 134-66.

6 This is why there is a section on 'preparations for and measures to expel epidemics' (*Quyi zhi shebei yu shishi* 驅疫之設備與實施) in the modern Chinese historical work by Deng Yunte 鄧雲特, *Zhongguo jiuhuang shi* 中國救荒史 [History of disaster relief in China] (Taipei: Taiwan Commercial Press, [1937] 1966), 357-65. See also Pierre-Etienne Will and R. Bin Wong, *Nourish the People: The State Civilian Granary System in China, 1650-1850* (Ann Arbor: Center for Chinese Studies, University of Michigan, 1991).

7 Chia-feng Chang, 'Aspects of Smallpox and Its Significance in Chinese History' (PhD diss., School of Oriental and African Studies, University of London, 1996); Angela Kiche Leung 梁其姿, 'Ming, Qing yufang tianhua cuoshi zhi yanbian' 明清預防天化措施之演變 [The development of preventive measures against smallpox during the Ming and Qing dynasties], in *Guoshi shilun: Tao Xisheng Xiansheng jiuzhi rongqing zhu shou lunwen ji* 國史釋論: 陶希聖先生九秩榮慶祝壽論文集 [Essays on Chinese history: Festschrift dedicated to Professor Tao Xisheng on his ninetieth birthday], ed. Yang Liansheng 楊聯陞 (Taipei: Shi huo chubanshe, 1987), 239-53.

8 Benedict, 'Bubonic Plague.' Examples of societies that provided coffins and repatriation of corpses are provided in Caroline Reeves, 'Grave Concerns: Bodies, Burial, and Identity in Early Republican China,' in *Cities in Motion: Interior, Coast, and Diaspora in Transnational China*, ed. Sherman Cochran and David Strand (Berkeley: Institute of East Asian Studies, University of California, Berkeley, 2007), 27-52.

9 Leung, 'Organized Medicine in Ming-Qing China,' 156.

10 Quoted in Susan Mann, *Local Merchants and the Chinese Bureaucracy, 1750-1850* (Stanford: Stanford University Press, 1987), 17-18.

11 Ibid. 'Liturgy,' from the Greek *leitourgia*, meaning public service, is used to indicate public service performed by local leaders on the state's behalf but at their own expense. See pages 12-13.

12 Frank Dikötter, *The Discourse of Race in Modern China* (London: Hurst, 1992), 99-111.

13 He Bingyuan 何炳元, 'Lun Zhongguo ji yi kai yizhi' 論中國急宜開醫智 [China should urgently propagate medical knowledge], *YXB* (July 1909): 49-50.

14 Rogaski, *Hygienic Modernity*.

15 Yang Suixi 楊燧熙, 'Wanguo weishengxue lun' 灣國衛生學論 [On international sanitation], *SXYYXB* 59 (1916): 108-9.

16 Wang Shouzhi 王壽芝, 'Yi Zhan' 醫戰 [Medical war], *SXYYXB* 7, 4 (1917): 27-29.

17 Li Jiafu 厲家福, 'Yishi weisheng yu guoshi zhi guanxi guan' 醫事衛生與國勢之關係觀 [A view of the relationship between national power and medicine and sanitation], *MGYXZZ* 2, 8 (1924): 424.

18 Charles E. Rosenberg, *No Other Gods: On Science and American Social Thought* (Baltimore: Johns Hopkins University Press, 1997), chap. 1.

19 Anon., 'Tongji dewen yixuetang weisheng yanshuo zeyao lu' 同濟德文醫學堂為生演說擇要錄 [Selections from a lecture on 'hygiene' at the German-language 'universal benefit' (Tongji) Medical School], *ZXYXB* 18 (1911): 4.

20 William C. Summers' book-length account of the Manchurian plague of 1910 appeared in print too late to be fully referenced here. See William C. Summers, *The Great Manchurian Plague of 1910-1911: The Geopolitics of an Epidemic Disease* (New Haven: Yale University Press, 2012).

21 Ramon H. Myers, 'Japanese Imperialism in Manchuria: The South Manchuria Railway Company, 1906-1933,' in *The Japanese Informal Empire in China, 1895-1937.* ed. Peter Duus, Ramon H. Myers, and Mark R. Peattie (Princeton: Princeton University Press, 1989), 101-32.

22 Cited in Carl F. Nathan, 'The Acceptance of Western Medicine in Early 20th-Century China: The Story of the North Manchurian Plague Prevention Service,' in *Medicine and Society in China*, ed. John Z. Bowers and Elizabeth Purcell (Philadelphia: Wm. F. Fell for the National Library of Medicine and the Josiah Macy Jr. Foundation, 1974), 58. See also Eli Chernin, 'Richard Pearson Strong and the Manchurian Epidemic of Pneumonic Plague, 1910-1911,' *Journal of the History of Medicine and Allied Sciences* 44 (1989): 296-319.

23 China Imperial Maritime Customs, *Decennial Reports of the Chinese Imperial Maritime Customs, Third Issue, 1902-1911.* (Shanghai: Statistical Department of the Inspectorate General of Customs, Shanghai, 1911), 13. See also Mark Gamsa, 'The Epidemic of Pneumonic Plague in Manchuria 1910-1911,' *Past and Present* 190 (2006): 147-83.

24 Gamsa, 'Epidemic,' 147-83.

25 Ibid., 152.

26 Lien-teh Wu, *Plague Fighter*, 37; Nathan, 'Acceptance of Western Medicine,' 58. Funding details from China Imperial Maritime Customs, *Decennial Reports*, 14.

27 Wu, *Plague Fighter*, 36; Nathan, 'Acceptance of Western Medicine,' 60.

28 Xiliang 錫良, 'Preface,' in *Dongsansheng yishi baogaoshu* 東三省疫時報告書 [Report on the plague in the three eastern provinces (i.e., Manchuria)] (n.p.: Viceroy's Office, 1911).

29 Nathan, 'Acceptance of Western Medicine,' 64.

30 Lien-teh Wu, 'Inaugural Address Delivered at the International Plague Conference, Mukden, 1911,' in *Manchurian Plague Prevention Service Memorial Volume, 1912-1932* (Shanghai: National Quarantine Service, 1934), 13-19.

31 Andrew Cunningham, 'Transforming Plague: The Laboratory and the Identity of Infectious Disease,' in *The Laboratory Revolution in Medicine*, ed. A.R. Cunningham and Perry Williams (Cambridge: Cambridge University Press, 1992), 209-44; Gamsa, 'Epidemic,' 166-71.

32 Wu, *Plague Fighter*, 76-77. For an account of the establishment of the Customs Service under foreign staff, see T. Roger Bannister, *A History of the External Trade of China, 1834-81, Together with a Synopsis of the External Trade of China, 1882-1931, Being an Introduction to the Customs Decennial Reports, 1922-1931*, Decennial Reports of the China Imperial Maritime Customs Service (Shanghai: Inspectorate General of Chinese Customs, 1931), 29-30.

33 Lien-teh Wu, *North Manchurian Plague Prevention Service Reports, 1911-1913* (Cambridge: Cambridge University Press, 1914), 1.

34 Nathan, 'Acceptance of Western Medicine,' 68.

35 Wu, *North Manchurian Plague Prevention*, 3, 8. See also Lien-teh Wu, 'Awakening the Sanitary Conscience of China,' *CMMJ* 29, 4 (1915): 222-29.

36 Nathan, 'Acceptance of Western Medicine,' 67, counted service delegations to at least twenty international conferences over eighteen years, details of which may also be found in Wu's autobiography, *Plague Fighter*.

37 Wong and Wu, *History of Chinese Medicine*, 602.

38 Yuwen Hou 毓汶侯, 'Shelun: Guanyu neiwubu yu bennian shuizai hou congshi fangyi zhi ganyan' 社論: 關於內務部於本年水災後從事放疫之感言 [Editorial: My feelings after observing how the Ministry of Internal Affairs dealt with epidemic prevention work after this year's floods], *MGYXB* 2, 10 (1924): 1.

39 Yuwen Hou 毓汶侯, 'Shelun: Ying yi zhongyang fangyichu gaishe wei chuanranbing yanjiusuo yi fuhe ming, shi zhi guanjian' 社論: 應以中央防疫處改設為傳染病研究所以符合名實之 [Editorial: A humble suggestion that the Central Epidemic Prevention Bureau should be reconstituted as the Institute of Infectious Diseases to match name and reality], *MGYXB* 2, 3 (1924): 1.

40 Yuwen Hou 毓汶侯, 'Shelun: Zhongyang yi sheli weishengyuan yi mou weisheng xingzheng zhi tongyi' 社論: 中央宜設立衛生院以某衛生行政之統 [Editorial: The government should establish a sanitation department in order to promote the unification of sanitary administration], *MGYXB* 2, 2 (1924): 1-3.

41 AnElissa Lucas, *Chinese Medical Modernization* (New York: Praeger, 1982), 60.

42 But see Michael Shiyung Liu, *Prescribing Colonization: The Role of Medical Practices and Policies in Japan-Ruled Taiwan, 1895-1945* (Ann Arbor, MI: Association for Asian Studies, 2009), 60-62.

43 Wong and Wu, *History of Chinese Medicine*, 602.

44 Lawrence M. Chen, *Public Health in National Reconstruction* (Nanjing: Council of International Affairs, 1937), 53.

45 Ka-che Yip, *Health and National Reconstruction in Nationalist China: The Development of Modern Health Services, 1928-1937* (Ann Arbor, MI: Association for Asian Studies, 1995), chap. 4. See also Arthur Kleinman, 'The Background and Development of Public Health in China: An Exploratory Essay,' in *Public Health in the People's Republic of China*, ed. Myron E. Wegman, Tsung-Yi Lin, and Elizabeth F. Purcell (New York: Josiah Macy, Jr. Foundation, 1973), 5-25; and (for the Nationalist government's own view of its achievements in this field) T'ang Leang-Li, ed., *Reconstruction in China: A Record of Progress and Achievement in Facts and Figures* (Shanghai: China United Press, 1935), 112-13. Accounts of individual projects may also be found in C.C. Chen, in collaboration with Frederica M. Bunga, *Medicine in Rural China: A Personal Account* (Berkeley and Los Angeles: University of California Press, 1989); and Charles W. Hayford, *To the People: James Yen and Village China* (New York: Columbia University Press, 1990).

46 Wang Jingwei 汪精衛, 'Xingzhengyuan Wang yuanzhang dui yixue zhi xiwang' 行政院汪院長對醫學之希望 [The head of the administrative yuan, Director Wang's, hopes for medicine], *CMJ* 20, 4 (1934): 453-55.

47 Li Ting-an, 'Summary Report on the Rural Public Health Practice in China,' *CMJ* 20, 9 (1934): 1113-32.

48 Yip, *Health and National Reconstruction*, chap. 4. There was a total of 1,098 *xian* (counties) across China at this time.

49 For Guangzhou, see Guangzhou shi weisheng ju 廣州市衛生局, *Guangzhou weisheng nianbao* 廣州衛生年報 [Annual report of the Department of Health of Canton Municipality] (Canton: n.p., 1926). For Tianjin, see Rogaski, *Hygienic Modernity*. Information about several other cities may be found in Deng Tietao 邓铁涛, ed., *Zhongguo fang yi shi* 中国防疫史 [History of epidemic prevention in China] (Nanning: Guangxi Science and Technology Press, 2006).

50 Yip, *Health and National Reconstruction*, 88-90. See also James C. Thomson, *While China Faced West: American Reformers in Nationalist China, 1928-1937* (Cambridge, MA: Harvard University Press, 1969), 58-63.

51 Clara Shepherd, 'The Present Situation: New Medicine in China,' *CR* 68 (1937):323-24 (emphasis added).

Chapter 6: Medical Lives

1 Wong and Wu, *History of Chinese Medicine*, 315-17.

2 Ibid., 439-40.

3 Ibid., 442.

4 W. Hamilton Jeffreys and James L. Maxwell, *The Diseases of China, Including Formosa and Korea* (London: John Bale and Danielson, 1911), 1.

5 Gordon, *Epitome*, xviii et seq. See also Desirée Cox-Maksimov, 'Foreign Bodies, Filthy Lands: Health, Disease and Sanitation on the China Coast in the Late 19th Century' (M.Phil, University of Cambridge, 1993).

6 Xu Shuangjun, 'Memories of Qiu Jin,' in Chen Xianggong 陈象恭, *Qiu Jin nianpu ji zhuanji ziliao* 秋瑾年谱及传记资料 [Annual chronicle and biographical materials on (the life of) Qiu Jin] (Beijing: Zhonghua shuju, 1983), 24. On Shimoda Utako and education for Chinese women in Japan, see Ono Kazuko, *Chinese Women in a Century of Revolution, 1850-1950* (Stanford: Stanford University Press, 1989), 54-59.

7 Three of her articles for the *Vernacular Journal* are reprinted at the front of the *Qiu Jin ji* 秋瑾集 [Collected works of Qiu Jin] (Beijing: Zhonghua shuju, 1960), 3-9.

8 Chen, *Qiu Jin nianpu*, 30-31.

9 Wong and Wu, *History of Chinese Medicine*, 449, 501, 556-58. See also Jane Hunter, *The Gospel of Gentility: American Women Missionaries in Turn-of-the-Century China* (New Haven: Yale University Press, 1984), 24.

10 Mary Backus Rankin, 'The Emergence of Women at the End of the Ch'ing: The Case of Ch'iu Chin,' in *Women in Chinese Society*, ed. Margery Wolf and Roxane Witke (Stanford: Stanford University Press, 1975), 39-66.

11 Li Juchen, *Flowers in the Mirror*, trans. Lin Tai-yi, UNESCO collection of representative works, Chinese series (London: Peter Owen, 1965), chap. 13.

12 See translations from the works of Kang and Liang in Ono Kazuko, *Chinese Women in a Century of Revolution, 1850-1950*, trans. Joshua A. Fogel, 23-46 (Stanford: Stanford University Press, 1989); Rankin, 'Emergence of Women,' 44.

13 Qiu Jin, *Qiu Jin ji*, 163-64.

14 Ibid., 164-75.

15 Ibid., 174.

16 The earliest advertisements I have found in the medical literature for milk products such as 'Lactogen' and 'Nestlé's Milk Food' date from around 1918, more than a decade after Qiu Jin published her *Course in Nursing*. This correlates well with Susan Glosser's study of the rise of the milk industry around Shanghai in the 1920s. See Glosser, *Chinese Visions of Family and State*, 138-55.

17 Qiu Jin, *Qiu Jin ji*, 15.

18 Ibid.

19 Zhou Fusheng 周服聖, 'Kanhuxue chanpoxue erzhe jun zu fu yiyao zhi suo bu ji Zhongguo wu ci mingchen bing wu ci jiaoyu ji ying ruhe fangxing zhishi ge tiao ju yi da' 看護學產婆學二者均足輔醫藥之所不及無此教育 [Although both nursing and midwifery extend medical provision, China has neither these titles nor education (in these subjects)], *YXB* 118 (1909): 4A-5B.

20 Tina Phillips Johnson, *Childbirth in Republican China: Delivering Modernity* (Lanham: Lexington Books, 2011).

21 He Dong 何东, chief editor, *Zhongguo geming shi renwu cidian* 中国革命史人物词典 [Biographical dictionary of China's revolutionary history] (Beijing: Beijing chubanshe, 1991), 420-21.

22 Chen Yuan, writing under the pseudonym Qianyi 謙益, 'Lun zhengfu duiyu Zheren zhi egan' 論政府對於浙人之惡感 [On the government's prejudice against Zhejiangese], reproduced in *Chen Yuan zaonian wenji* 陳垣早年文集 [The early writings of Chen Yuan], comp. Chen Zhichao 陳智超, 93-95 (Taipei: Zhongyang yanjiu yuan Zhongguo wenzhe yanjiusuo, 1992).

23 Liu Naihe 刘乃和, 'Chen Yuan tongzhi qinfen de yi sheng' 陳垣同志勤奮的一生 [The industrious life of Comrade Chen Yuan], Manuscript copy of unnamed book extract, kindly supplied by Zhao Pushan (dated 1981), 89.

24 See Chen Zhichao's biographical Preface to Chen, *Chen Yuan zaonian wenji*, 3-12.

25 Zhao Pushan 趙璞珊, 'Chen Yuan xiansheng he yixue shi' 陈垣先生和医学史 [Mr Chen Yuan and the history of medicine], in *Essays to Commemorate the 110th Anniversary of the Birth of Director Chen Yuan* (Beijing: Beijing Shifan Daxue chubanshe, 1990), 17. My thanks to the late Professor Zhao Pushan for generously giving me a copy of this work as well as photocopies of several original articles by Chen Yuan. On the South China Medical College, see Wong and Wu, *History of Chinese Medicine*, 545-46.

26 Information gained from the articles reproduced in Chen, *Chen Yuan zaonian wenji.*

27 Ssu-yü Teng and John K. Fairbank, *China's Response to the West: A Documentary Survey, 1839-1923* (Cambridge, MA: Harvard University Press, 1954), 136.

28 Gwei-djen Lu and Joseph Needham, 'A History of Forensic Medicine in China,' *Medical History* 32 (1988): 357-400.

29 Chen Yuan, 'Zou she jianyan li yi zixing dao Yue' 奏設檢驗吏已咨行到粵 [The memorial for the establishment of coroners arrives in Guangdong], *YXWSB* 9 (1909): n.p., in Chen, *Early Writings of Chen Yuan*, 284-85.

30 Chen Yuan, 'Lun Jiang Du kaoshi yisheng' 論江督考試醫生 [On the Yangzi governor's medical examination], *YXWSB* 3, 4 (1909): n.p., in Chen, *Early Writings of Chen Yuan*, 181-91.

31 Even by his own accounts, the total number of medical works Ding produced vary. In Ding Fubao, *Chouyin jushi zizhuan* 疇隱居士自傳 [Autobiography of the lay Buddhist of mathematical mysteries] (hereafter *Autobiography*) (Shanghai: Gulin jingshe chubanshe, 1948), 55, the figure eighty-three is mentioned, but a running total of the number of medical books published annually in Ding's publishing ventures, as recorded in Ding Fubao, *Chouyin jushi ziding nianpu* 疇隱居士自訂年普 [Annalistic autobiography of the lay Buddhist of mathematical mysteries] (hereafter *Annals*) (Shanghai: Shanghai yixue shuju, ca. 1937), gives the larger number of ninety-five. The figure of eighty-three may refer to the titles published as 'Ding Fubao's medical collection,' the remainder being works and translations by other authors published by him.

32 See Pei-yi Wu, *The Confucian's Progress: Autobiographical Writings in Traditional China* (Princeton: Princeton University Press, 1990) for a discussion of the different forms of Chinese autobiography.

33 Ding, *Annals*, 10A.

34 Barry Keenan, 'Lung-men Academy in Shanghai and the Expansion of Kiangsu's Educated Elite, 1865-1911,' in *Education and Society in Late Imperial China*, ed. B.A. Elman and A. Woodside (Berkeley and Los Angeles: University of California Press, 1994), 499.

35 Ding, *Annals*, 10A.

36 Zhao Pushan 趙璞珊, 'Zhao Yuanyi he tade bishu yishu' 趙元益和他的筆述醫書 [Zhao Yuanyi and his paraphrasings of (Western) medical works], *Zhongguo keji shiliao* 中國科技史料 [China historical materials of science and technology] 12, 1 (1991): 69-74. Zhao Pushan quotes part of Ambassador Xue's diary to the effect that he dispatched Zhao Yuanyi and an interpreter to Berlin to learn about Koch's new vaccine against tuberculosis. See also Li Yun 李云, chief editor, *Zhongyi renming cidian* 中醫人名辭典 [Biographical dictionary of Chinese medicine] (Beijing: Guoji wenhua chubangongsi, 1988), 616.

37 Sheng, also associated with the 'self-strengthening movement,' and the inventor of the 'official supervision and merchant management' formula for China's early

industrial enterprises, had just been awarded the upper second rank in the imperial bureaucracy and the title of junior guardian of the heir apparent in recognition of his role in keeping South China out of the Boxer uprising in 1900. See Albert Feuerwerker, *China's Early Industrialization: Sheng Hsuan-huai (1844-1916) and Mandarin Enterprise* (Cambridge: Harvard University Press, 1958), 72.

38 Ding, *Annals*, 15A.

39 The Translation Bureau of the Metropolitan University was the continuation, under a different name, of the old Tongwen Guan or School of Foreign Languages, founded in 1863. Both the Tongwen Guan and the Metropolitan University had been badly damaged and forced to close during the Boxer Rebellion of 1900, and Ding Fubao's invitation coincided with the reopening of the university as part of the Qing government's reforms during the era of the New Policies, 1901-10, and the transfer of the Tongwen Guan's functions to the university's translation bureau. See Knight Biggerstaff, *The Earliest Modern Government Schools in China* (Ithaca, NY: Cornell University Press, 1961), 94-139.

40 Ding, *Annals*, 17B.

41 Ibid., 19A; Zhao Pushan, 'Ding Fubao he ta zaoqi bianzhu fanyi de yishu' 丁福保和他早期编著翻译的医书 [Ding Fubao and his early medical translations and compilations], *Zhong, xi yi jiehe zazhi* 中西医结合杂志 [Journal for the integration of Chinese and Western medicine] 10, 4 (1990): 248-49.

42 See 'Jiang Du kaoshi yisheng zhangcheng' 江督考試醫生章程 [Regulations for the lower Yangzi governor's medical examinations], *SXYYXB* 1 (1908): 16-17. The same issue also reported the concern of the Bureau of Civil Administration (*Minzhengbu* 民政部) in Beijing over standards of practice in that city. According to the report, the bureau was planning an investigation of standards of medical practice in and around the capital. See page 53.

43 Ding, *Annals*, 19A. The full text of the first four questions, and Ding's answers to the first three, are reproduced in 'Nanyang yike kaoshi wenti' 南洋醫科考試問題 [The questions from the southern provinces medical examination], *SXYYXB* 16 (1909): n.p. (Ding reproduces all his answers in Ding, *Autobiography*, 32-48.)

44 Lianchen He, 'Editorial,' *SXYYXB* 3 (1908): 1.

45 *SXYYXB* 15 (1909): 18. Letter from Ding Fubao dated Xuantong Year 1 (1909), seventh month, twenty-sixth day.

46 I rely on the account of this dispute given by Zhao, *Jindai Zhong-, Xiyixue lunzheng shi*, 77-81.

47 Notice that the term 'Sino-western' (*zhong-xi*) in the names of Ding's society and its journal mirror the common Chinese term of this period for the Western medicine practised in Japan, 'Eastern-western medicine' (*dong-xi yi*).

48 Zhao, *Jindai Zhong-, Xiyixue lunzheng shi*, 80.

49 Chang'an was the imperial capital for most of the period from the unification of China in 221 BCE to the An Lushan Rebellion during the Tang dynasty in 756 CE.

Ding is therefore saying that he doesn't know where to place his political loyalties. See Ding, *Autobiography*, 14.

50 Ding, *Annals*, 70B.

51 Cited in Lu Zhaoji, 'Yidai xuezhe Ding Fubao' 代学者丁福保 [Scholar of his age Ding Fubao], *CJMH* 15, 2 (1985): 92-95.

52 Ding Fubao, 'Fakanci' 發刊詞 [Foreword], *Guoyao xinsheng* 國藥新聲 [The new voice of national drugs] 1, 1 (1939): 1-2.

53 Fubao Ding, *Zhongyao qianshuo* 中藥淺說 [Simple Chinese pharmacy], Everyman's Library (reprint) (Taipei: Commercial Press [Taiwan]: 1966 [1940?]). Ding published at least another five titles of this type, which are listed in his *Autobiography* of 1948.

54 Reprinted in Ding, *Annals*, 32B-33B.

55 Adapted from Bridie J. Andrews, 'Tuberculosis and the Assimilation of Germ Theory in China, 1895-1937,' *Journal of the History of Medicine and Allied Sciences* 52, 1 (1997): 114-57, with permission.

56 Zhao Hongjun 赵洪钧, 'Zhang Xichun nianpu' 张锡纯年谱 [Annual chronicle of (the life of) Zhang Xichun], *CJMH* 21, 4 (1991): 214-18.

57 Zhang Xichun 張錫純, *Yixue zhong Zhong can xi lu* 醫學衷中參西錄 [The assimilation of Western to Chinese in medicine] (Shijiazhuang: Hebei kesue jishu chubanshe, 1918), 11-21.

58 The Five Phases (or Agents, or Elements) along with *yin* and *yang*, form the conceptual framework of Chinese correlative cosmology. Accessible introductions may be found in Ted Kaptchuk, *The Web That Has No Weaver: Understanding Chinese Medicine*, 2nd ed. (London: Rider, 2000), app. H; and Nathan Sivin, *Traditional Medicine in Contemporary China* (Ann Arbor: Center for Chinese Studies, University of Michigan, 1987), 70-80.

59 Zhang, *Yixue zhong Zhong can xi lu*, 14, 19.

60 Ibid., 18-20.

61 For examples, see Hanson, *Speaking of Epidemics*, chap. 8.

62 Zhao, 'Zhang Xichun nianpu,' 216.

63 Volker Scheid, *Currents of Tradition in Chinese Medicine, 1626-2006* (Seattle: Eastland Press, 2007).

64 Biographical details from: Lü Simian's preface to Xie Guan 謝觀, *Zhongguo yixue yuan liu lun* 中國醫學源流論 [The origin and development of Chinese medicine] (Fuzhou: Fujian kexue jishu chubanshe, 1935); Chen Daoqin 陈道瑾 and Xue Weitao 薛渭涛, eds., *Jiangsu lidai yiren zhi* 江苏历代医人志 [Records of Jiangsu physicians throughout history] (Nanjing: Jiangsu Science and Technology Press, 1985), 377-78; Li Yun 李云, ed., *Zhongyi renming cidian* 中医人名辞典 [Biographical dictionary of Chinese medicine] (Beijing: Guoji wenhua chubangongsi, 1988), 898-99; and Chen Cunren 陈存仁 in Zhang Zanchen 张赞臣, *Zhongguo lidai yixue shilue* 中国历代医学史略 [Sketch history of Chinese medicine], 2nd ed. (Shanghai: Zhongyi shuju, 1954), 51-66.

65 Jessie Gregory Lutz, *China and the Christian Colleges, 1850-1950* (Ithaca, NY: Cornell University Press, 1971), 90-91.

66 Zhang Shangjin 张尚金, ed., *Wujin xianzhi* 武进县志 [Gazetteer of Wujin County] (Shanghai: Shanghai People's Press, 1988), 1930-31.

67 Chen, in Zhang, *Zhongguo lidai yixue shilue,* 61.

68 Li Jian 李建, 'Quanguo yiyao tuanti zonglianhehui de jianli ji qi huodong lishi diwei' 全国医药团体总联合会的建立及其历史地位 [The establishment, activities, and historical position of the National Union for Chinese Medicine], *Zhongguo keji shiliao* 中国科技史料 [China historical materials of science and technology] 14, 3 (n.d.): 67-75. For a vivid account of the 'chaotic medical situation in Shanghai' as described by Western-style doctor Pang Jingzhou in 1931, see Lei, 'When Chinese Medicine Encountered the State,' 106-16.

69 For a compelling description of the pervasiveness of native-place associations, see Elizabeth J. Perry, *Shanghai on Strike: The Politics of Chinese Labor* (Stanford: Stanford University Press, 1993), chap. 2.

70 This incident is what historian Sean Lei refers to as the crucial moment 'when Chinese medicine encountered the state.' It is described at length in his PhD dissertation of the same name and also in Scheid, *Currents of Tradition in Chinese Medicine,* 200-20.

71 Chen, in Zhang, *Zhongguo lidai yixue shilue,* 58.

72 Ibid., 58-60.

73 Xie, *Zhongguo yixue yuan liu lun,* 113.

74 Olive Checkland, *Humanitarianism and the Emperor's Japan, 1877-1977* (Basingstoke: Macmillan, 1994), 45-50.

75 Surgeon-General Baron Tadanori Ishiguro, 'The Red Cross in Japan,' in *Fifty Years of New Japan,* ed. Count Shigenobu Okuma (London: Smith, Elder, 1909), 307-22.

76 Chen Yuan 陳垣, 'Riren yi xin shijie, yishu bi Han' 日人以新世界醫術逼韓 [Japanese use new global medicine to close in on Koreans], in Chen, *Chen Yuan zaonian wenji,* 293-95.

Chapter 7: New Medical Institutions

 1 Although it might seem strange that Chinese students should have turned to Japan so soon after the war, the fact that this was the case has been amply documented by Douglas R. Reynolds, *China, 1989-1912: The Xinzheng Revolution and Japan* (Cambridge, MA: Council on East Asian Studies, Harvard University, 1993). Reynolds describes the period from 1898 to 1907 as a 'Golden Decade' in China's relationship with Japan.

 2 See the contributions of Timothy Lenoir and Paul Weindling to A.R. Cunningham and Perry Williams, eds., *The Laboratory Revolution in Medicine* (Cambridge: Cambridge University Press, 1992).

3   Shi Quansheng 史全生, ed., *Zhonghua minguo wenhua shi* 中華民國文化史 [Cultural history of the Republic of China] 1:420-21. See also Wong and Wu, *History of Chinese Medicine,* 604-6.

4   Wong and Wu, ibid., 605.

5   Statistics from Jiang Huiming 將晦鳴, 'Zhongguo yixue jiaoyu zhi qianzhan hougu' 中國醫學教育之前瞻後顧 [On the history and future prospects of medical education in China], *ZXYY* 1, 1 (1935): 50-65.

6   For a full account of this significant event in the political and disease history of China, see William C. Summers, *The Great Manchurian Plague of 1910-1911: The Geopolitics of an Epidemic Disease* (New Haven: Yale University Press, 2012).

7   Wu Liande 伍連德, 'Lun Zhongguo ji yi mou jin yixue jiaoyu' 論中國急宜謀進醫學教育 [Why China should urgently promote medical studies], *ZXYXB* 5, 10 (1915): 1-5.

8   Yan Fu wrote a series of essays on Herbert Spencer in 1895; Zhang Binglin and Zeng Guangquan published an introduction to his thought in 1898 in the reformist journal *Changyanbao* 昌言報. In 1902, Yan Fu had his translation of Spencer's *The Study of Sociology* published, and two further works describing Spencer's sociology appeared in 1903. See Dikötter, *Discourse of Race in Modern China,* 101-2.

9   From Lu Xun's *Zhongguo dizhi lüe lun* 中國地質略論 [Brief outline of Chinese geology], cited in Akira Nagazumi, 'The Diffusion of the Idea of Social Darwinism in East and Southeast Asia,' *Historia Scientiarum* 24 (1983): 9. Further examples of the influence of social Darwinism on the attitudes of the famous reformers Liang Qichao, Kang Youwei, and Tan Sitong towards medicine are given in Croizier, *Traditional Medicine in Modern China,* chap. 3. The influence of Japanese eugenic thought on Chinese reformers is studied extensively in Chung, *Struggle for National Survival.* As noted previously, the idea of degeneration was also current in Western society at this time.

10   See, for instance, Ye Zuzhang 葉租章, 'To Cure the Nation, First Cure the People, to Cure the People First Cure Medical Theories,' *ZXYXB* 3 12 (1913): 1-2; Li Jiafu 厲家福, 'Yishi weisheng yu guoshi zhi guanxi guan' 醫事衛生與國勢之關係觀 [A view of the relationship between national power and medical affairs], *MGYXZZ* 2, 8 (1924): 424. This theme is explored in more detail in Liping Bu, 'Social Darwinism, Public Health, and Modernization in China, 1895-1925,' in *Uneasy Encounters: The Politics of Medicine and Health in China, 1900-1937,* ed. Iris Borowy (Frankfurt am Main: Peter Lang, 2009), 96-98.

11   Hou Yuwen 侯毓文, 'Duiyu Riren suo li Qingdao yixuexiao zhi wo jian' 對於日人所立青島醫學校之我見 [My opinion of the establishment by Japanese of Qingdao Medical School], *MGYXZZ,* October 1924.

12   Jiang, 'Zhongguo yixue jiaoyu,' tables opposite page 54; and Zhen and Fu, *Zhongguo yixue shi,* 510-11.

13   'Neizhengbu zhiding guanli yishi zanxing guize' 內政部指定管理醫士暫行規則 [Ministry of Internal Affairs enacts provisional regulations governing medical

scholars], *SXYYXB* 12, 4 (1922): 65A-66B; and 'Neizhengbu zhiding guanli yishi zanxing guize 內政部指定管理醫師暫行規則 [Ministry of Internal Affairs enacts provisional regulations governing physicians], *SXYYXB* 12, 4 (1922): 66B-71B.

14 Zhang et al., *Minguo yiyao weisheng fagui xuanbian*.

15 Xiaoqun Xu, *Chinese Professionals and the Republican State: The Rise of Professional Associations in Shanghai, 1912-1937* (Cambridge: Cambridge University Press, 2001), 147-48.

16 Editorial, 'Wuneng wuze zhi jiaoyu dangju' 無能無責之教育當局 [The incompetent and irresponsible educational authorities,' *MGYXZZ* 3, 10 (1925): 437-40. Volker Scheid writes that the college never in fact received government recognition, but this exchange demonstrates the importance of institutional recognition at the time, whatever the outcome. See Scheid, *Currents of Tradition in Chinese Medicine*, 236.

17 See Douglas R. Reynolds, 'Training Young China Hands: Tōa Dōbun Shoin and Its Precursors, 1886-1945,' in *The Japanese Informal Empire in China, 1895-1937*, ed. R.H. Myers and M.R. Peattie (Princeton: Princeton University Press, 1989), 259-61.

18 Hou Yuwen 侯毓文, 'Wo panwang yu women yijie tongrende' 我盼望與我們醫界同人的 [Editorial: My hopes for my medical colleagues], *MGYYXB* 3, 7 (1924): 1.

19 E Meng 萼夢 (pseud.), 'Wusa yihou jiaoyujie, zhi da juewu' 五卅以後教育界之大覺悟 [The great awakening of the educational world after the May 30th incident],' *SSYB*, 28 August 1925, 1.

20 Wong and Wu, *History of Chinese Medicine*, 767.

21 Wu Lien-teh, 'Medical Registration in China,' *CMJ* (English section) 14, 6 (1928): n.p.

22 Wu Lien-teh's editorials, 'Harsh Legislation and Its Results,' and 'The Future of Our Association' in *CMJ* (English section) 15, 6 (1929): n.p.

23 'Medical Bodies Combine,' *NCH*, 26 April 1932, 143.

24 *Zhonghua yixue hui gaikuo baogao* 中華醫學會改擴報告 [Brief report of the National Medical Association], *CMJ* (Chinese section), 18, 1 (1932): 175-83.

25 See the reports of the opening addresses to the conference in *CMJ* 20, 4 (1934): 456-58. On the centrality of dissection to the epistemic authority of modern medicine in China, see David Luesink, 'Dissecting Modernity: Anatomy and Power in the Language of Science in China' (PhD diss., University of British Columbia, 2012).

26 James Y.C. Yen to F.S. Brockman, YMCA, 9 March 1928, and 'From Report Letters Dated June 10 and October 30, 1935' [to the YMCA's New York office], in Yale China Missions Archive, RG 8, Hersey Papers. The China Mission Association commissioned Dr. Li Tingan to survey the existing rural public health provision in China in 1934. His report showed that there were seventeen rural health centres in China, of which only three were not at least receiving partial help from 'some other agency' than the local or national government. See the full report in Ting-an Li, 'Summary Report on the Rural Public Health Practice in China,' *CMJ* 20, 9 (1934): 1113-32.

27 'The Hospitals of China,' in *CR* 68 (1937): 466-68.

28   Eliot Freidson, *Profession of Medicine: A Study of the Sociology of Applied Knowledge* (New York: Dodd, Mead, 1972), 72.

29   A voluntary medical registration scheme was implemented by the Shanghai Municipal Council in the 1930s, and a compulsory one was implemented in the French Settlement at Shanghai in 1930, but this is as far as the enforcement of medical standards seems to have come by 1937. See Anon., 'New Rules for Doctors: Registration Required by the F.M.C. [French Municipal Council],' *NCH* 16 December 1930, 375.

30   Xu, *Chinese Professionals and the Republican State*, 155-56.

31   Wu Lien-teh, 'The Private Medical Practitioner in Relation to Public Health,' in *Reports, National Quarantine Service, Series V, 1934*, ed. Wu Lien-teh and Wu Chang-yao (Shanghai: National Quarantine Service, 1934), 109-14.

32   Frederick W. Maze, *Circular 4304* (2nd ser.)(Quarantine: Development of, in China; Connexion of Customs with; to be Handed over to National Quarantine Bureau of Ministry of Health; I.G.'s instructions. Quarantine and Port Sanitary Matters One of the Rights of a Sovereign State) (Shanghai: Shanghai Office of the Inspectorate General of Customs, 1931), 582-97.

33   Ibid.; Lien-teh Wu, 'History of the National Quarantine Service,' in *Reports, National Quarantine Service, Series II, 1931*, edited by Wu Lien-teh and Wu Chang-yao, 7-8 (Shanghai: National Quarantine Service, 1931).

34   Maze, *Circular 4304*. See also Wu Lien-teh, 'Quarantine Practice in China before 1930,' in *Reports, National Quarantine Service, Series II, 1931*, edited by Wu Lien-teh and Wu Chang-yao, 21-22 (Shanghai: National Quarantine Service, 1931). See also J.K. Fairbank, *Trade and Diplomacy on the China Coast: The Opening of the Treaty Ports, 1842-1854* (Cambridge, MA: Harvard University Press, 1953); Gordon, *Epitome*.

35   This happened, for instance, in Fuzhou in 1926-27. See Maze, *Circular 4304*, 587; Wu, 'Quarantine Practice,' 21-22.

36   Tse-hsiung Kuo, *Technical Co-operation between China and Geneva* (Nanking: Council of International Affairs, 1936), 1-10; F. Norman White, *The Prevalence of Epidemic Disease and Port Health Organisation and Procedure in the Far East* (Geneva: The Health Committee of the League of Nations, 1923. C.H. 130).

37   James C. Thomson Jr., *While China Faced West: American Reformers in Nationalist China, 1928-1937* (Cambridge, MA: Harvard University Press, 1969), 16.

38   League of Nations, *Proposals of the National Government of the Republic of China for Collaboration with the League of Nations on Health Matters* (Geneva: League of Nations Health Organization, 1930. C.H. 842).

39   C.L. Park, 'Report on the Quarantine Needs of the Port of Shanghai, in *National Quarantine Service Reports, Series I.*, ed. Lien-teh Wu (Shanghai: National Quarantine Service, Republic of China, 1931), 58-91.

40   'China's Quarantine Service,' *NCH*, 24 June 1930, 484; Wu, *Plague Fighter*, 407-11.

41 'China and the League of Nations: Agreement over Collaboration in Studying and Solving Health Problems; Measures for Port Quarantine,' *NCH*, 18 March 1930, 424.

42 Ibid.

43 As noted in an investment prospectus for 1930s China, thinly disguised as a reference work: 'Twelve out of the nineteen leading personalities in the Government have received specialized education abroad.' See T'ang Leang-Li, ed., *Reconstruction in China: A Record of Progress and Achievement in Facts and Figures* (China Today series) (Shanghai: China United Press, 1935), 3.

44 Another, smaller source was the Salt Administration after the establishment of a Sino-foreign inspectorate in 1913 did much to 'modernize' collection of the salt gabelle. See S.A.M. Adshead, *The Modernization of the Chinese Salt Administration, 1900-1920,* Harvard East Asian Series 53 (Cambridge, MA: Harvard University Press, 1970), 60-126.

45 Wu Lien-teh, 'Lun Zhongguo ji yi mou jin yixue jiaoyu' 論中國急宜謀進醫學教育 [Why China should urgently promote medical studies], *ZXYXB* 10 (1915): 1-5. The relationship between the reinvestment of the authority to conduct medical inspections on shipping and to impose quarantine restrictions and the Chinese government's 'rights recovery' movement is also made explicit by the Chinese historian Yang Shangchi. See Yang Shangchi 杨上池, 'Woguo shouhui jianyi zhuquan dou-zheng' 我国收回检疫主权斗争 [China's struggle to regain control over quarantine inspection], *ZHYSZZ* 20, 1 (1990): 25-26, and 'Sanshi niandai de quanguo haigang jianyi guanlichu yu Wu Liande boshi' 三十年代的全国海港检疫管理处于伍连德博士 [Dr. Wu Liande and the Chinese Maritime Customs quarantine inspection stations in the 1930s], *ZHYSZZ* 18, 1 (1988): 29-32.

46 'Chinese Health Service: Representatives of Shipping Companies Entertained to Dinner' *NCH*, 16 December 1930, 375; Wu, *Plague Fighter,* 413-15.

47 'Reorganisation of the quarantine services at Chinese ports,' *Quarterly Bulletin of the Health Organisation of the League of Nations* 5, 4 (1936): n.p.

48 Wu, *Plague Fighter,* 438-39.

49 Thomson, *While China Faced West,* 14.

50 Croizier, *Traditional Medicine in Modern China,* 59-68.

51 Nathan Sivin, 'Text and Experience in Classical Chinese Medicine,' in *Knowledge and the Scholarly Medical Traditions,* ed. D. Bates (Cambridge: Cambridge University Press, 1995), 177-204.

52 Hanson, *Speaking of Epidemics,* chap. 7; Scheid, *Currents of Tradition in Chinese Medicine.*

53 Liu Xiaobin 刘小斌 and Deng Tietao 邓铁涛, 'Guangdong jindai de zhongyi jiaoyu' 广东近代的中医教育 [Chinese-medical education in modern Guangdong], *ZHYSZZ* 12, 3 (1982): 133-38.

54 Ren Xigeng 任錫庚, *Tai yi yuan zhi* 太醫院誌 [Annals of the Imperial Medical Academy] (n.p.: n.p., 1923), 1A-1B.

55   Zhu Chao 朱潮, chief editor, *Zhong, wai yixue jiaoyu shi* 中外医学教育史 [History of medical education in China and elsewhere] (Shanghai: Shanghai Yike Daxue chubanshe, 1988), 55-56.

56   Ibid., 56; Ren, *Taiyiyuan zhi*, 1A-1B. For an extended study of the role of the Imperial Medical Academy in the late Qing, see Che-chia Chang, "The Therapeutic Tug of War: The Imperial Physician-Patient Relationship in the Era of Empress Dowager Cixi, 1874-1908" (PhD diss., University of Pennsylvania, 1998).

57   Zhu, *Zhong wai yixue jiaoyu shi*, 55.

58   Ibid., 80-81; Li, *Zhongyi renming cidian*, 513; Li Jingwei 李经纬, chief editor, *Zhongyi renwu cidian* 中医人物词典 [Biographical dictionary of Chinese medicine] (Shanghai: Shanghai cishu chubanshe, 1988), 308-9.

59   Zhu, *Zhong, wai yixue jiaoyu shi*, 81-82.

60   Elman, *On Their Own Terms*, 426, translates *qixue* as 'pneumatics,' but 'physics' seems more likely here. In Neo-Confucianist thought, *qixue* meant a study of cosmology, and it was a branch of natural philosophy.

61   Jerome Ch'en, *China and the West: Society and Culture, 1815-1937* (London: Hutchinson, 1979), 69.

62   Reynolds, *China*, 131-50; Marianne Bastid, *Educational Reform in Early Twentieth-Century China*, 2nd ed. (Ann Arbor: Center for Chinese Studies, University of Michigan, 1988), 1-92. A succinct description of the eight-legged essay is given by Benjamin Elman, 'Eight-Legged Essay: *Baguwen*,' in *Berkshire Encyclopedia of China*, ed. Linsun Cheng (Great Barrington: Berkshire Publishing, 2009), 695-98.

63   Bastid, *Educational Reform*, 34-36.

64   Zhao, *Jindai Zhong-, Xiyixue lunzheng shi*, 82. Similarly token concessions to Chinese medicine had been made at the Beiyang Medical College, founded in 1881.

65   Reynolds, *China*, 149.

66   Ibid. See also Hiroshi Abe, 'Borrowing from Japan: China's First Modern Educational System,' in *China's Education and the Industrialized World: Studies in Cultural Transfer*, ed. Ruth Hayhoe and Marianne Bastid (New York: M.E. Sharpe, 1987), 58-70; Ichiko Chūzō, 'Political and Institutional Reform, 1901-1911,' in *The Cambridge History of China*, vol. 11, ed. J.K. Fairbank and Kwang-ching Liu, chap. 7 (Cambridge: Cambridge University Press, 1980); Wolfgang Franke, *The Reform and Abolition of the Traditional Chinese Examination System* (Cambridge, MA: Harvard University Press, 1963), 59-70; Biggerstaff, *Earliest Modern Government Schools in China*.

67   Elizabeth Sinn, *Power and Charity*, 62-63.

68   Liu and Deng, 'Guangdong jindai de zhongyi jiaoyu,' 133-38.

69   Xie Weinan, 謝煒南, 'Guangdong yixue qiuyishe kao' 廣東醫學求益社考 [The 'Medical Pursuits Society' in Guangdong], *ZHYSZZ* 20, 2 (1990): 86-90. 'Medical Pursuits Society' is Xie's own translation, so I retain it in the translated title.

70   Ibid., 88.

71   Liu and Deng, 'Guangdong jindai de zhongyi jiaoyu,' 135.

72 Xu, *Chinese Professionals and the Republican State*, 131-32.

73 Yanggu Xie, 阳谷谢, ed., *Bai nian Beijing zhongyi* 百年北京中医 [One hundred years of Chinese medicine in Beijing] (Beijing: Huaxue gongye chubanshe, 2007), 35-36.

74 Croizier, *Traditional Medicine in Modern China*, 69.

75 In addition to Croizier's (1968) treatment of the subject, this interpretation of the meeting has been given by Yu Shenchu 俞慎初, *Zhongguo yixue jianshi* 中国医学简史 [Outline of history of Chinese medicine] (Fuzhou: Fujian kexue jishu chubanshe, 1983), 390.

76 Zhao, *Jindai Zhong-, Xiyixue lunzheng shi*, 142.

77 The news section of the *SXYYXB* records that, on the twenty-fourth day of the Chinese tenth month, the director of the Imperial Medical Academy Zhang Shenyuan, Imperial Physician Jin Shun, and two other physicians were all dismissed from office. Ren, *Taiyiyuan zhi*, 3B, 11B also notes that the Bureau of New (i.e., Western) Medicine was established in 1908, though there is no indication of whether this was before or after the Guangxu emperor's demise. There was to be a four-year course, but the school folded after the 1911 revolution. The separate account given in Dan Shikui 單士魁, 'Qingdai tai yi yuan' 清代太醫院 [The Qing dynasty Imperial Medical Academy], *Gugong bowuyuan yuankan* 故宮博物院院刊 [Palace museum journal] 3 (1985): 49-53, suggests that the introduction of Western medicine into the Imperial Academy may have occurred before the death of the emperor since the suggestion came from Director Zhang Shenyuan, one of the officials dismissed after the emperor's death.

78 These curricula, and those of several other Chinese-medical schools of the period, are summarized in Zhao, *Jindai Zhong-, Xiyixue lunzheng shi*, 165-68; and in Zhen and Fu, *Zhongguo yixue shi*, 499-502. Further examples are given in Zhu, *Zhong, wai yixue jiaoyu shi*, 90-98.

79 See the article by Zhou Fengru 周逢儒 in *SXYYXB* 12 1, (1922): 79-82 to this effect.

80 Anon., 'Huizhang Shanxi Yan dujun jian shengzhang diyici kaihui yanshuo' 會長山西閻督軍兼省長第一次開會演說 [Opening address of the chairman, Shanxi warlord and provincial governor Yan (Xishan)], *YXZZ* 1, 1 (1921): 11-14.

81 Ibid.

82 Zhou Xiaonong 小農周, 'Lun neijing yiben dongwen bu zu shi' 論內景譯本東文不足恃 [On the unreliability of anatomical translations from Japanese], *SXYYXB* 50 (1915): 34.

83 Examples of such letters may be found in *SXYYXB* 55 (1916): 94; and *SXYYXB* (n.s.) 7, 5 (1917): 15.

84 Qiu Jisheng 裘吉生, ed., *Zhen ben yi shu jicheng* 珍本醫書集成 [Compilation of valuable medical works] (Shanghai: Shijie, shuju, 1936), 4.

85 Cao Bingzhang 曹炳章, ed., *Zhongguo yixue da cheng* 中國醫學大城 [Great achievements of Chinese medicine] (Changsha: Yuelu shuju, 1994 [1936]), 3.

86 Ibid., 2.

87   Andrew Cunningham and Perry Williams, 'Introduction,' in Cunningham and Williams, *Laboratory Revolution in Medicine*, 1-12.

88   Jean-Pierre Drège, 'Les aventures de la typographie, et les missionnaires protestants en Chine au XIXe siècle,' *Journal asiatique* 280, 3-4 (1992): 279-305; Christopher A. Reed, *Gutenberg in Shanghai* (Vancouver: UBC Press, 2004), chap. 1.

89   Song Daren 宋大仁 and Shen Jingfan 沈警凡, 'Quanguo yiyao qikan diaocha ji' 全國醫藥期刊調查記 [Results of a national survey of medical periodicals], *ZXYY* 1, 1 (1935): 120-33; ibid., *ZXYY* 1, 3 (1935): 279-88.

90   This Shanghai journal was devoted to explaining the new Western medicine and was published from 1904 as the organ of the Medical Research Society, of which He Lianchen was a member, as was Ding Fubao. Its aims would have been similar to those under consideration here, but the journal is listed by Song and Shen (1935) as a Western-medical publication. In this period, however, such distinctions would have been impressionistic and would not have implied the exclusion of medical alternatives from discussion.

91   He Lianchen, 'Fakanci' 發刊詞 [Editorial foreword], *SXYYXB* 1, 1 (1908): 1A-2B.

92   Ibid.

93   Nedostup, *Superstitious Regimes*, chap. 6.

94   Duara, *Rescuing History from the Nation*, 79.

95   Qiu Qingyuan, Biographical note on the back of a photographic frontispiece depicting He Lianchen.

96   Song Chengjia 宋承家, 'Shaoxing xian jingchasuo bugao di shiyi hao' 紹興縣警察所布告第十一號 [Proclamation 11 from the Shaoxing county police station], *SXYYZB* (n.s.) 7, 3 (1917): 45

97   Fan Tianqing 范天磐, 'Fakanci, 發刊詞 [Editorial foreword], *GYPL* 1, 1 (1933): 1-18.

98   Xu Zhaonan 徐召南, 'Yixue gaige xiaolun' 醫學改革小論 [A note on medical reform], *SSYB* 3, 3 (1925): 1-2.

99   Chen Bangxian 陳邦賢, *Zhongguo yixue shi* 中國醫學史 [History of Chinese medicine] (Shanghai: Shanghai yixue shuju, 1919), cited in Zhao, *Jindai Zhong-, xiyixue lunzheng shi*, 206.

100 Yun Tieqiao 惲鐵樵, *Wu xing wei si shi zhi daimingci* 五行為四時之代名辭 [The Five Phases are pronouns/synonyms for the four seasons], in *Zhongyi xin lun huibian* [Compilation of new essays in Chinese medicine], ed. Wang Shenxuan (Shanghai: Shanghai shudian, 1932), 34; Yun Tieqiao, 'Qun jing jian zhi lu' 群經見智錄 [Record of wisdom observed in the medical classics], in *Jindai zhongyi zhenben ji* 近代中医珍本集, 医经分册 [Valuable works of modern Chinese medicine, medical classics volume], comp. Lu Zheng 陸拯, 513-80 (Hangzhou: Zhejiang kexue jishu chubanshe, 1990). See also Wu Yunbo 吳云波, 'Yun Tieqiao shengping he xueshu sixiang' 惲鐵樵生平和學術思 [The life and academic thought of Yun Tieqiao], *ZHYXZZ* 2 (1991): 88-93.

101 Xie Guan 謝觀, ed., *Zhongguo yixue da cidian* 中國醫學大辭典 [Encyclopaedic dictionary of Chinese medicine] (Shanghai: Commercial Press, 1921).

102 Zhang, *Zhongguo lidai yixue shilüe*, 54.

103 Wang Yunwu 王雲五, *Shangwu yinshuguan yu xin jiaoyu nianpu* 商務印書館與新教育年普 [Annual chronicle of the Commercial Press and modern education] (Taipei: Commercial Press, 1973), 69.

104 Jerry Norman, *Chinese* (Cambridge: Cambridge University Press, 1988), 170-73.

105 Chen Cunren, in Zhang, *Zhongguo lidai yixue shilüe*, 54.

106 Ibid.

107 Liu Yeqiu 刘叶秋, *Zhongguo zidian shilüe* 中国字典史略 [A brief history of Chinese dictionaries] (Beijing: Zhonghua shuju, 1983), 233-43.

108 Wang Yunwu, another native of Wujin County, had been editor-in-chief at the Commercial Press since 1922, was a keen supporter of the vernacularization movement, and ensured that the Commercial Press invested heavily and early in printing books in the vernacular. The four-corner indexing system was consistent with Wang's interests in the vernacular and in the National Phonetic alphabet since it enabled students to locate characters in a dictionary by their shape alone, without having to identify the correct radical or even to count the number of strokes. The new index was, however, probably foisted on Xie Guan as part of Wang's editorial policy since Xie had shown little interest in any of these new developments.

109 Fan Tianqing 范天磐, 'Shudian wangzu zhi Zhongguo yixue da cidian' 數典忘祖之中國醫學大辭典 [The historical ignorance of the encyclopaedic dictionary of Chinese medicine], *GYPL* 1, 2 (1933): 35-51.

110 Bruno Latour, 'Give Me a Laboratory and I Will Raise the World,' in *Science Observed*, ed. Karin D. Knorr-Cetina and Michael Mulkay (London: Sage, 1983), 141-70.

111 Nedostup, *Superstitious Regimes*, 206-19.

112 Croizier, *Traditional Medicine in Modern China*, 92-93.

113 Sinn, *Power and Charity*.

114 Xi Gao, 'Between the State and the Private Sphere: The Chinese State Medicine Movement, 1930-1949,' in *Science, Public Health and the State in Modern Asia*, ed. Liping Bu, Darwin Stapleton, and Ka-che Yip (London: Routledge, 2012),117-30.

115 Cochran, *Chinese Medicine Men*.

Chapter 8: From New Theories to New Practices

1 This section is adapted from Bridie J. Andrews, 'From Case Records to Case Histories: The Modernisation of a Chinese Medical Genre, 1912-49,' in *Innovation in Chinese Medicine*, ed. Elisabeth Hsu (Cambridge: Cambridge University Press, 2001), 324-36. With permission.

2 Reproduced in Shi Qi 施杞 and Su Mincai 肃敏材, eds., *Zhongguo bing'an xue* 中国病案学 [Chinese-medical case histories] (Shanghai: Zhongguo da baike quanshu chubanshe, 1994), 153.

3 I am grateful to Judith Farquhar for suggesting that it would be useful to see just how much information can be squeezed out of such minimal case records.

4　Charlotte Furth, Judith T. Zeitlin, and Ping-Chen Hsiung, eds., *Thinking with Cases: Specialist Knowledge in Chinese Cultural History* (Honolulu: University of Hawai'i Press, 2007).

5　Judith Farquhar, 'Time and Text: Approaching Chinese Medical Practice through Analysis of a Published Case,' in *Paths to Asian Medical Knowledge*, ed. Charles Leslie and Allan Young (Berkeley and Los Angeles: University of California Press, 1992), 62-73.

6　Scheid, *Currents of Tradition in Chinese Medicine*.

7　From Ding Ganren 丁甘仁, 'Housha zheng zhi gai yao' 喉痧症治概要：治案 [Essentials of throat-pox, symptoms and treatment: Treatment records], in *Zhongguo lidai yian xuan* 中国历代医案选 [Selected medical cases from Chinese historical sources], ed. Wang Xinhua 王新华 (Nanjing: Jiangsu Science and Technology Press, 1993), 150.

8　I have been unable to satisfactorily versify the rhyming couplet at the end: suggestions include 'Cases of throat-pox will get better / If the patient is a sweater' (Christopher Cullen, with thanks) or 'In throat pox there's no need to fret / If the patient can be made to sweat.'

9　One *fen* is one-tenth of a *qian*, which is one-tenth of a Chinese ounce, or *liang*. International weight units were introduced by the Republican government in China. By this scale, one *fen* equals one gram, one *qian* equals ten grams, and one *liang* equals one hundred grams. The kilogram is called *gong jin*. In the most common Chinese weight system before this, there were sixteen *liang* to one *jin*.

10　From He Lianchen 何廉臣, *Quanguo ming yi yan an lei bian* 全国名医验案按类编 [Classified case histories by famous Chinese physicians] (Fuzhou: Fujian kexue jishu chubanshe, 2002 [1927]), 382-83.

11　Zhao, *Jindai Zhong-, Xiyixue lunzheng shi*, 62-64. For brief biographies of He Lianchen and Ding Ganren, see Zhang Xiaoping 张笑平, ed., *Xiandai Zhongyi gejia xueshuo* 现代中医各家学说 [Doctrines of modern Chinese-medical physicians] (Beijing: Zhongguo Zhongyiyao chubanshe, 1991), 41-47 and 32-40. Ding Ganren's career is explored in detail in Scheid, *Currents of Tradition in Chinese Medicine*, chaps. 9-11.

12　See his preface in He, *Quanguo ming yi yan an lei bian*.

13　For evidence of this scientism and associated vilification of Chinese medicine, see Croizier, *Traditional Medicine in Modern China*.

14　Shi Jinmo, *Shi Jinmo yian* 施今墨醫案 [Shi Jinmo's case records], in *Jindai zhongyi zhenben ji: Yian fence* 近代中医珍本集：医案分册 (Collection of valuable modern Chinese medical works: Medical records volume), ed. Lu Zheng 陆拯 (Hangzhou: Zhejiang kexue jishu chubanshe, 1987 [1940]), 971.

15　Hinrichs, T.J., 'The Catchy Epidemic: Theorization and Its Limits in Han to Song Period Medicine,' *East Asian Science, Technology and Medicine* (forthcoming, 2014).

16　Hanson, *Speaking of Epidemics*.

17 This brief summary of the nosological principles of the two schools is necessarily somewhat cavalier. For an account of how the different theories developed over time, see Zhen and Fu, *Zhongguo yixue shi*, 305-9.

18 Lou Jie 婁杰, 'Wenbing zhinan' 溫病指南 [A compass for warmth diseases], in Lu Zheng 陆拯, ed., *Jindai zhongyi zhenben ji: wenbing fence* 近代中医珍本集: 溫病分册 [Collection of valuable modern Chinese medical works: Warmth diseases volume] (Hangzhou: Zhejiang kexue jishu chubanshe, 1987 [1903]), 485.

19 See, for example, the historical summary in the preface to Wan Yousheng 万友生, *Han, wen tongyi lun* 寒温统一论 [On the unification of cold and warmth] (Shanghai: Shanghai kexue jishu chubanshe, 1988).

20 'Abbreviated Constitution of the Shaoxing Medical Association,' *SXYYXB* 12 (1909): 13-15.

21 Zhang, *Yixue zhong Zhong can Xi lu*, 3. Publication dates of successive installments are noted in the editor's preface. Zhang is almost certain to have learned most of his Western medicine from Japanese medical textbooks since he was living in Shenyang, the capital of the Japanese 'informal empire' in Manchuria at this time.

22 '*Zhenci, huojiu, jiu fei jujun zhi suo yi.*' See Zhen and Fu, *Zhongguo yixue shi*, 334.

23 Ma Kanwen 马堪文, 'Qing Daoguang di jin zhenjiu yu taiyiyuan kao' 清道光帝禁针灸于太医院考 [An investigation into the banning of acupuncture from the Imperial Medical Academy by the Daoguang Emperor], *Shanghai zhongyi zazhi* 上海中医杂志 [Shanghai journal of traditional Chinese medicine] 4 (2002): 38-40.

24 Gwei-djen Lu and Joseph Needham, *Celestial Lancets: A History and Rationale of Acupuncture and Moxa* (Cambridge: Cambridge University Press, 1980), 160. Xu's book is titled *Yixue yuanliu lun* 醫學源流論 [On the origins and course of medicine].

25 Christopher Cullen, 'Patients and Healers in Late Imperial China: Evidence from the *Jinpingmei*,' *History of Science* 31, 2 (1993): 99-150.

26 I thank Tim Boon, curator of the London Science Museum's oriental collection, for access to this material, and Dr. Chris Wolff of Darwin College, Cambridge, for lending me his personal collection of Chinese surgical instruments.

27 Chen Cunren 陳存仁, ed., *Huanghan yixue congshu* 皇漢醫學從書 [Sino-Japanese medical collection] (Shanghai: Shijie, shuju, 1936).

28 Huang Shuze 黄树则, chief editor, 'Cheng Dan'an (1899-1957),' in *Zhongguo xiandai mingyi zhuan* 中国现代名医传 [Biographies of famous modern Chinese physicians] (Beijing: Kexue puji chubanshe, 1984), 152-57.

29 The earliest edition I have had access to is Cheng Dan'an, *Xiuding Zhongguo zhenjiu zhiliaoxue* 修訂中國針灸治療學 [Chinese acupuncture and moxibustion therapeutics, rev. ed.) (Shanghai: Qianqingtang shuju, 1932).

30 Ibid., 35.

31 Wang Weiyi's work, including overseeing the casting of the first two bronze figures for teaching of acupoints, is described in Gwei-djen Lu and Joseph Needham,

Celestial Lancets: A History and Rationale of Acupuncture and Moxa (Cambridge: Cambridge University Press, 1980), 130-35.

32 Asaf Moshe Goldschmidt, *The Evolution of Chinese Medicine: Song Dynasty, 960-1200* (New York: Routledge 2008).

33 Wang Weiyi's life and work is described further in Fu Weikang 傅维康, chief ed., *Zhenjiu tuina xue shi* 针灸推拿学史 [History of acupuncture, moxibustion and massage] (Shanghai: Shanghai guji chubanshe, 1991), 133-41.

34 Zhen and Fu, *Zhongguo yixue shi,* 453. Lu and Needham, *Celestial Lancets,* 22, also commend Cheng as a pioneer of the scientification of acupuncture. They note that the first book to combine Western-anatomical and acupuncture charts appeared in 1906.

35 Cheng, *Xiuding Zhongguo zhenjiu zhiliaoxue,* 36-39.

36 Ibid., 39-48

37 Xie Yongguang 谢永光, 'Woguo diyi jia zhenjiu jiaoyu jigou' 我国第一家针灸教育机构 [China's first teaching organization for acupuncture and moxibustion], *ZHYSZZ* 20, 4 (1990): 216-17.

38 Ibid.

39 Liang Fanrong 梁繁荣, chief editor, *Zhenjiu tuina xue cidian* 针灸推拿学辞典 [Dictionary of acupuncture, moxa and massage] (Beijing: People's Health Press, 2006), 461.

40 Taylor, *Chinese Medicine,* chap. 2.

Chapter 9: Conclusions

1 John R. Watt, *Saving Lives in Wartime China, 1928-1945* (Leiden: Brill, 2013), chap. 3.

2 Quoted in Taylor, *Chinese Medicine,* 16.

3 Ibid., 17-19; Zhu Lian, 'Zhenjiu liaofa de zhongyaoxing ji qi yuanli' 针灸疗法的重要性及其原理 [The importance and principles of acupuncture therapy], *Renmin Ribao* 人民日报 [People's daily], 17 February 1951.

4 Rogaski, *Hygienic Modernity,* chap. 5.

5 Wataru Iijima, 'On the Japanese "Imperial Medicine": A Case Study in Colonial Taiwan, 1895-1945,' Society for the Social History of Medicine Conference titled 'Medicine and the Colonies,' Oxford, 3 July 1996.

6 Taylor, *Chinese Medicine,* 36-44; Volker Scheid, *Chinese Medicine in Contemporary China* (Durham, NC: Duke University Press, 2002), 69-75.

7 Taylor, *Chinese Medicine,* 45-49.

8 Scheid, *Chinese Medicine in Contemporary China,* 70-74; Rogaski, *Hygienic Modernity,* 293-98. Nathan Sivin has translated the first section of one of these textbooks for Western-style physicians, the *Xinbian Zhongyixue gaiyao* [Revised outline of Chinese medicine] of 1972, in his *Traditional Medicine in Contemporary China,* 203-440.

9 Scheid, *Chinese Medicine in Contemporary China,* 75.

10 Elisabeth Hsu, *The Transmission of Chinese Medicine* (Cambridge: Cambridge University Press, 1999), 177-86.

11 Some of the first textbooks compiled after the end of the Cultural Revolution omitted mention of the Five Phases altogether. See, for example, Shenyang College of Pharmacy, *Zhongyixue jichu* [Fundamentals of Chinese medicine], National textbooks for higher-level colleges of medicine and pharmacy (Beijing: Renmin weisheng chubanshe, 1978).

12 Xiaoping Fang, Barefoot Doctors and Western Medicine in China. (Rochester: University of Rochester Press, 2012).

13 Hsu, *Transmission of Chinese Medicine*, 21-57.

14 Mei Zhan, *Other-Worldly: Making Chinese Medicine through Transnational Frames* (Durham, NC: Duke University Press, 2009), 150-51.

15 Personal communication.

16 Sean Hsiang-Lin Lei, 'How Did Chinese Medicine Become Experiential? The Political Epistemology of Jingyan,' *Positions* 10, 2 (2002): 333-64.

17 Zhan, *Other-Worldly*, 37-38.

18 Ibid., chap. 3.

19 Linda L. Barnes, 'The Psychologizing of Chinese Healing Practices in the United States,' *Culture, Medicine and Psychiatry* 22, 4 (1998): 413-43.

20 Kim Taylor, 'Divergent Interests and Cultivated Misunderstandings: The Influence of the West on Modern Chinese Medicine,' *Social History of Medicine* 17, 1 (2004): 93-111.

21 Burke, *Cultural Hybridity*, 34-65.

22 Rogaski, *Hygienic Modernity*, 10-12.

23 Barry Buzan, 'Culture and International Society,' *International Affairs* 86, 1 (2010): 1-26. Quote at 8, citing Shogo Suzuki, *Civilization and Empire: China and Japan's Encounter with European International Society* (London: Routledge, 2009).

24 Ibid.

25 Marwah Elshakry, 'When Science Became Western: Historiographical Reflections,' *Isis* 101 (2010): 98-109.

26 See Charlotte Furth, *Ting Wen-chiang: Science and China's New Culture* (Cambridge: Harvard University Press, 1970).

27 Benjamin A. Elman, 'Rethinking the Twentieth-Century Denigration of Traditional Chinese Science and Medicine in the Twenty-First Century' (paper presented at the 6th International Conference on the New Significance of Chinese Culture in the Twenty-First Century titled 'The Interaction and Confluence of Chinese and Non-Chinese Civilization,' Prague, Czech Republic, 1 November 2003).

Bibliography

Andrews, Bridie, J. 'From Case Records to Case Histories: The Modernisation of a Chinese Medical Genre, 1912-49.' In *Innovation in Chinese Medicine*, 324-36. Cambridge: Cambridge University Press, 2001.

–. 'Tuberculosis and the Assimilation of Germ Theory in China, 1895-1937.' *Journal of the History of Medicine and Allied Sciences* 52, 1 (1997): 114-57.

Anon. 'Conference Report of the Medical Missionary Conference Held at Shanghai, April 19-23 1907: Discussion on Dr. McCartney's Paper, "The Fevers of West China."' *CMJ* 21, 3 (1907): 163-64.

–. 'Editorial.' *CMMJ* 7, 2 (1893): 110.

–. 'Progress in China: The Wheels Move Slowly in the Dragon's Empire.' *New York Times*, 11 March 1892.

–. 'Tongji dewen yixuetang weisheng yanshuo zeyao lu' [Selections from a lecture on 'hygiene' at the German-language 'Universal Benefit' (Tongji) Medical School]. *ZXYXB* 18 (1911): 4.

–. *Zhongguo shuili shigao* [A draft history of Chinese waterworks]. Beijing: Shuili dianli chubanshe, 1989.

–. 'Zhonghua yixue hui gaikuo baogao' [Summary report on the National Medical Association]. *NMJC* (Chinese section) 18, 1 (1932): 175-83.

Arikha, Noga. *Passions and Tempers: A History of the Humours*. New York: HarperCollins, 2007.

Balme, Harold. *China and Modern Medicine: A Study in Medical Missionary Development*. London: United Council for Missionary Education, 1921.

Bannister, T. Roger. *A History of the External Trade of China, 1834-81, Together with a Synopsis of the External Trade of China, 1882-1931, Being an Introduction to the Customs*

Decennial Reports, 1922-1931. Decennial Reports of the China Imperial Maritime Customs Service. Shanghai: Inspectorate General of Chinese Customs, 1931.

Barnes, Linda L. 'The Psychologizing of Chinese Healing Practices in the United States.' *Culture, Medicine and Psychiatry* 22, 4 (1998): 413-43.

Bartholomew, James R. *The Formation of Science in Japan: Building a Research Tradition.* New Haven: Yale University Press, 1989.

Bastid, Marianne. *Educational Reform in Early Twentieth-Century China.* Center for Chinese Studies, University of Michigan, 1988.

Benedict, Carol. 'Bubonic Plague in Nineteenth Century China.' PhD diss., Stanford University, 1992.

–. *Bubonic Plague in Nineteenth-Century China.* Stanford: Stanford University Press, 1996.

Bensky, Dan, and Randall Barolet. *Chinese Herbal Medicine: Formulas and Strategies.* 1st ed. Seattle: Eastland Press, 1990.

Biggerstaff, Knight. *The Earliest Modern Government Schools in China.* Ithaca, NY: Cornell University Press, 1961.

Bivins, Roberta. *Alternative Medicine? A History.* Oxford: Oxford University Press, 2007.

Borowy, Iris, ed. *Uneasy Encounters: The Politics of Medicine and Health in China, 1900-1937.* Frankfurt am Main: Peter Lang, 2009.

Bowers, John Z. *Western Medical Pioneers in Feudal Japan.* Baltimore: Johns Hopkins University Press, 1970.

Bu, Liping. 'Social Darwinism, Public Health, and Modernization in China, 1895-1925.' In *Uneasy Encounters: The Politics of Medicine and Health in China, 1900-1937,* ed. Iris Borowy, 93-124. Frankfurt am Main: Peter Lang, 2009.

Bullock, Mary B. *An American Transplant: The Rockefeller Foundation and Peking Union Medical College.* Berkeley: University of California Press, 1980.

Burke, Peter. *Cultural Hybridity.* Cambridge: Polity, 2009.

Burns, Susan. 'Nanayama Jundo- at Work: A Village Doctor and Medical Knowledge in Nineteenth-Century Japan.' *East Asian Science, Technology and Medicine* 29 (2008): 62-82.

Buzan, Barry. 'Culture and International Society.' *International Affairs* 86, 1 (2010): 1-26.

Chadwick, Edwin. 'On the Prevention of Epidemics.' In *Transactions of the Brighton Health Congress,* 24-47. London: E. Marlborough, 1881.

Chang, Che-chia. 'The Therapeutic Tug of War: The Imperial Physician-Patient Relationship in the Era of Empress Dowager Cixi, 1874-1908.' PhD diss., University of Pennsylvania, 1998.

Chang, Chia-feng. 'Aspects of Smallpox and Its Significance in Chinese History.' PhD diss., School of Oriental and African Studies, University of London, 1996.

Chang, K.C., ed. *Food in Chinese Culture: Anthropological and Historical Perspectives.* New Haven: Yale University Press, 1977.

Chao, Yuan-ling. *Medicine and Society in Late Imperial China: A Study of Physicians in Suzhou, 1600-1850.* New York: Peter Lang, 2009.

Chau, Adam Yuet. *Miraculous Response: Doing Popular Religion in Contemporary China.* Stanford: Stanford University Press, 2006.

Checkland, Olive. *Humanitarianism and the Emperor's Japan, 1877-1977.* Basingstoke: Macmillan, 1994.

Chen Cunren. *Huanghan yixue congshu* [Sino-Japanese medical collection]. Shanghai: Shijie, shuju, 1936.

Chen Daoqin and Weitao Xue. *Jiangsu lidai yiren zhi* [Records of Jiangsu physicians throughout history]. Nanjing: Jiangsu Science and Technology Press, 1985.

Chen, Hsi-Yuan. *Confucian Encounters with Religion: Rejections, Appropriations, and Transformations.* New York: Routledge, 2006.

Chen, Ping. *Modern Chinese: History and Sociolinguistics.* Cambridge: Cambridge University Press, 1999.

Chen, Xianggong. *Qiu Jin nianpu ji zhuanji ziliao* [Annual chronicle and biographical materials on Qiu Jin]. Beijing: Zhonghua shuju, 1983.

Chen Yuan. 'Riren yi xin shijie, yishu bi Han' [Japanese use New World medicine to close in on Koreans]. In *Chen Yuan zaonian wenji* [The early writings of Chen Yuan], 293-95. Taipei: Academia Sinica, 1992.

Chernin, Eli. 'Richard Pearson Strong and the Manchurian Epidemic of Pneumonic Plague, 1910-1911.' *Journal of the History of Medicine and Allied Sciences* 44 (1989): 296-319.

China Imperial Maritime Customs. *Decennial Reports of the Chinese Imperial Maritime Customs, Third Issue, 1902-1911.* Statistical Department of the Inspectorate General of Customs, Shanghai, 1911.

Cho, Philip S. "Ritual and the Occult in Chinese Medicine and Religious Healing: The Development of Zhuyou Exorcism." PhD diss., University of Pennsylvania, 2005.

Chuan, S.H. "Chinese Patients and Their Prejudices." *CMJ* 31, 6 (1917): 504-10.

Chung, Yuehtsen Juliette. *Struggle for National Survival: Eugenics in Sino-Japanese Contexts, 1896-1945.* New York: Routledge, 2002.

Cochran, Sherman. *Chinese Medicine Men: Consumer Culture in China and Southeast Asia.* Cambridge, MA: Harvard University Press, 2006.

Conner, Alison W. 'Lawyers and the Legal Profession during the Republican Period.' In *Civil Law in Qing and Republican China,* ed. Kathryn Bernhardt and Philip C. Huang, 215-48. Stanford: Stanford University Press, 1994.

Conrad, Lawrence I., Michael Neve, Vivian Nutton, Roy Porter, and Andrew Wear. *The Western Medical Tradition, 800 BC to AD 1800.* Cambridge: Cambridge University Press, 1995.

Cox-Maksimov, Desirée. 'Foreign Bodies, Filthy Lands: Health, Disease and Sanitation on the China Coast in the Late 19th Century.' M.Phil, University of Cambridge, 1993.

Crellin, J.K. *A Social History of Medicines in the Twentieth Century: To Be Taken Three Times a Day*. Binghamton: Pharmaceutical Products Press, 2004.

Croizier, Ralph C. 'The Ideology of Medical Revivalism in Modern China.' In *Asian Medical Systems: A Comparative Study in Non-Western Cultures*, ed. Charles Leslie, 341-54. Berkeley: University of California Press, 1977.

–. *Traditional Medicine in Modern China: Science, Nationalism and the Tensions of Cultural Change*. Cambridge, MA: Harvard University Press, 1968.

Cullen, Christopher. 'Patients and Healers in Late Imperial China: Evidence from the Jinpingmei.' *History of Science* 31, 2 (1993): 99-150.

Cunningham, A.R., and Perry Williams, eds. *The Laboratory Revolution in Medicine*. Cambridge: Cambridge University Press, 1992.

Deng Tietao, ed. *Zhongguo fang yi shi* [History of epidemic prevention in China]. Nanning: Guangxi Science and Technology Press, 2006.

Deng Yunte. *Zhongguo jiuhuang shi* [History of disaster relief in China]. Taipei: Taiwan Commercial Press, 1966.

Dikötter, Frank. *The Discourse of Race in Modern China*. London: Hurst, 1992.

Duara, Prasenjit. *Rescuing History from the Nation: Questioning Narratives of Modern China*. Chicago: University of Chicago Press, 1995.

Dudgeon, John. 'The Chinese Arts of Healing.' *CR* 2, 70 (1869-70): 163-66; 183-86; 267-71; 293-98; 332-39.

–. *Chinese Healing Arts: Internal Kung-Fu*. Ed. William R. Berk. Burbank, CA: Unique Publications, 1986.

–. *The Diseases of China; Their Causes, Conditions, and Prevalence, Contrasted with Those in Europe*. Glasgow: Dunn and Wright, 1877.

Editorial. 'Diseases of China.' *Lancet* 110, 2821 (1877): 439-40.

–. 'An Obstacle to Sanitary Progress.' *CMJ* 34, 5 (1920): 523-24.

Elman, Benjamin A. 'Eight-legged Essay: *Baguwen*.' In *Berkshire Encyclopedia of China*, ed. Linsun Cheng, 695-98. Great Barrington: Berkshire Publishing, 2009.

–. *On Their Own Terms: Science in China, 1550-1900*. Cambridge, MA: Harvard University Press, 2005.

–. 'Rethinking the Twentieth-Century Denigration of Traditional Chinese Science and Medicine in the Twenty-First Century." Paper presented at the 6th International Conference on the New Significance of Chinese Culture in the Twenty-First Century, titled 'The Interaction and Confluence of Chinese and Non-Chinese Civilization,' Prague, Czech Republic, 1 November 2003.

Elshakry, Marwah. 'When Science Became Western: Historiographical Reflections.' *Isis* 101 (2010): 98-109.

Englund, Harri, and James Leach. 'Ethnography and the Meta-Narratives of Modernity.' *Current Anthropology* 41, 2 (2000): 225-48.

Ewart, William. *Res Medica, Res Publica: The Profession of Medicine: Its Future Work and Wage*. London: St. George's Hospital, 1907.

Ewen, Jean. *China Nurse, 1932-39*. Toronto: McClelland and Stewart, 1981.

Fan, Ka-wai. 'Discussion on Scientification of Acupuncture in Hong Kong in 1950s: With Special Reference to Zhu Lian's *The New Acupuncture*.' *Asian Culture and History* 3, 2 (2011): 2-8.

Fan Tianqing. 'Shudian mangzu zhi "Zhongguo yixue da cidian"' [The historical ignorance of the 'Encyclopedic dictionary of Chinese medicine']. *GYPL* 1, 2 (1933): 35-51.

Fan Xingzhun. *Zhongguo yufang yixue sixiang shi* [History of preventative medical thought in China]. Beijing: Renmin weisheng chubanshe, 1955.

Fang, Xiaoping. 'Barefoot Doctors and Western Medicine in China. Rochester: Rochester University Press, 2012.

Farquhar, Judith. '"Medicine and the Changes Are One": An Essay on Divination Healing with Commentary.' *Chinese Science* 13 (1996): 107-34.

Feuerwerker, Albert. *China's Early Industrialization: Sheng Hsuan-huai (1844-1916) and Mandarin Enterprise*. Cambridge, MA: Harvard University Press, 1958.

Freidson, Eliot. *Professional Powers: A Study of the Institutionalization of Formal Knowledge*. Chicago: University of Chicago Press, 1986.

Fujikawa, Y. *Japanese Medicine*. English ed., trans. from the 1911 German, Clio Medica. New York: Paul B. Hoeber, 1934.

Fukuoka, Maki. *The Premise of Fidelity: Science, Visuality, and Representing the Real in Nineteenth-Century Japan*. Stanford: Stanford University Press, 2012.

Furth, Charlotte. *A Flourishing Yin: Gender in China's Medical History, 960-1665*. Berkeley: University of California Press, 1997.

–. *Ting Wen-chiang: Science and China's New Culture*. Cambridge, MA: Harvard University Press, 1970.

Furth, Charlotte, Judith T. Zeitlin, and Ping-Chen Hsiung. *Thinking with Cases: Specialist Knowledge in Chinese Cultural History*. Honolulu: University of Hawai'i Press, 2007.

Gamsa, Mark. 'The Epidemic of Pneumonic Plague in Manchuria 1910-1911.' *Past and Present* 190 (2006): 147-83.

Gao, Xi. "Between the State and the Private Sphere: The Chinese State Medicine Movement, 1930-1949." In *Science, Public Health and the State in Modern Asia*, ed. Liping Bu, Darwin H. Stapleton, and Ka-Che Yip, 117-30. New York: Routledge, 2012.

–. *Dezhen zhuan: Yige yingguo chuanjiaoshi yu wan Qing yixue jindaihua* [Biography of John Dudgeon: A British missionary and the modernization of late Qing medicine]. Shanghai: Fudan University Press, 2009.

Garrett, Shirley S. *Social Reformers in Urban China: The Chinese YMCA, 1895-1926*. Harvard East Asian Series. Cambridge, MA: Harvard University Press, 1970.

Glosser, Susan L. *Chinese Visions of Family and State, 1915-1953*. Berkeley: University of California Press, 2003.

Goldschmidt, Asaf Moshe. *The Evolution of Chinese Medicine: Song Dynasty, 960-1200*. Abingdon: Routledge, 2008.

Gordon, Andrew. *A Modern History of Japan: From Tokugawa Times to the Present*. Oxford: Oxford University Press, 2009.

Gordon, C.A. *An Epitome of the Reports of the Medical Officers of the China Imperial Maritime Customs Service, from 1871-1882*. London: Baillière, Tindall and Cox, 1884.

Gray, Jack. *Rebellions and Revolutions: China from the 1800s to the 1980s*. Oxford: Oxford University Press, 1990.

Greenish, Henry George. *Materia Medica: Being an Account of the More Important Crude Drugs of Vegetable and Animal Origin: Designed for Students of Pharmacy and Medicine*. London: J. and A. Churchill, 1924.

Guangzhou shi weisheng ju. *Guangzhou weisheng nianbao* [Annual report of the Department of Health of Canton Municipality). Canton: Canton Department of Health, 1926.

Hale White, W. *Materia Medica, Pharmacy, Pharmacology and Therapeutics*. London: J. and A. Churchill, 1892.

Hanson, Marta. *Speaking of Epidemics in Chinese Medicine: Disease and the Geographic Imagination in Late Imperial China*. London: Routledge, 2011.

Harrison, Henrietta. 'The Experience of Illness in Early Twentieth-Century Rural Shanxi.' *East Asian Science, Technology and Medicine* 33 (2014): forthcoming.

He Bingyuan. 'Lun Zhongguo ji yi kai yizhi' [China should urgently propagate medical knowledge].' *YXB* (July 1909): 49-50.

He Lianchen. *Quanguo ming yi yan an lei bian* [Classified case histories by famous Chinese physicians]. Fuzhou: Fujian kexue jishu chubanshe, 1927.

Henderson, James. 'The Medicine and Medical Practice of the Chinese.' *JNCBRAS* 1 (1864): 61-105.

–. *Shanghai Hygiene: Or, Hints for the Preservation of Health in China*. Shanghai: Presbyterian Mission Press, 1863.

Hinrichs, T.J., 'The Catchy Epidemic: Theorization and Its Limits in Han to Song Period Medicine.' *East Asian Science, Technology and Medicine* (forthcoming).

Howard-Jones, Norman. *The Scientific Background of the International Sanitary Conferences, 1851-1938*. WHO History of International Public Health. Vol. 1. Geneva: World Health Organization, 1975.

Hsiung, Ping-chen. *A Tender Voyage: Children and Childhood in Late Imperial China*. Stanford: Stanford University Press, 2007.

Hsu, Elisabeth. *The Transmission of Chinese Medicine*. Cambridge: Cambridge University Press, 1999.

Huang, Philip C. *Code, Custom, and Legal Practice in China*. Stanford: Stanford University Press, 2001.

Hume, Edward H. *Doctors East, Doctors West: An American Physician's Life in China*. New York: W.W. Norton, 1946.

Hymes, Robert P. 'Not Quite Gentlemen? Doctors in Sung and Yuan.' *Chinese Science* 8 (1987): 9-76.

Iijima, Wataru. 'On the Japanese "Imperial Medicine": A Case Study in Colonial Taiwan, 1895-1945.' Paper presented at the Society for the Social History of Medicine Conference titled 'Medicine and the Colonies,' Oxford, 3 July 1996.

Jannetta, Ann. *The Vaccinators: Smallpox, Medical Knowledge, and the 'Opening' of Japan*. Stanford: Stanford University Press, 2007.

Jansen, Marius B. 'Japan and the Chinese Revolution of 1911.' In *The Cambridge History of China*, 339-74, vol. 11, pt. 2: Cambridge University Press, 1980.

Jeffreys, W. Hamilton, and James L. Maxwell. *The Diseases of China, Including Formosa and Korea*. London: John Bale and Danielson, 1911.

Jiang Huiming. 'Zhongguo yixue jiaoyu zhi qianzhan hougu' [On the history and future prospects of medical education in China]. *Zhong-xi yiyao* [Sino-Western medicine and pharmacy] 1, 1 (1935): 50-65.

Jin Shiying. 'Jindai Zhong, Ri liang guo de zhongyi jiaoliu' [Modern Sino-Japanese exchanges in Chinese medicine]. *ZHYSZZ* 22, 2 (1992): 106-12.

–. 'Riben fan feizhi hanfang yu Zhongguo fan feizhi zhongyi zhi douzheng ji qi bijiao' [Comparison of the Japanese and Chinese opposition to the abolition of traditional medicine]. *Zhonghua yishi zazhi* [Chinese journal of medical history], 1 (1993): 45-51.

Johnson, Tina Phillips, *Childbirth in Republican China: Delivering Modernity*. Lanham: Lexington Books, 2011.

Johnston, William. "Of Doctors, Women, and the Knife of Hope: The Surgical Treatment of Breast Cancer in Early Modern Japan." In *History of Ideas in Surgery*, ed. Yosio Kawakita, Shizu Sakai, and Yasuo Otsuka, 153-80. Proceedings of the 17th International Symposium on the Comparative History of Medicine – East and West. Tokyo: Ishiyaku EuroAmerica, 1997.

Kaptchuk, Ted. *The Web That Has No Weaver: Understanding Chinese Medicine*. 2nd ed. London: Rider, 2000.

Katz, Paul. *Demon Hordes and Burning Boats: The Cult of Marshal Wen in Late Imperial Chekiang*. New York: State University of New York Press, 1995.

[Kerr], J.G.K. 'Chinese Materia Medica.' *CMMJ* 1, 2 (1887): 79-80.

Kiang, M.D., Peter. 'Chinese Drugs of Therapeutic Value to Western Physicians.' *CMJ* 37, 9 (1923): 742-46.

Kleinman, Arthur. *Writing at the Margin*. Berkeley: University of California Press, 1997.

–. *Patients and Healers in the Context of Culture: An Exploration of the Borderland between Anthropology, Medicine and Psychiatry*. Berkeley: University of California Press, 1980.

Kleiweg de Zwaan, Dr. J.P. *Völkerkundliches und Geschichtliches über die Heilkunde der Chinesen und Japaner* [Ethnographic and historical study of Chinese and Japanese healing]. Haarlem: De Erven Loosjes, 1917.

Koo, Linda Chih-ling. *Nourishment of Life: Health in Chinese Society*. Hong Kong: The Commercial Press, 1982.

Kuhn, Philip A. *Soulstealers: The Chinese Sorcery Scare of 1768.* Cambridge, MA: Harvard University Press, 1990.

Latour, Bruno. *We Have Never Been Modern.* Cambridge, MA: Harvard University Press, 1993.

Lei, Sean Hsiang-Lin. 'From "Changshan" to a New Anti-malarial Drug: Re-networking Chinese Drugs and Excluding Chinese Doctors.' *Social Studies of Science* 29, 3 (1999): 323-58.

–. 'How Did Chinese Medicine Become Experiential? The Political Epistemology of Jingyan.' *Positions* 10, 2 (2002): 333-64.

–. 'When Chinese Medicine Encountered the State: 1910-1949.' Chicago: University of Chicago, Committee on the Conceptual Foundations of Science, 1999.

Lennox, W.G. 'A Self-Survey by Mission Hospitals in China.' *CMJ* 46, 5 (1932): 484-534.

Leung, Angela Ki Che. 'Ming, Qing Yufang Tianhua Cuoshi Zhi Yanbian' [The development of preventive measures against smallpox during the Ming and Qing dynasties]. In *Guoshi Shilun: Tao Xisheng Xiansheng jiuzhi rongqing zhu shou lunwen ji* [Treatises on national history: Festschrift for Mr. Tao Xisheng's 90th birthday], 239-53. Taipei: n.p., 1987.

–. 'Organized Medicine in Ming-Qing China: State and Private Medical Institutions in the Lower Yangzi Region.' *Late Imperial China* 8, 1 (1987): 134-66.

–. "Women Practicing Medicine in Pre-modern China." In *Chinese Women in the Imperial Past: New Perspectives,* 101-34. Leiden: Brill, 1999.

Levy, Dore J. *Ideal and Actual in* The Story of the Stone. New York: Columbia University Press, 1999.

Li Jiafu. 'Yishi weisheng yu guoshi zhi guanxi guan' [A view of the relationship between national power and medical affairs]. *MGYXZZ* 2, 8 (1924): 424.

Li Jian. 'Quanguo Yiyao Tuanti Zonglianhehui De Chuanli Ji Qi Huodong Lishi Diwei' [The establishment, activities, and historical position of the National Union for Chinese Medicine]. *Zhongguo Keji Shiliao* [China historical materials of science and technology] 14, 3 (n.d.): 67-75.

Li, Jingwei, chief editor. *Zhongyi renwu cidian* [Biographical dictionary of Chinese medicine]. Shanghai: Shanghai cishu chubanshe, 1988.

Li, Shang-jen. 'Eating Well in China: British Medical Practitioners on Diet and Personal Hygiene at Nineteenth-Century Chinese Treaty Ports.' In *Health and Hygiene in Chinese East Asia,* ed. Angela Ki Che Leung and Charlotte Furth, 109-31. Durham, NC: Duke University Press, 2010.

–. 'Jiankang de daode jingji – Dezhen lun Zhongguoren shenghuo xiguan he weisheng' [Moral economy and health: John Dudgeon on hygiene in China]. *Zhongyang yanjiuyuan lishi yuyan yanjiusuo jikan* [Bulletin of the Institute of History and Philology, Academia Sinica] 76, 3 (2005): 467-509.

Li Yun, ed. *Zhongyi renming cidian* [Biographical dictionary of Chinese medicine]. Beijing: Guoji wenhua chubangongsi, 1988.

Liang Fanrong 梁繁荣, chief editor. *Zhenjiu tuina xue cidian* 针灸推拿学辞典 [Dictionary of acupuncture, moxa and massage]. Beijing: People's Health Press, 2006.

Liu, Lydia H. *The Clash of Empires: The Invention of China in Modern World Making.* Cambridge, MA: Harvard University Press, 2006.

Liu, Michael Shiyung. *Prescribing Colonization: The Role of Medical Practices and Policies in Japan-ruled Taiwan, 1895-1945.* Ann Arbor, MI: Association for Asian Studies, 2009.

Liu, Xun. *Daoist Modern: Innovation, Lay Practice, and the Community of Inner Alchemy in Republican Shanghai.* Cambridge, MA: Harvard University Asia Center, 2009.

Liu Yeqiu. *Zhongguo zidian shilüe* [A brief history of Chinese dictionaries]. Beijing: Zhonghua shuju, 1983.

Lo, Ming-Cheng M. *Doctors within Borders: Profession, Ethnicity, and Identity in Colonial Taiwan.* Berkeley: University of California Press, 2002.

Lock, Margaret M. *East Asian Medicine in Urban Japan.* Berkeley: University of California Press, 1980.

Lu, Gwei-djen, and Joseph Needham. 'Hygiene and Preventive Medicine in Ancient China.' In *Clerks and Craftsmen in China and the West: Lectures and Addresses on the History of Science and Technology*, ed. Joseph Needham, 340-78. Cambridge: Cambridge University Press, 1970.

Lu, Xun. *Selected Works of Lu Hsun.* Vol. 1. Beijing: Foreign Languages Press, 1956.

Lu Yuanlei. *Shanghan Lun jin shi* [Modern exposition of the *Treatise on Cold-damage*]. Beijing: Renmin weisheng chubanshe, 1931.

Lutz, Jessie Gregory. *China and the Christian Colleges, 1850-1950.* Ithaca, NY: Cornell University Press, 1971.

Ma Boying, Xi Gao, and Zhongli Hong. *Zhong, wai yixue wenhua jiaoliu shi* [The history of intercultural communication in medicine between China and foreign countries]. Shanghai: Wenhui Press, 1993.

Macpherson, Kerrie L. *A Wilderness of Marshes: The Origins of Public Health in Shanghai, 1843-1893.* East Asian Historical Monographs. Oxford: Oxford University Press, 1987.

Mann, Susan. *Local Merchants and the Chinese Bureaucracy, 1750-1850.* Stanford: Stanford University Press, 1987.

Marks, Harry M. *The Progress of Experiment.* Cambridge: Cambridge University Press, 1997.

Masini, Federico. *The Formation of the Modern Chinese Lexicon and Its Evolution toward a National Language: The Period from 1840 to 1898. Journal of Chinese Linguistics,* Monograph series 6. Berkeley: Project on Linguistic Analysis, 1993.

McDougall, Bonnie, S., and Kam Louie. *The Literature of China in the Twentieth Century.* New York: Columbia University Press, 1999.

Medical History Committee of the Shanghai Branch of Chinese Medical Association. 'Yu Yunxiu xiansheng zhuanlüe he nianpu' [Biographical sketch and chronology of the life of Mr Yu Yunxiu]. *ZHYSZZ* 2 (1954): 81-84.

Morris, Andrew D. *Marrow of the Nation: A History of Sport and Physical Culture in Republican China*. 1st ed. Berkeley: University of California Press, 2004.

Myers, Ramon H. 'Japanese Imperialism in Manchuria: The South Manchuria Railway Company, 1906-1933.' In *The Japanese Informal Empire in China, 1895-1937*, 101-32. Princeton: Princeton University Press, 1989.

Nakamura, Ellen Gardner. *Practical Pursuits: Takano Choei, Takahashi Keisaku, and Western Medicine in Nineteenth-Century Japan*. Cambridge, MA: Harvard University Asia Center, 2005.

Nathan, Carl F. 'The Acceptance of Western Medicine in Early 20th-Century China: The Story of the North Manchurian Plague Prevention Service.' In *Medicine and Society in China*, ed. John Z. Bowers and Elizabeth Purcell, 55-75. Philadelphia: Wm. F. Fell for the National Library of Medicine and the Josiah Macy Jr. Foundation, 1974.

Nedostup, Rebecca. *Superstitious Regimes: Religion and the Politics of Chinese Modernity*. Cambridge, MA: Harvard University Asia Center, 2010.

Oberländer, Christian. 'The Modernization of Japan's Kanpo Medicine, 1850-1950.' In *East Asian Science: Tradition and Beyond; Papers from the Seventh International Conference for the History of Science in East Asia, Kyoto, 2-7 August 1993*, ed. Keizo Hashimoto, Cathérine Jami, and Lowell Skar, 141-46. Osaka: Kansai University Press, 1993.

–. *Zwischen Tradition und Moderne: Die Bewegung für den Fortbestand der Kanpō-Medizin in Japan* [Between tradition and modernity: The movement for the continuation of kanpō medicine in Japan]. Stuttgart: F. Steiner, 1995.

Okuma, Count Shigenobu. *Fifty Years of New Japan*. London: Smith, Elder, 1909.

Pan, Guijuan, and Zhenglun Fan. *Riben hanfang yixue* [Japanese kanpō medicine]. Beijing: Zhongguo Zhongyiyao chubanshe, 1994.

Patterson, B.C., MD. 'Correspondence: Substitute for Cataplasma Kaolini (USP).' *CMJ* 37, 2 (1923): 201.

People's Daily Online. 'Constitution of the People's Republic of China,' 22 March 2004. http://english.people.com.cn/constitution/constitution.html.

Perry, Elizabeth J. *Shanghai on Strike: The Politics of Chinese Labor*. Stanford: Stanford University Press, 1993.

Peter, W.W. 'Appeal by Joint Council on Public Health Education in China.' *CMJ* 31, 1 (1917): 57-59.

Pittman, Don Alvin. *Toward a Modern Chinese Buddhism*. Honolulu: University of Hawai'i Press, 2001.

Pompe van Meerdervoort, J.L.C. 'Dissection of a Japanese criminal.' *JNCBRAS* 2, 1 (1860): 85-91.

Porter, Dorothy. *The History of Public Health and the Modern State*. The Wellcome Institute Series in the History of Medicine. Amsterdam: Rodopi, 1994.

Porter, Dr. H.D. 'From China.' In *The Medical Arm of the Missionary Service: Testimonies from the Field,* ed. E. K. Alden, 37-41. Boston: American Board of Commissioners for Foreign Missions, 1894.

Pusey, James Reeve. *China and Charles Darwin.* Cambridge, MA: Harvard University Press, 1983.

Qin Danwei. 'Chi Yu Yunxiu yijiao xitong boyi' [A denunciation of Yu Yunxiu's disagreements with the medical school system *San san yi bao* [Double three medical journal] 3, 12 (1925): 1-2.

Qiu Jisheng. 'Shaoxing zhi yi su' [Medical customs of Shaoxing]. In *Qiu Jisheng yi wenji* [Medical writings of Qiu Jisheng], ed. Jisheng Qiu, 8-18. Beijing: Renmin weisheng chubanshe, 2006.

Ranzaburō, Otori. 'The Acceptance of Western Medicine in Japan.' *Monumenta Nipponica* 19, 3-4 (1964): 20-40.

Read, B.E. 'Correspondence: Substitute for Cataplasma Kaolini (USP).' *CMJ* 37, 3-4 (1923): 340.

Read, B.E., and C.O. Lee. "Chinese Inorganic Materia Medica." *CMJ* 39, 1 (1925): 23-32.

Reed, Christopher A. *Gutenberg in Shanghai.* Vancouver: UBC Press, 2004.

Reeves, Caroline. 'The Changing Nature of Philanthropy in Late Imperial and Republican China.' *Papers on Chinese History, Harvard University* 5 (1996): 79-97.

–. 'Grave Concerns: Bodies, Burial, and Identity in Early Republican China.' In *Cities in Motion: Interior, Coast, and Diaspora in Transnational China,* ed. Sherman Cochran and David Strand, 27-52. Berkeley: Institute of East Asian Studies, University of California, 2007.

Renshaw, Michelle. *Accommodating the Chinese: The American Hospital in China, 1880-1920.* New York: Routledge, 2005.

Reynolds, Douglas R. *China, 1989-1912: The Xinzheng Revolution and Japan.* Cambridge, MA: Council on East Asian Studies, Harvard University, 1993.

Rogaski, Ruth. *Hygienic Modernity: Meanings of Health and Disease in Treaty Port China.* Berkeley: University of California Press, 2004.

Rosen, George. *A History of Public Health.* Expanded edition, with an introduction by Elizabeth Fee. Baltimore: Johns Hopkins University Press, 1993.

Rosenberg, Charles E. *No Other Gods: On Science and American Social Thought.* Baltimore: Johns Hopkins University Press, 1997.

Rothstein, William G. *American Physicians in the 19th Century: From Sects to Science.* Baltimore: Johns Hopkins University Press, 1972.

Scheid, Volker. *Chinese Medicine in Contemporary China.* Durham, NC: Duke University Press, 2002.

–. *Currents of Tradition in Chinese Medicine, 1626-2006.* Seattle: Eastland Press, 2007.

–. 'Kexue and Guanxixue: Plurality, Tradition and Modernity in Contemporary Chinese Medicine.' In *Plural Medicine, Tradition and Modernity, 1800-2000,* ed. Waltraud Ernst, 130-52. Abingdon: Routledge, 2002.

Screech, Timon. *The Lens within the Heart: The Western Scientific Gaze and Popular Imagery in Later Edo Japan.* Honolulu: University of Hawai'i Press, 2002.

Shahar, Meir. *The Shaolin Monastery: History, Religion, and the Chinese Martial Arts.* 1st ed. Honolulu: University of Hawai'i Press, 2008.

Shapiro, Hugh L. 'The View from a Chinese Asylum: Defining Madness in 1930s Peking.' PhD diss., Harvard University, History and East Asian Languages, 1995.

Shenyang College of Pharmacy. *Zhongyixue Jichu* [Fundamentals of Chinese medicine]. National Textbooks for Higher-Level Colleges of Medicine and Pharmacy. Beijing: Renmin weisheng chubanshe, 1978.

Shepherd, Clara. 'The Present Situation: New Medicine in China.' *CR* 68 (1937): 323-24.

Shi Shiqin. *Zhongyi chuan Ri shi lüe* [A brief history of the transmission of Chinese medicine to Japan]. Wuchang: Huazhong shifan daxue chubanshe, 1991.

Sinn, Elizabeth. *Power and Charity: The Early History of the Tung Wah Hospital, Hong Kong.* Hong Kong: Oxford University Press, 1989.

Sivin, Nathan. *Traditional Medicine in Contemporary China.* Ann Arbor, MI: Center for Chinese Studies, University of Michigan, 1987.

Slinn, Judy. 'The Development of the Pharmaceutical Industry.' In *Making Medicines: A Brief History of Pharmacy and Pharmaceuticals,* ed. Stuart Anderson, 155-74. London: Pharmaceutical Press, 2005.

Smith, Richard J. *Fortune-Tellers and Philosophers: Divination in Traditional Chinese Society.* Boulder, CO: Westview Press, 1991.

Society for National Medicine. *Jianghu yishu mizhuan* [Transmitted secrets of 'rivers-and-lakes' medicine]. Hong Kong: Li Li Publishing Co., 1954.

Song Daren and Jingfan Shen. 'Quanguo yiyao qikan diaocha ji' [Results of a national survey of medical periodicals]. *Zhong, Xi yiyao* [Chinese and Western medicine and pharmacy] 1, 1 (1935): 120-33. And ibid., vol. 1, no. 3, pp. 279-88.

Summers, William C. *The Great Manchurian Plague of 1910-1911: The Geopolitics of an Epidemic Disease.* New Haven: Yale University Press, 2012.

T'ang, Leang-Li. *Reconstruction in China: A Record of Progress and Achievement in Facts and Figures.* Shanghai: China United Press, 1935.

Tadanori Ishiguro, Surgeon-General Baron. 'The Red Cross in Japan.' In *Fifty Years of New Japan,* ed. Count Shigenobu Okuma, 307-22. London: Smith, Elder, 1909.

Taylor, Kim. *Chinese Medicine in Early Communist China, 1945-63: A Medicine of Revolution.* Abingdon: RoutledgeCurzon, 2005.

–. 'Divergent Interests and Cultivated Misunderstandings: The Influence of the West on Modern Chinese Medicine.' *Social History of Medicine* 17, 1 (2004): 93-111.

Ter Haar, B.J. *The White Lotus Teachings in Chinese Religious History.* Honolulu: University of Hawai'i Press, 1992.

Thomson, James C. *While China Faced West: American Reformers in Nationalist China, 1928-1937.* Cambridge, MA: Harvard University Press, 1969.

Tretiakov, Sergei. *A Chinese Testament: The Autobiography of Tan Shih-hua*. New York: Simon and Schuster, 1934.

Tsukahara, Togo. *Affinity and Shinwa Ryoku: The Introduction of Western Chemical Concepts in Early Nineteenth-Century Japan*. Amsterdam: J.C. Gieben, 1993.

Unschuld, Paul U. *Forgotten Traditions of Ancient Chinese Medicine: The I Hsüeh Yüan Liu Lun of 1757 by Hsü Ta-Ch'un*. Brookline, MA: Paradigm Publications, 1990.

–. *Medicine in China: Historical Artifacts and Images*. Illustrated edition. Munich: Prestel, 2000.

–. *Medicine in China: A History of Ideas*. Berkeley: University of California Press, 1985.

Van de Ven, Hans J. *War and Nationalism in China, 1925-1945*. Abingdon: RoutledgeCurzon, 2003.

Wang Shenxuan. *Zhongyi xin lun huibian* [Compilation of new essays in Chinese medicine]. Shanghai: Shanghai shudian, 1932.

Wang Shouzhi. 'Yi zhan (Medical War).' *SXYYXB* 7, 4 (1917): 27-29.

Wang Yunwu. *Shangwu yinshuguan yu xin jiaoyu nianpu* [Annual chronicle of the Commercial Press and modern education]. Taipei: (Taiwan) Commercial Press, 1973.

Watt, John R. *Saving Lives in Wartime China, 1928-1945*. Leiden: Brill, 2013.

Will, Pierre-Etienne, and R. Bin Wong. *Nourish the People: The State Civilian Granary System in China, 1650-1850*. Ann Arbor, MI: Center for Chinese Studies, University of Michigan, 1991.

Wong, K. Chimin, and Lien-teh Wu. *History of Chinese Medicine*. Vol. 2. Shanghai: Southern Materials Center, Taipei, 1936.

Woo, Dr. S.M. 'Health Work in Amoy.' *CMJ* 32 (1918): 289-91.

Wright, David. 'Careers in Western Science in Nineteenth-Century China: Xu Shou and Xu Jianyin.' *Journal of the Royal Asiatic Society of Great Britain and Ireland* 5, 1 (1995): 49-90.

Wu, Lien-teh. 'The Future of Medical Research in the Orient.' *NMJC* (English section) 8, 4 (1922): 286-90.

–. 'Inaugural Address Delivered at the International Plague Conference, Mukden, 1911.' In *Manchurian Plague Prevention Service Memorial Volume, 1912-1932*, ed. Wu Lien-teh, 13-19. Shanghai: National Quarantine Service, 1934.

–. *North Manchurian Plague Prevention Service Reports, 1911-1913*. Cambridge: Cambridge University Press, 1914.

–. *Plague Fighter: The Autobiography of a Modern Chinese Physician*. Cambridge: Heffers, 1959.

Wu, Yi-Li. *Reproducing Women: Medicine, Metaphor, and Childbirth in Late Imperial China*. Berkeley: University of California Press, 2010.

Wujastyk, Dominik. 'Medical Error and Medical Truth: The Placebo Effect and Room for Choice in Ayurveda.' *Health, Culture and Society* 1, 1 (2011): 221-31.

Xie, Yanggu, ed. *Bai nian Beijing zhongyi* [One hundred years of Chinese medicine in Beijing]. Beijing: Huaxue gongye chubanshe, 2007.

Xie Guan. *Zhongguo yixue yuan liu lun* [The origin and development of Chinese medicine]. Fuzhou: Fujian kexue jishu chubanshe, 1935.

Xiliang. 'Preface.' In *Dongsansheng yishi baogaoshu* [Report on the plague in the three eastern provinces (i.e., Manchuria)]. N.p.: Viceroy's Office, 1911.

Xu, Xiaoqun. *Chinese Professionals and the Republican State: The Rise of Professional Associations in Shanghai, 1912-1937*. Cambridge: Cambridge University Press, 2001.

Yang, Mayfair Mei-hui, ed. *Chinese Religiosities: Afflictions of Modernity and State Formation*. 1st ed. Berkeley: University of California Press, 2008.

Yang, Shangchi. 'Sanshi niandai de quanguo haigang jianyi guanlichu yu Wu Liande boshi' [Dr. Wu Liande and the Chinese maritime customs quarantine inspection stations in the 1930s]. *ZHYSZZ* 18, 1 (1988): 29-32.

–. 'Woguo shouhui jianyi zhuquan douzheng' [China's struggle to regain control over quarantine inspection]. *ZHYSZZ* 20, 1 (1990): 25-26.

Yang, Suixi. 'Wanguo weishengxue lun' [On international sanitation]. *SXYYXB* 59 (1916): 108-9.

Yip, Ka-che. 'Disease and the Fighting Men: Nationalist Anti-Epidemic Efforts in Wartime China, 1937-1945.' In *China in the Anti-Japanese War, 1937-1945: Politics, Culture, and Society*, ed. David P. Barrett and Larry N. Shyu, 171-201. New York: Peter Lang, 2001.

–. *Health and National Reconstruction in Nationalist China: The Development of Modern Health Services, 1928-1937*. Ann Arbor, MI: Association for Asian Studies, 1995.

Yu, Xinzhong. 'Qingdai Jiangnan de minsu yiliao xingwei shenxi' [Analysis of folk healing behaviour in Qing dynasty Jiangnan.' In *Qing yilai de jibing, yiliao he weisheng* [Disease, medicine and hygiene since the Qing], ed. Xinzhong Yu, 91-108. Beijing: Sanlian, 2009.

Yu, Yongyan. 'Jindai zhongyi fangzhi baihoubing shilüe' [A brief history of prevention and treatment of diphtheria in modern TCM]. *ZHYSZZ* 34, 2 (2004): 79-82.

Yu, Yunxiu. 'Yixue geming de guoqu gongzuo, xianzai xingshi he weilai de celue' [The past work of the medical revolution, its present state and future strategy]. *CMJ* 20, 1 (1934): 11-23.

–. *Yixue geming lun: Chuji* [On the medical revolution: Part one]. Vol. 3. Shanghai: Yushi yanjiushi, 1928.

Zhan, Mei. *Other-Worldly: Making Chinese Medicine through Transnational Frames*. Durham, NC: Duke University Press, 2009.

Zhang Qimin. 'Xiandai yixue zhi guanjian' [The key to modern medicine]. *Xiandai guoyi* [Modern national medicine] 2, 6 (1932): 5-10.

Zhang Shangjin, ed. *Wujin xianzhi* [Gazetteer of Wujin County]. Shanghai: Shanghai People's Press, 1988.

Zhang Xiaoping, ed. *Xiandai Zhongyi gejia xueshuo* [Doctrines of modern Chinese-medical physicians]. Beijing: Zhongguo zhongyiyao chubanshe, 1991.

Zhang Xichun. *Yixue zhong Zhong can Xi lu* [The assimilation of Western to Chinese in medicine]. Reprint. Shijiazhuang: Hebei kesue jishu chubanshe, (1918) 1984.

Zhang Zaitong, chief editor: *Minguo yiyao weisheng fagui xuanbian* [Compilation of medical and sanitary laws and regulations during the Republic, 1912-1948]. Taian: Shandong University Press, 1990.

Zhang Zanchen. *Zhongguo lidai yixue shilüe* [Sketch history of Chinese medicine]. 2nd ed. Shanghai: Zhongyi shuju, 1954.

Zhang Zhongjing, Craig Mitchell, Ye Feng, and Nigel Wiseman. *Shāng Hán Lùn: On Cold Damage, Translation and Commentaries*. Taos: Paradigm Publications, 1999.

Zhao Hongjun. *Jindai Zhong, Xi yi lunzheng shi* [History of the controversies between Chinese and Western medicine in modern times]. Hefei: Anhui Science and Technology Press, 1989.

–. 'Zhang Xichun nianpu' [Annual chronicle of (the life of) Zhang Xichun]. *ZHYSZZ* 21, 4 (1991): 214-18.

Zhen Zhiya and Weikang Fu, eds. *Zhongguo yixue shi* [History of Chinese medicine]. Beijing: Renmin weisheng chubanshe, 1991.

Zhu Lian. 'Zhenjiu liaofa de zhongyaoxing ji qi yuanli' [The importance and principles of acupuncture therapy]. *Renmin Ribao* [People's daily], 17 February 1951.

Zhu Weiju. *Bingli fahui* [Pathology elucidated]. Mr. Zhu's Medical Collection. Shanghai: n.p., 1931.

Index

Contemporary Chinese Studies

Glen Peterson, *The Power of Words: Literacy and Revolution in South China,*
1949-95

Wing Chung Ng, *The Chinese in Vancouver, 1945-80: The Pursuit of Identity*
and Power

Yijiang Ding, *Chinese Democracy after Tiananmen*

Diana Lary and Stephen MacKinnon, eds., *Scars of War: The Impact of*
Warfare on Modern China

Eliza W.Y. Lee, ed., *Gender and Change in Hong Kong: Globalization,*
Postcolonialism, and Chinese Patriarchy

Christopher A. Reed, *Gutenberg in Shanghai: Chinese Print Capitalism,*
1876-1937

James A. Flath, *The Cult of Happiness: Nianhua, Art, and History in Rural*
North China

Erika E.S. Evasdottir, *Obedient Autonomy: Chinese Intellectuals and the*
Achievement of Orderly Life

Hsiao-ting Lin, *Tibet and Nationalist China's Frontier: Intrigues and*
Ethnopolitics, 1928-49

Xiaoping Cong, *Teachers' Schools and the Making of the Modern Chinese*
Nation-State, 1897-1937

Diana Lary, ed., *The Chinese State at the Borders*

Norman Smith, *Resisting Manchukuo: Chinese Women Writers and the*
Japanese Occupation

Hasan H. Karrar, *The New Silk Road Diplomacy: China's Central Asian*
Foreign Policy since the Cold War

Richard King, ed., *Art in Turmoil: The Chinese Cultural Revolution, 1966-76*

Blaine R. Chiasson, *Administering the Colonizer: Manchuria's Russians under*
Chinese Rule, 1918-29

Emily M. Hill, *Smokeless Sugar: The Death of a Provincial Bureaucrat and the*
Construction of China's National Economy

Kimberley Ens Manning and Felix Wemheuer, eds., *Eating Bitterness: New*
Perspectives on China's Great Leap Forward and Famine

Helen M. Schneider, *Keeping the Nation's House: Domestic Management and the Making of Modern China*

James A. Flath and Norman Smith, eds., *Beyond Suffering: Recounting War in Modern China*

Elizabeth R. VanderVen, *A School in Every Village: Educational Reform in a Northeast China County, 1904-31*

Norman Smith, *Intoxicating Manchuria: Alcohol, Opium, and Culture in China's Northeast*

Juan Wang, *Merry Laughter and Angry Curses: The Shanghai Tabloid Press, 1897-1911*

Richard King, *Milestones on a Golden Road: Writing for Chinese Socialism, 1945-80*

David Faure and Ho Ts'ui-P'ing, eds., *Chieftains into Ancestors: Imperial Expansion and Indigenous Society in Southwest China*

Yunxiang Gao, *Sporting Gender: Women Athletes and Celebrity-Making during China's National Crisis, 1931-45*

Peipei Qiu with Su Zhiliang and Chen Lifei, *Chinese Comfort Women: Testimonies from Imperial Japan's Sex Slaves*

Julia Kuehn, Kam Louie, and David M. Pomfret, eds., *Diasporic Chineseness after the Rise of China: Communities and Cultural Production*

Printed and bound in Canada by Friesens

Set in Myriad and Sabon by Artegraphica Design Co. Ltd.

Copy editor: Joanne Richardson

Proofreader: Frank Chow

Indexers: Noeline Bridge

Cartographer: Eric Leinberger